THE PARENTAL
ALIENATION SYNDROME

ABOUT THE AUTHOR

Linda J. Gottlieb received her MSW from Adelphi University School of Social Work in 1980 and two weeks later entered their DSW program with a specialization in family therapy. In order to allow her immediate entrance into the doctoral program, the school had waived their requirement for a two-year work experience post the MSW degree. Upon completing eighteen DSW credits, she resolved to pursue a clinical rather than a research direction. In 1994, she entered the extern program in family therapy at the Minuchin Center for the Family, where she studied for nine years. She was personally trained by Salvador Minuchin, M. D., the world renowned, highly respected child psychiatrist and founder of structural family therapy, one of the schools of family systems therapy. From 2003–2007, she served on the faculty of the Minuchin Center, at which time she provided training in structural family therapy to mental health therapists.

Throughout her professional career, Mrs. Gottlieb has been providing treatment services to families of varying compositions and orientations, from all cultural backgrounds, and presenting diverse issues. She has 40 years of experience handling a variety of family issues, relationship problems, and crisis situations.

Mrs. Gottlieb first appreciated the child's instinctual, profound, and intense desire for a relationship with each of her/his parents as a result of her 24 years of professional work experience in adoption and foster care. She initially began her career helping families as a caseworker and subsequently as a psychiatric social worker in New York City's foster care system. She concluded her foster care experience as Assistant Director of Foster Care and Adoption for Nassau County, New York, at which time she transitioned into the mental health field. Her first position in mental health was as a supervisor at South Shore Child Guidance Center, Freeport, New York, where she designed, operationalized, and supervised the Pathways program, a home-based, crisis intervention service to prevent the psychiatric hospitalization of children.

Since 1996, Mrs. Gottlieb has been in private practice on Long Island, New York and practices exclusively as a Family/Relationship Therapist. Drawing on her experiences in child welfare and her training at the Minuchin Center, she recognizes the critical importance of both parents to the emotional, cognitive, social, and physical development of their children. Matrimonial lawyers, attorneys for the child, and personnel in Nassau and Suffolk County Supreme and Family Courts are a source of referrals because they recognize her effectiveness in helping parents using a nonadversarial approach to settle their differences in the best interests of their children and thereby develop a healthy, civil, and respectful shared parenting relationship.

The following is Mrs. Gottlieb's treatment philosophy:

> I will support the family in uncovering its hidden strengths and talents, and I will encourage family members and/or partners to discover with each other new pathways to problem resolution. As a family therapist, I believe in the power of family members to heal each other out of the love they have for each other. I am a catalyst, as I help people in intimate relationships to change each other and to achieve the goals and hopes that they share together.

THE PARENTAL ALIENATION SYNDROME

A Family Therapy and Collaborative Systems Approach to Amelioration

By

LINDA J. GOTTLIEB, LMFT, LCSW

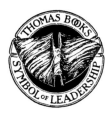

CHARLES C THOMAS · PUBLISHER, LTD.
Springfield · Illinois · U.S.A.

Published and Distributed Throughout the World by

CHARLES C THOMAS • PUBLISHER, LTD.
2600 South First Street
Springfield, Illinois 62704

© 2012 by CHARLES C THOMAS • PUBLISHER, LTD.

ISBN 978-0-398-08735-7 (hard)
ISBN 978-0-398-08736-4 (paper)
ISBN 978-0-398-08737-1 (ebook)

Library of Congress Catalog Card Number: 2011044157

Printed in the United States of America
MM-R-3

Library of Congress Cataloging-in-Publication Data

Gottlieb, Linda J.
 The parental alienation syndrome: a family therapy and collabora-
tive systems approach to amelioration / by Linda J. Gottlieb
  p. cm.
 Includes bibliographical references and index.
 ISBN 978-0-398-08735-7 (hard) -- ISBN 978-0-398-08736-4 (pbk.)
-- ISBN 978-0-398-08737-1 (ebook)
 1. Parental alienation syndrome. 2. Family therapy. I. Title.

RJ506.P27G68 2012
618.92'89–dc23
                                    2011044157

To my husband, Dan, who has complemented me for 37 years.
I could not have undertaken this adventure, this demanding endeavor,
without his understanding, patience, and love. Knowing me as well as
he does, he graciously tolerated my determination to complete this task
with the dedication and commitment that it deserves. I love him for this.
But I love him even more because he embraced, loved, and reared
my son as if he were biologically his.

To my son, Jeffrey, the light of my life. We are so proud of him.
Not primarily because he is professionally successful;
but because he is humanely successful.

In memory of my father, Irving Kase, who left us too soon but not before
I had the opportunity to discover the loving, dedicated, nurturing,
and inspiring father whom he always had been. I relish the time
when we found our way back to each other.

In memory of Joe, my son's father, whose devotion to Jeffrey
always enabled him to cooperate and collaborate with me
in a shared parenting arrangement.

To my stepmother, Sylvia, whose commitment to and
nurturing of my father added precious years to his life.

And finally, to those who have lost family ties.
May you all be as fortunate as I to reconnect.

PREFACE

This book is an outgrowth of the declarations by all too many alienated parents who had shared with me their desperation, hopelessness, and profound agonies concerning their lost children. Repeatedly I have heard their helpless laments, "I want to tell my story. I want to get it out there so that those with the authority and influence can do something–something to correct how they minimize, discount, and frequently abet the alienation." These parents unreservedly told their sagas, clinging to a glimmer of hope that doing so might somehow reconnect them to their lost children. Despite the humiliation, the slander, the abuse, and the maltreatment that each alienated parent had endured, they almost unanimously would have preferred that her/his saga be transparent and identities disclosed so that their children might come to see the light. (I clarified my obligation to protect the anonymity of each who has been herein discussed.) Although some judged that their revelations would be little more than a desperate gesture, it was something that they nonetheless felt impelled to do. But one alienated parent articulated, "Where there is life, there is hope."

The alienated parents whose sagas are herein told (however well disguised) further hoped that publicizing the very real existence of the PAS, along with its insidiousness, may **spare** other parents as well as **the children** from the agony of an alienation. To that cause, they hoped that the revelation of their painful sagas would impact the professionals in the systems which intervene in the family.

And so out of their pain as well as their hope, this book came to be. Those who told their sagas would not want the reader to conclude that conveying hopelessness about the PAS is the book's primary purpose. They, instead, wished to impart to the reader their hopefulness that the PAS can be reversed and ultimately undone. Indeed, that was the treatment outcome for many of those who are discussed herein. So more particularly, this is a book about change, hope, reuniting, and faith–faith in the healing power of the family. It is about what Nichols referred to as " The enormous potential for satisfaction and emotional refueling in family life . . . the rich possibilities of family life, and family therapy's special powers to liberate those possibilities" (pp. 10, 13).

INTRODUCTION

I have heard it stated so many times–time after time–like a broken record, the opening remark from alienating parents conveying the identical message: I want my child to have a relationship with (the other parent)–IF ONLY (the other parent) would stop hitting our child, yelling at our child, saying hurtful things to our child, keeping our child up too late at night, not monitoring our child's homework, taking our child to inappropriate movies, failing to take our child to play dates, continuing to embarrass our child in front of friends with silly remarks, being too strict, or being too permissive, if only. . . . There is always an "if only" which is fabricated, embellished, and/or distorted.

The stories are repetitive: horrific tales of manufactured child abuse; referrals to child protective services (CPS) resulting in suspension of visits between targeted parents and their children; meritless reports to police alleging domestic violence resulting in orders of protection which slander and stigmatize targeted parents; exclusionary tactics preventing the targeted parent's involvement in their children's medical, educational and social lives and activities; depletion of the targeted parent's resources due to the legal fees required to defend herself/himself against frivolous allegations and to obtain legal enforcement of her/his parental rights.

These agonizing sagas are identical; only the names change.

This book is a portrayal of these sagas, resulting from a family interactional pattern called parental alienation syndrome–herein referred to as the PAS. The PAS is an insidious, devastating, bewildering, and commonly unrecognizable form of child abuse. It is a syndrome that often goes by no name for those who are victimized by it; for the therapists who treat it; for forensic evaluators who assess for it; for the child protective workers who investigate it; for the law enforcement system which becomes ensnared in it; and for the judicial system which adjudicates it.

And yes, I could have been counted among those unknowing therapists when I initially faced such a situation some 15 years ago. I have discovered much about this syndrome in subsequent years. I know now that what I had observed and treated is a specific syndrome, with symptoms and behaviors that repetitively and universally occur in all of its young victims and which stems from a common etiology–the malicious programming of an alienating parent.

It was because of the pioneering work of child psychiatrist, Richard Gardner, that this syndrome gained recognition. In his 1985 article, "Recent Trends in Divorce and Custody Litigation," Dr. Gardner first labeled this family interactional pattern as the PAS after having observed for years recurring situations in which children presented as being happily alienated from a formerly-loved and loving parent. Finding no justification for this "happy" alienation, Dr. Gardner concluded that the combination of symptoms repetitively observed in these children, along with a recurring programming of the child by a parent against the targeted parent, formed the basis of a syndrome. He called it the *Parental Alienation Syndrome* (PAS). And although I, too, deem this condition to be a syndrome based on my observations and treatment of more than two hundred children afflicted with it, I do not wish to become distracted by a game of semantics. I will take no issue with the reader who still wishes to shun the label of syndrome–after having read the book–in describing this "condition" of a child being lost to one parent due to a malicious programming by the other parent. I just request that the reader keep an open mind with respect to the issue.

Although there are chapters in this book which will likely interest a general audience, such as alienated parents and adult child victims of the PAS, I am primarily addressing those who are in the helping professions, such as therapists, children's lawyers, judges, matrimonial attorneys, parent coordinators/educators, forensic evaluators, child protective staff, law enforcement personnel–and rescuers. Yes, the professional rescuer, who believes that a child must be saved from a parent–from one of only two people in the child's entire lifetime who will love her/him unconditionally.

Rescued from a parent? Rescued, why? Rescued from bogus allegations, from fabricated abuses, from fictionalized tales in service of deprecating and humiliating the targeted parent. These falsehoods are created by one person– the alienating parent–and then they are introjected, rehashed and embellished upon by the child whom she/he has co-opted.

The following are stories about parents who were driven from the lives of their children. They are dedicated, nurturing, supportive, loving and appropriate parents who have been libeled, vilified, demeaned, and humiliated–not only by their alienating former partners–but tragically also by the professionals in the mental health, child protection, law enforcement, and judicial systems–by the very systems which are meant to support children. These are not, therefore, stories about parents who are alienated from their children due to neglect and/or abuse on their part. (Even in the cases of abuse and neglect, I discovered from my years working in New York's foster care system that children still voraciously yearn for relationships with their parents.)

Based on the limited number of cases presented here, the reader might erroneously conclude that I am indicating that the alienator is typically the mother. Although the early literature on the PAS maintained that the mother is almost four times more likely to pursue a course of alienation than is the father, the most recent literature contends that it more closely approximates 50/50. Indeed, in his latter years just prior to his death, Dr. Gardner (2002) revised his belief that it is the mother who is the predominate alienator, and he, too, concluded that the behavior approaches 50/50 (p. 1). It is not the position of this author/therapist that the mother is primarily to blame for what has happened to the family. Divorce and custody issues are exceedingly complicated, and many factors contribute to the mutual incivility and meanness that often occur during these proceedings. I am unequivocal–the PAS is **NOT** a syndrome endemic to women based on genetics or on some psychological deficiency or for some other reason. The PAS is an opportunistic syndrome, and it is generally the mother who is afforded this opportunity. The opportunity arises because the judicial system in this country is more likely to grant residential custody to the mother, even if joint legal custody is simultaneously granted. And access to the child by the alienator–as well as lack of access by the alienated parent–is the environment which permits the PAS to thrive. It is not possible, therefore, to rule out the potential of fathers for assuming the alienating role in equal numbers to mothers were they to obtain residential custody more frequently. Indeed, many of my esteemed colleagues whom I interviewed for this book asserted that fathers have been equally zealous in pursuing a crusade of alienation against the mother when afforded the opportunity as the residential parent.

The message, however, which I wish to impart to the multidisciplinary professions which intervene in the lives of children, is that children require both parents for their optimal development, and indeed, for escaping serious emotional and behavioral issues that often lead to crippling dysfunction and to a failure in becoming self-sufficient and functioning members of society. This is also the professional judgment of highly esteemed family therapists, psychologists, psychiatrists, forensic evaluators, and social workers who have developed expertise in the areas of child custody.

Raymond Havlicek, Ph.D., is one of these esteemed experts, and he was interviewed for this book on 4/11/11. (A video of the interview and written comments are in possession of the author.) Dr. Havlicek is a forensic and clinical psychologist who is a Diplomat of the American Board of Professional Psychology and a Fellow at the American Academy of Clinical Psychology. He is a founding member of the Parent Coordinator Association of New York. Dr. Havlicek has completed hundreds of child custody evaluations for Supreme and Family Courts throughout New York State. He has been consulted by CPS to do evaluations for that agency. He is currently developing an educational program for upstate New York judges concerning issues of child custody and parental alienation. He specializes in family reunification, domestic violence treatment, validation for sex abuse, and assessment and treatment of parental alienation. Indeed, my research regarding Dr. Havlicek's credibility and expertise in these areas derived from other sources and from one of his forensic evaluations that assessed for the presence of parental alienation and became a precedent-setting case when it was upheld on appeal in New York's highest court, the Court of Appeals. This landmark case led to the standard that grants judges the authority to order, in a probable alienation case, a case manager to oversee and counsel the progress at remedying the alienation.

My first contact with Dr. Havlicek was for this interview for this book. He impressed me with his knowledge, his competency, his commitment, his creativity, and his compassion. Dr. Havlicek emphatically upholds the fulfillment of the child's need and desire "to have both parents appropriately and meaningfully involved in her/his life." Addressing the child's requirement for a relationship with both parents—even if one has problems, just as long as they do no harm to the children—he asserted, "The trust that children place in **BOTH** parents is to their mental health what the foundation is to a building. If you undermine that trust, there is no stability."

Amy Baker holds a Ph.D. in developmental psychology with a specialization in early social and emotional development. She is the Director of Research at the Vincent J. Fontana Center for Child Protection at the New York Foundling. She has conducted one qualitative study on adults who experienced the PAS as children, at least two studies using standardized measures on adults who also had this experience, several studies on parents who had the experience of the other parent interfering with their relationship with their child, and one survey of custody evaluators. She is widely recognized and highly respected as a forensic evaluator for determining the presence of the PAS. In her 2007 research study entitled, *Adult Children of Parental Alienation Syndrome,* Dr. Baker makes a foremost, enlightening contribution to the knowledge base of the PAS by corroborating its existence; by describing the course of its progression; by exploring the tactics employed by the alienating parent; by delineating (as a result of her interviews with adult child-victims of the PAS) its lifelong detrimental impact; and finally by summarizing the various therapeutic approaches recommended by those who engage in its treatment. She has been invited by numerous professionals throughout the country and in Canada to conduct trainings on the PAS. She has commented on the PAS in numerous multimedia forums such as *Good Morning America, Help Me Howard, The Joy Behar Show* and has commented about the PAS in *U.S. News & World Report,* in the *Daily News,* and in *The New York Times.* Most recently, she was a keynote speaker at the Canadian symposium on the PAS held in New York, New York in October, 2010.

My first contact with Dr. Baker was her interview for this book, but I have been impressed with the meticulousness of her writings and research on the PAS, her commitment to helping those who have been afflicted by it, and by her extraordinary efforts at exposing and combating it. Dr. Baker was interviewed for this book on 5/6/2011. (An audio of the interview and written comments are in possession of the author.) Dr. Baker affirmed:

> Kids really want a relationship with the rejected parent. This is what I believe. Their consciousness is complicated that on one level they are nasty and rejecting children; and on another level, they still want their rejected parent in their life. This is an eye opener for the rejected parents who have gone through this. I keep telling them that their child is in there and that they should not to listen to the brittle shell.

Barbara Burkhard, Ph.D., co-founded Child and Family Psychological Services, P.C., Smithtown, New York in 1999 with Jane Albertson-Kelly, Ph.D. This agency provides research-informed therapy for children and families. It has a contract with Suffolk County Department of Social Services (DSS) to provide therapeutic child/parent visits and evaluations of parents who have been accused of abuse and neglect. They also receive referrals from Suffolk County Supreme and Family Courts for custody evaluations, therapeutic visitation, reunification therapy, and forensic mental health evaluations and risk assessments. These may include problems related to high conflict divorce such as parental alienation. They further receive referrals for sex abuse validations as well as referrals to provide therapy for children who are victims of crime. Prior to co-founding this agency, both Dr. Burkhard and Dr. Kelly worked for a community agency which treated abused and neglected children.

I have known Dr. Burkhard for two years as a result of our collaboration on a number of cases. I can unequivocally confirm her reputation throughout Suffolk County for thoroughness, dedication, professionalism, fairness, and compassion. Her capabilities cannot be overstated. I met Dr. Kelly for the first time when I interviewed her for this book. It was immediately obvious to me why she and Dr. Burkhard instantly connected when they first met at their previous work location. Dr. Kelly is enthusiastic, optimistic, committed, and compassionate. The doctors are currently involved in research projects related to their work with children from high conflict divorce. One of these is a collaboration with Dr. Baker regarding the differences between PAS children and other children in other types of treatment due to high conflict divorce.

I interviewed Dr. Burkhard for this book on 1/26/2011 and Dr. Kelly on 2/1/2011. (Video recordings and written comments are in possession of the author.) Both Dr. Burkhard and Dr. Kelly affirmed that children generally benefit from a relationship with each parent with respect to the attainment of healthy long-term relationships and for their optimal social, psychological, and cognitive development. These doctors maintain that children, even those who have experienced documented abuse, generally crave a relationship with each parent; expressions to the contrary may be questionable and should raise a red flag.

As a family therapist, I could not agree more with these respected doctors regarding the importance of both parents playing an active role in their children's lives–especially in situations when the parents are apart. In order to support the goal for each parent to provide a meaningfully and substantial involvement in the lives of their children, I affirm that the resolution to custody requires an arrangement for joint legal custody with physical custody that maximizes the time that nonresidential parents have with their children. It is my professional opinion that the customary visitation arrangement for nonresidential parents to visit every other weekend and one night during the week is not sufficient to maintain a consequential relationship with their children. Although I have heard matrimonial attorneys as well as children's attorneys assert that the child needs the consistency of the same residence, I deem this assumption to be nonsense. I cannot be convinced that the consistency with one's bed trumps consistency with a parent! I further submit that this typical visitation arrangement is based on custom and has no basis in any scientific research about optimal child development and child rearing. In fact, the opposite is the case, and I refer the reader to the book, *Fatherneed*, by Kyle Pruitt, Ph.D. (2000), which documents the extensive compilation of the research summarized by Yale University about the importance of fathers to their children. (We have already been inundated with information about the importance of mothers to their children.)

In all too many states, the burden of proof is that joint custody must be shown to be preferable to sole custody. This must be reversed: the burden of proof must be to demonstrate that sole custody is preferable. I wish to impress upon my fellow professionals who are concerned with children that our customary adversarial framework to child custody decisions serves only to maintain and encourage an already contentious relationship between the parents. Such an approach does not and cannot render a judgment that is in the best interests of the child. Each professional who influences custody decisions must advocate for a position which promotes cooperation and shared parenting and which rejects an adversarial framework. This adversarial framework undermines healthy family functioning and optimal child rearing. Each of these professionals must impart to the parents the message that anything less than a cooperative and compromising parental relationship is unacceptable. These systems which intervene in the lives of children must be committed to the position that, except in the rare cases of the social deviancy of a parent, children need their parents to maintain a civil, respectful shared parenting relationship that includes a meaningful, ongoing relationship with the nonresidential parent. Parents who fail to meet this minimum standard must receive a categorical message from each of these systems, particularly the legal system, that they will suffer severe consequences. The professionals treating children are well aware of the severe consequences which children suffer for this failure. These professionals must cease responding impulsively to their clients/patients. The mental health professional must be disabused of the belief that the presenting parent is the sole holder of the family's truths, and they must thereby not convey to the presenting parent, "Don't worry. I will help you protect your child from their worthless and abusive other parent. I will allow your child to vent her/his anger for and fear of the other parent, and I will inform the court of these feelings." The matrimonial attorney must cease from conveying to the client, "I will make this as nasty and adversarial as I legally (but certainly not morally) am able to do. In the meantime, don't say a word to your estranged spouse, not even when it comes to parenting the children. And avoid participating in co-parenting counseling." Child protection staff must not rush to judgment and conclude that a child is expressing her/his own words and feelings when she/he becomes "hysterical" about the prospects of visiting with the nonresidential parent. And law enforcement personnel must be more neutral and evenhanded when called to the scene of a domestic incident. They too frequently assume that the father is the obstructionist, who must prove himself to be innocent.

Each professional system which impacts custody and visitation decisions must develop policies which encourage the parents to engage in a collaborative approach to their conflicts; and should a parent facilitate an alienation, these systems must be prepared to impose real penalties.

This book will make recommendations to the mental health, child protection, law enforcement, and judicial systems as to how they can change their respective professions to the issue of child custody and visitation. I have reviewed the suggestions from the many multidisciplinary professionals interviewed for this book in order to recommend the changes that will mitigate the adversarial nature of child custody proceedings and to encourage that decisions affecting children support the equal importance of each parent to the child. The parents must be educated to recognize that it is in the child's best interest when they collaborate in parenting. And the book will also document how a family systems approach is an exceedingly effective treatment modality of the PAS family while simultaneously substantiating why an individually oriented approach is generally ineffective and quite frequently detrimental to the child and to the family system as a whole.

I trained to be a family therapist under the auspices of Dr. Salvador Minuchin, the world-renowned and highly respected child psychiatrist, my mentor. It was his unyielding conviction that family members heal each other out of the love they have for each other. I have been practicing on this basis for the past 17 years. I am, therefore, not the healer but rather the catalyst who encourages the family members to engage with each other to heal each other. It is out of this belief system that I present in this book my unyielding conviction of the necessity for shared parenting of the child.

In keeping with my family therapy training at the Minuchin Center for the Family, I was educated to assess the power between the two members of the parental dyad as being roughly equal and subject to amelioration by a trained family therapist when that homeostasis is no longer functional—assuming that neither parent's power is enhanced by a professional rescuer. My family therapy education also taught me that the relationships among the family members are complementary or reciprocal. That is, the behavior of each individual family member is a function of and is maintained by the interactions with other family members. For example, if one parent is underfunctioning, that signifies that the other parent is overfunctioning, and this reciprocity maintains the homeostasis of the system. Another example of the complementarity of family relationships would be a couple who relates more as parent and child than like husband and wife: the first partner could not play the role of the parent if the second partner did not act like an irresponsible child; and the second partner could not play the role of a child if the first partner refused to act like an omniscient parent. They have co-created each other. Each family member's behavior is related to the behaviors of the other family members. Independent behavior, therefore, does not exist when one lives in intimate relationships with other people. We all react to and are proactive upon each family member.

How does this pertain to the PAS? I intend to formulate a systemic interpretation of the relationships which occur during divorce; that is, the relationships between the family and the larger social systems with which the family interacts and in the relationship between the alienating and the alienated parents. Much of the current literature on PAS characterizes this relationship by portraying the alienating parent as the aggressor and an abuser and the alienated parent as a victim who is the recipient of abuse and too passive to remedy her/his situation. However, a systemic orientation compels me to pose the following question: is it the aggression of the alienating parent that makes the alienated parent a victim or does the passive inclination of the alienated parent permit the alienating parent to victimize her/him? If the reader is wondering whether this is a chicken or egg question, the reader would be correct.

My systemic approach to assessing PAS families allows me to view the alienating and alienated parents in a very different light than is portrayed in most of the literature on the PAS. As the reader continues in this book, I suggest that attention be paid to this distinction: namely that there is an essential difference between being a victim and allowing oneself to be victimized. I am not talking about, for example, a woman who has been abducted off the streets by a stranger and held in captivity against her will. I am talking about adults who are choosing to live with each other in intimate relationships over a protracted period of time in which the behaviors of each are predictable and known to the other. Clearly each of the adults in the previous statement has made a choice. Victims, however, do not see themselves as having options, and this is a disempowering self-perception. There are major implications for treatment depending upon which formulation is made about the relationship between the alienating and the alienated parents; that is, how we perceive the family map.

The reader should not interpret this analysis to mean that my intent is to blame the alienated parent for her/his plight. I would not assert this anymore than I would declare that a woman who has been physically abused by her partner is to blame for the abuse. I am merely maintaining that the alienated parent has options to ameliorate her/his situation, just as the abused woman can choose to leave her partner. What the reader should conclude from this book is that the alienated parent becomes a victim as a result of the confluence of the authority of the aforementioned larger systems, which solidify, intensify, and perpetuate the power imbalance between the alienating and alienated parents. It is when the professionals in these systems are co-opted by the alienating parent—their susceptibility perhaps being a result of their biases, preconceived ideas, ignorance, inattention, and/or self-interest—that the alienated parent finds herself/himself at a severe disadvantage in custody and visitation proceedings. This disadvantageous situation is akin to tying a bowling ball around a runner's leg and expecting her/him to be able to compete in a track meet. The playing field instead must be leveled by these powerful systems, which must examine how to remedy its respective participation in the escalation of the power imbalance between the alienated and alienating parents.

At the same time, I will not pathologize the alienating parent and rush to advocating measures to eliminate connections to her/his children. To do so would be isomorphic with the deprecation and rejection of the alienated parent. Labels serve only to constrict options and eliminate hope. For professionals who help the family (and consequently children), we must reject unhealthy and ineffective family interactional behaviors and not reject individuals. This is certainly what the child wants and needs. The goal must be to ameliorate behaviors which are detrimental to children by encouraging healthy transactional patterns between the participants in the executive/parental subsystem and between the parent/child subsystems in recognition of the importance of both parents to healthy and successful child rearing. Such a perspective signifies that, first and foremost, the remedying of the dysfunctional interactions between the alienating and the alienated parents must be the critical area for attention, thereby demonstrating respect for the ability of the family members to heal each other. But this can be achieved **only if** the larger aforementioned systems guarantee to the family therapist a level playing field upon which to encounter the family. These systems must encourage a collaborative rather than an adversarial approach to child custody decisions. Accomplishing this would truly restore balance to the justice system when adjudicating child custody issues and ameliorating the PAS.

So what exactly is the PAS? Come travel with me on a journey to the twilight zone; to Kafka-esque trials; to a no-mans land where hate and fear must be carefully taught.

ACKNOWLEDGMENTS

I wish to extend my deep appreciation to all who came forward to disclose their painful, traumatic tales. I recognize how difficult it was for each of them to relive, re-experience, and reveal their alienation.

I am extending profound appreciation to my **mentor, Salvador Minuchin, MD**, for the invaluable year of supervision he graciously extended to me on his own time. I believe that this supervisory experience was the peak of my family therapy training experience which helped me to "really get" its unique, magical, and inspiring approach to producing change and to become an effective catalyst who enables family members to heal each other. I further lack adequate words to extend to him my deep gratitude for having invested his time in reading the *introduction to this book* as well as the *chapter on treatment* and for providing invaluable feedback on both.

Special thanks also to **Patricia Minuchin, Ph.D.**, whose one caveat to me, "Don't forget all your training at the Minuchin Center for the Family when you write this book," provided the framework for the book's final conception.

Further acknowledgements are extended to the faculty members of the **Minuchin Center for the Family** for each one's investment to teach me Structural Family Therapy:

Ema Genijovich, Lic.   Daniel Minuchin, MA, LMFT
David E. Greenan, EdD, LMFT   George Simon, MS, LMFT

The following is a list of the attorneys, mental health therapists, forensic evaluators, and a pediatrician who graciously granted an interview for this book. I extend to them my gratitude for the time they invested and detracted from their heavy practices to impart their knowledge and suggestions in the hopes of remedying this destructive family interactional pattern known as Parental Alienation Syndrome. I chose to interview these professionals primarily because of my professional experiences with them and because I was impressed by their passion, commitment, expertise, and willingness to go above and beyond their profession's mandates in order to obtain resolutions that not only satisfy their obligations to their respective clients but also achieve a solution in the best interests of the child.

The Professional Interviewees are Listed in Alphabetical Order

Amy Baker, Ph.D.

Barbara Burkhard, Ph.D.

Costas Constantatos, M.D.

Dorothy A. Courten, J.D.

Susan DeNatale, J.D.

Raymond Havlicek, Ph.D.

Joshua B. Hecht, J.D.

Robert Hiltzik, J.D.

Jane Kelly, Ph.D.

Paul Levitt, J.D.

Jeannemarie Massetti, R-L/ACSW

Francine H. Moss, J.D.

Robert Previto, J.D.

Susan Saltz, J.D.

Chaim Steinberger, J.D.

Evie Zarkadas, J.D.

Additional appreciation to Richard Sauber, Ph.D. for taking the time to read a draft copy of this book and provide feedback.

DISCLAIMER

I have employed diligent measures to conceal the identity and protect the anonymity of each person cited in this book–exclusive of those professionals who were interviewed. In the furtherance of protecting anonymity, the nature of some of my diligent measures will remain clandestine. But one measure I will make clear: the altering of recognizable and idiosyncratic information in the quotes and in the case descriptions. For example, the locations in which events had occurred were changed and objects were substituted for comparable ones. To illustrate this point, an amusement park will become a movie theater; a trip to London would be mentioned as a trip to Paris; an iPad might replace a Playstation; a trip to the science museum might be cast as a trip to the Planetarium; a trip to Disneyland becomes a trip to Sea World; a scooter will be portrayed as a rocking horse, and so on. The changes in no way altered, minimized, or intensified the significance of the case material being portrayed.

Should you believe that you recognize yourself in one of the case descriptions, do not become too excited. Because PAS children and alienators so closely resemble each other–in that their behaviors, vocabulary, expressions, thinking, and beliefs bare such striking similarity to those of every other PAS child and alienator–the likelihood that you have mistaken yourself for another would be of high probability. Furthermore, in my attempts to avoid redundancy, for every child I cited, there were likely at least four others who were so strikingly similar that I chose not to include them. By my calculations, therefore, the reader would have a better chance of winning the powerball lottery than being mentioned in this book.

CONTENTS

THE PARENTAL ALIENATION SYNDROME

Chapter 1

DEFINITION OF PARENTAL ALIENATION SYNDROME

What's in a name?
—Shakespeare, *Romeo and Juliet*

Dr. Richard Gardner (1985) is appropriately acknowledged as being the first to have labeled the parental alienation as a syndrome based on a clearly defined grouping of symptoms with a common etiology—a syndrome characterized by eight symptoms in the child at the instigation of the brainwashing/programming of a parent against the other parent. This family interactional pattern can therefore be characterized as a cross-generational coalition between the parent and the child(ren) to the disparagement and rejection of the other parent. Gardner (1998, 2001) further elaborated on how to identify and treat the PAS in these referenced books, which are just two of his many additional contributions on the subject.

But Gardner is frequently incorrectly credited for being the first to have identified the occurrence of this coalition (generally in less severity) which family systems therapists confront when problematical families present for treatment at all stages in the life cycle, not only during high conflict divorce situations. Indeed, Leona Kopetski, M.S.S.W (2006) had been independently publicizing as early as the 1970s her observations of and conclu-sions about this family transactional pattern occurring in high conflict divorce cases, and her experience of these families was astonishingly similar to that of Gardner's. She assessed these families to be highly disturbed (pp. 378–389). Wallerstein and Kelly (1980) are also credited with having initially identified this cross-generational coalition, which they described in their book, *Surviving the Breakup: How Children and Parents Cope with Divorce.* In this seminal research about the effects of divorce on children, they describe a pattern of behavior in which an irate parent and a child join together in a coalition to disengage from and minimize the other parent. The authors asserted that this coalition produces disturbances in the child (pp. 77–80).

Wallerstein and Kelly, however, are far from being the earliest to recognize this dysfunctional family interactional pattern. It was actually in the 1950s that the psychiatrists who subsequently founded the various schools of family systems therapy who began to identify a cross-generational coalition which they had observed occurring when their hospitalized psychiatric patients were visiting with their families. These psychiatrists subsequently labeled this interaction as the perverse or pathological triangle, and they defined it as a dysfunctional cross-generational coalition between a parent who had requested the allegiance of the psychiatric patient in that parent's dispute with the other parent. Intervening to remedy this devastating consequence to their patients, these psychiatrists made the facilitation of healthy family interactional patterns as the focus of their treatment. The extensive experience that family systems therapists have had in treating this interactional pattern is the basis for my recommendation that a systems modality is the treatment of choice for the PAS family. The effectiveness of this treatment modality will be exemplified in a later chapter in which I present my treatment summaries of 16 PAS families. In the meantime, I will return to the definition of the PAS and establish the credibility of the man who first identified it.

Gardner was for many years, until his death in 2003, Clinical Professor of Child Psychiatry at the College of Physicians and Surgeons at Columbia University. He was certified in psychiatry and child psychiatry by the American Board of Psychiatry and Neurology and a life Fellow of the American Psychiatric Association and a Fellow of the American Academy of Child and Adolescent Psychiatry and the American Academy of Psychoanalysis. Dr. Gardner is recognized as one of the leading innovators in the field of child psychiatry, and he authored more than 40 books and 250 articles, which are deemed by mental health professionals as extremely valuable to their practices. He is universally regarded by the PAS-aware professional throughout the world as an expert in identifying and treating Parental Alienation Syndrome. Based on his years of observations of hundreds of cases in his professional practice, Gardner developed the

widely accepted criteria for diagnosing for the presence of the PAS. Subsequent to his initial article and first book regarding the etiology of the syndrome and delineating its manifestations, he refined and expanded his knowledge base about the PAS, which he published in additional books and articles; developed strategies for intervention and treatment; and testified as a forensic evaluator regarding the PAS in hundreds of custody/visitation trials.

Gardner (1998) defined the PAS as:

> a disorder that arises primarily in the context of child-custody disputes. Its primary manifestation is the child's campaign of denigration against a parent, a campaign that has no justification. It results from the *combination* of a programming (brainwashing) parent's indoctrinations and the child's own contributions to the vilification of the target parent. (p. xx)

Although there is an initial programming by the alienating parent, the diagnosis of PAS cannot be made without the addition of the child's contributions to the vilification, humiliation, and rejection of the targeted parent. In other words, until and unless the child is co-opted by the alienator into adopting the alienator's perceptions of the targeted parent, then the PAS is not present. The alienator's introjected perceptions, however, form the basis of the child's justifications to maltreat the targeted parent. The PAS therefore occurs within the context of the family system in that it could not occur without an alienating parent's instigation, is actively promoted and maintained by an alienating parent, must be accepted and executed by the child, and has a targeted parent as the recipient of the humiliation, denigration, and abuse. The alienating parent's programming alone is not sufficient to account for the PAS; nevertheless, the programming and alienating maneuvers have the potential to produce the PAS because children can resist the induction by a parent upon whom they are dependent only for just so long. Early intervention is therefore critical when confronted with the PAS.

Gardner (1998) determined that the PAS can be diagnosed by eight characteristic primary symptoms, almost all being present to a significant degree in severe cases with fewer symptoms present and to lesser degrees in moderate and mild cases (p. xxv). The diagnosis is made on the basis of the symptomatology in the child, as reflected in the child's expressions of feelings, thoughts, attitudes, and behaviors demonstrated about and towards the targeted parent.

The PAS is almost unanimously accepted as a syndrome by those professionals who are familiar with it–the acceptance being based on the universality of situations in which all or almost all of the eight symptoms are observed and in which they share the common etiology of a programming by an alienating parent. *The Diagnostic and Statistical Manual of Mental Disorders,* 4th ed. (APA, 2002) states that a condition rises to the level of a syndrome as follows:

> Each of the mental disorders is conceptualized as a clinically significant behavioral or psychological syndrome or pattern that occurs in an individual and that is associated with present distress (e.g., a painful symptom) or disability (i.e., impairment in one or more areas of functioning) or with a significantly increased risk of suffering death, pain, disability, or an important loss of freedom. . . . Whatever its original course, it must currently be considered a manifestation of behavioral, psychological, or biological dysfunction in the individual. (p. xxi)

It is the experience of the diagnosticians familiar with the PAS that the cluster of eight symptoms coupled with the programming by an alienating parent are universally present to some degree when the PAS is indicated. In other words, the predominance of

the eight symptoms and the programming, when taken together, are inescapably predictive of the PAS and do not account for any other syndrome. In sum, the PAS is one of the most easily identified and recognizable syndromes. Gardner (1998) asserts:

> This consistency results in PAS children resembling one another. It is because of these considerations that the PAS is a relatively "pure" diagnosis that can easily be made by those who are not somehow blocked from seeing what is right in front of them. (p. xxv)

In her 2002 doctoral dissertation, *Parental Alienation Syndrome in Court Referred Custody Cases,* Janelle Burrill, Ph.D., concluded, "The findings from this study's 30 cases with 59 children does appear to support the existence of PAS . . . the criticism and denial of PAS by practitioners is unjustified" (p. 75). Her dissertation validates the conclusions reached by Gardner in that she evaluated the 30 cases for the presence of the PAS based on Gardner's eight symptoms. Burrill continued, "The data from this study appears to support Dr. Gardner's observations of PAS published in 1985" (p. 78). Her observations further substantiate how the programming of the alienating parent influences the PAS child. Burrill declared:

> Children's negative behaviors towards the alienated parent increase in severity as the negative behaviors and hostility of the alienating parent increase. The results of this data are significant . . . the behaviors observed in the severe cases manifest exactly as described by Gardner. (p. 78)

Richard Warshak, Ph.D., a highly esteemed psychologist who is widely accepted as an expert in identifying and treating the PAS, summed up as follows the empirical support for Gardner's observations when he referenced Slobogin's case for the PAS having met the *Frye* test. Warshak (2006) stated:

> Taken together, the frequency of reports in the clinical literature, the close similarity of reported cases to Gardner's descriptions, and the reference section of the APA guidelines, lend support to the validity of PAS in terms of its utility to a sizeable group of experienced practitioners in the field. (p. 357)

Empirical evidence for Gardner's diagnosis of the PAS is further supported in a 12-year study of 700 families, published by the American Bar Association section of Florida Family Law. This exhaustive study lends considerable credibility to Gardner's diagnosis of the PAS based on the universality of his eight characteristic symptoms, which were observed in the children. The study further concluded that, in divorce situations, parental alienation, the programming of a child against the other parent, occurs regularly, 60 percent of the time, and sporadically another 20 percent (Clawar & Rivlin, 1991, pp. 174–180).

These are staggering statistics—especially given the current divorce rate that exceeds 52 percent—and clearly portend societal disruption if this tidal wave is not stemmed.

Many other forensic evaluators and therapists throughout the world have utilized Gardner's criteria to assess for the presence of the PAS in their cases, and they, too, have observed the repetitiveness and universality of his eight characteristic symptoms whenever there is an unjustified humiliation and rejection of a parent. A fraction of the esteemed therapists, evaluators, and attorneys who have experienced the PAS in their practices are referenced in this book.

Dr. Havlicek stated to me in his interview that he not only has unequivocally concluded that the PAS is a valid syndrome; he has also found that alienation "is prevalent to some degree in about 75 percent of all di-

vorce cases." He defined parental alienation as "an unreasonable rejection of a parent. The extent of the child's resistance to a relationship with that parent is out of proportion to reality. The child's view is not supported by anything that the parent has done. It is a campaign of denigration that is initiated by the custodial parent."

Dr. Baker stated in her interview for this book that, in her professional opinion, this family dynamic which Gardner labeled the PAS "absolutely" exists. She indeed has concluded that it is a syndrome which she described as follows:

> I believe it is a syndrome using the definition that it is a collection of symptoms with a common etiology; that is, the eight behaviors as identified by Dr. Gardner are a cluster of symptoms that tend to go together, and when you see one in a child, you tend to see the others. The common etiology is the exposure to parental alienation strategies.

Based on her research and her forensic work, she diagnoses for the presence of the PAS based on four characteristics, paraphrased as follows: (1) the child had a previously amicable relationship with the now rejected parent; (2) there is an absence of abuse and neglect on the part of the now rejected parent; (3) there is evidence that the other parent is exhibiting, intentionally or otherwise, many of the 17 alienating behavioral strategies identified in her research which have the effect on the child to succumb to rejection of the other parent; these strategies promote a psychological rupture between the child and the other parent; (4) the child is exhibiting many of the eight behavioral symptoms of alienation as identified by Gardner. Dr. Baker summed up in our interview by stating, "If all four of these characteristics exist together, I'm willing to conclude that alienation is a dynamic that is present in the particular case."

Nevertheless, there are the naysayers who dispute, not the existence of the phenomenon of the alienation–which is accepted and characterized even by the naysayers to be an unreasonable rejection of a formerly loved and loving parent–but rather that it does not rise to the level of a syndrome. These skeptics assert that it lacks a common etiology. Most notably, the credible naysayers are Janet Johnston, Ph.D., (2001) and Joan Kelly, Ph.D., to whose systems critique of the PAS I must respond. I will leave it principally to my PAS-aware colleagues, including Gardner, who have responded to their other criticisms of the syndrome label. I will just briefly summarize their rebuttals.

In his article, "Response to Kelly/ Johnston Article," Gardner (2002) disputes their contention that the PAS lacks widespread support in the scientific community. He asserted, to the contrary, that it has past the Frey test in a court of law in Florida and in other legal jurisdictions; that it has been recognized in numerous peer reviewed writings, which he cites in his rebuttal; and that it has been replicated by numerous professionals worldwide through observations in their practices (pp. 6–10). Gardner disputed their argument that the PAS cannot be considered a syndrome because it had not been accepted into in the *DSM-IV,* the latest edition. He emphasized that it takes many years for a syndrome to be accepted, and the PAS was only in the nascent stages of its documentation when the *DSM-IV* was published in 1994. As he pointed out, it took Asperger's syndrome 37 years for acceptance into the *DSM* after its symptoms were first noted, and Tourette's syndrome took 95 years (pp. 193– 195).

I should also like to emphasize that there are political as well economic factors that hinder acceptance. For example, the Nation-

al Organization of Women is opposing its acceptance as a syndrome, and some insurance companies have expressed their objections as it would become another diagnosis which they will be required to cover.

I also leave it primarily to Warshak (2001) in his very thorough and persuasive article entitled, "Current Controversies Regarding Parental Alienation Syndrome," to rebut further the nonsystems objections to the syndrome label of Johnston, Kelly and others. He very ably disputes the assertions that the PAS has not been significantly substantiated and corroborated by mental health professionals through their clinical observations in their practices, that it has not been meaningfully documented in peer-reviewed literature, and that there has not been adequate scientific foundation to rise to the level of a syndrome (pp. 36–43). Please refer to this article for his extensive review of professional corroboration for the existence of the PAS. Warshak further argues persuasively that the reformulation by Kelly and Johnston (2001) from the PAS model to their "alienated child" (AC) model (pp. 2–4) is a distinction without a difference. He firstly punctuates that they accept two of Gardner's three criteria for the syndrome, namely that of the child's malicious rejection and denigration of the targeted parent and that of the child's feelings and beliefs being utterly out of proportion to anything which that parent did (31–36). What Kelly and Johnston (2001) did not adopt in their AC model from Gardner's PAS model is the role played by their "aligned parent" (pp. 3–7) as opposed to Gardner's almost identically named alienating parent, who facilitates the creation of the alienation. I will soon be returning to this issue in my systems rebuttal of their systems critique of the syndrome label. Warshak elaborated in his article about how closely the child's symptoms in the AC model adhere to Gardner's eight symptoms (pp. 32–36). Johnston (2001) described this as follows: "An alienated child is defined as one who expresses, freely and persistently, unreasonable negative feelings and beliefs (such as anger, hatred, rejection, and/or fear) toward a parent that are significantly disproportionate to the child's actual experience with that parent" (p. 3).

Warshak (2001) further disputed the authors' contention that hatred and maltreatment of a parent is sometimes an age-appropriate/stage-specific development of the child's maturation process or can be a response to traumatic events, such as to high conflict divorce. Indeed, he documented that such hostility to a parent is seriously harmful to children. He asserted that the authors confuse this for the normalcy of children switching their closeness to each parent as they progress through their developmental stages. But this clearly does not signify that the other parent is rejected or degraded–only that it is normal for children to regulate distance and closeness with each parent at different developmental stages or due to a significant event (pp. 30–33).

Indeed, I concur that "alliances" (meaning closeness) are not pathological when they are flexible–changing over time and under different circumstances **and** never to the rejection and humiliation of the other parent. It is when a coalition between the child and the same parent becomes rigid over time that it has the potential to lead to an alienation. I strongly urge that the disbelievers read Warshak's article in its entirety for an in-depth rebuttal to the most prominent, nonsystems objections to the label of a syndrome.

Before I articulate my systems criticisms, I must briefly add my voice to those who assert that Johnston, Kelly, and other naysayers, themselves, lack scientific substantiation of their objections to the syndrome label.

In her above referenced article, Johnston (2001) stated:

> The first problem is that PAS focuses almost exclusively on the alienating parent as the etiological agent of the child's alienation. This flies in the face of clinical observations that shows [*sic*] that, in a high-conflict divorce, many parents exhibit indoctrinating behaviors but only a small proportion of children become alienated. In other cases, it has been observed that some children (especially adolescents) develop unjustified animosity, negative beliefs and fears of a parent in the apparent absence of alienating behaviors by a parent. It would appear that alienating behavior by a parent is neither a sufficient nor a necessary condition for a child to become alienated. (pp. 1–2)

It is interesting to me that Johnston accords greater validity to her observations than she does to those observations of Gardner or to those of the numerous other professionals who have encountered the PAS phenomenon in their practices either as therapists, forensic evaluators, or matrimonial attorneys. What does she mean when she states, "It has been observed?" By whom has it been observed and by how many? Where is the peer-reviewed literature and research to support the "it has been observed"? When she states, "It flies in the face of clinical practice," to whose and how many clinical practices is she referring? And what did she mean by "apparent absence of alienating behaviors by a parent"? Is she rejecting Gardner's criteria of a parent facilitating the alienation on the basis of something that is "apparent" and that is not research informed? Indeed, Johnston (2001) provides a "cautionary" note about the unsubstantiation by the widespread scientific community of the ideas expressed in this article when she stated:

> The ideas and views expressed in this paper are largely based on the clinical insights and

practical experience of working with the broad array of high conflict divorcing families by a small task force of experienced mental health professionals. There is critical need for more systematic research into this subject (*supra* note 2).

Nevertheless, Johnston's assertions about their observations are stated in such a take-it-for granted/matter-of-fact manner that the implication is that the observations of the **small** task force members are irrefutable and commonly accepted by in the larger scientific community. To the contrary, the literature summarized by Warshak utterly disputes their observations, as do Baker's research and the anecdotal experiences of numerous professionals, including this therapist. These professionals, along with the ones interviewed for this book, confirm a high degree of alienation, as much as 75–80 percent of all divorce cases, and occurring at the instigation of an alienating parent. It appears that Johnson's "alienated child" model has far less substantiation and corroboration from the anecdotal experiences of mental health professionals, from empirical support, and from other research informed studies than does Gardner's PAS model.

Also refuted by the therapists interviewed for the book is Johnston's assertion that the unjustified loathing of alienated children for their targeted parent can be considered normal child development under certain circumstances, such as in a divorce situation. Johnston stated, "We argue that it is critical to differentiate the alienated child (who persistently refuses and rejects visitation because of unreasonable negative views and feelings) from other children will also resist contact with a parent after separation but for a variety of normal developmentally expectable reasons" (p. 3). I emphatically dispute that enmity for and rejection of a parent is ever indicative of healthy child develop-

ment. The progression of an alienation from the mild stage to the severe stage is such an abnormal development that it no more belongs on the same continuum as the child's healthy developmental progress towards separation/individuation than does an Axis II diagnosis belong on Axis I. This analysis is completely misguided. It would have been helpful in this article if Johnston had therefore provided a comprehensive and precise definition of alienation to make this assertion and because she concluded that "only a small proportion of children become alienated" (p. 2) in a divorce situation. It seems that her criteria for determining an alienation is primarily the presence of visit refusal (p. 3). This is a narrow definition of the alienated child, being far from inclusive of their behaviors, attitudes, and emotional state. Indeed, it appears that Johnston assesses that the child who becomes fully "alienated" from a parent after separation/divorce travels on the same continuum that pertains to a child who is developing normally in the process of readjusting over time her/his closeness and distance to each parent after divorce (pp. 3, 6). She does not seem to appreciate that the alienation is pathological from its inception and therefore necessitates a separate continuum as it traverses through the mild to severe stages.

I will explain my systems rebuttal of Johnston's systems critique of the PAS. I do find myself in the seemingly contradictory position of concurring with her position that a family systems modality is the treatment of choice for these families while simultaneously supporting the position that Gardner is correct in defining as a syndrome the highly dysfunctional family transactional pattern of an alienation.

My principal criticisms of Johnston are her failure to apply systems principles consistently and to apply systems theory in its entirety to her critique of Gardner's classification of alienation as a syndrome. To begin with, suppose I grant her position that the aligned parent did not cause or did not principally initiate the alienation. This I will stipulate: systems theory refutes emphasis on linear causation in favor of recognizing that there is a reciprocity of behaviors among family members. (What Dr. Salvador Minuchin labeled as their complementarity.) As such, Johnston is aware that systems theory is instead concerned with how each individual member is involved in the **maintenance** of the dysfunctional transactional patterns and symptoms which are occurring in the family system. The question must then be raised as to why Johnston does not concede that the aligned parent must be playing a role in the **maintenance of the alienation**–such role being no better exemplified than by her/his failure to encourage and support the relationship and visits between the other parent and their child; that is, to be proactive in assuring that the other parent is offered the opportunity to be involved in their child's life. Moreover, in the typical alienation case, the alienated parent no longer lives with the family and has frequently had no contact with the child for upwards of months and frequently years, so it is improbable that the alienated parent is playing any role in symptom maintenance. The only conclusion that can be reached, therefore, is that the alienating parent is primarily responsible for the maintenance of the alienation. Focusing on symptom maintenance and on the current family constellation (which is most likely comprised of **only** the aligned parent and children) are the critical dynamics that Johnston conveniently obfuscates but which are, nonetheless, the philosophical underpinnings of a systemic diagnosis of family dysfunction. Thus, there is no escaping the conclusion that the aligned parent is, at the very least, culpable for the maintenance of the alienation.

So if the behavior of the aligned parent is not the primary cause of the alienation in Johnston's AC model, who and what is the cause? Johnston (2001) declares that many factors contribute, and they include the family's history of events, developmental stages, interactional patterns, and even the individual personality characteristics of the child influence the child's susceptibility to a brainwashing. She expressed it this way, "They are responding to complex and frightening dynamics within the divorce process itself, to an array of parental behaviors, and as a result of their own early developmental vulnerabilities which have rendered them susceptible" (p. 4). She further elaborated upon this last factor when she stated, "Children who are temperamentally vulnerable (anxious, fearful, dependent, or emotionally troubled) are those that [*sic*] are less able to withstand the inordinate stress inherent in being in the middle of a high-conflict divorce. Instead they are more likely to be drawn into an alienated stance" (p. 7). This last variable characterizing the child as "temperamentally vulnerable" is an intrapsychic concept and is therefore quite peculiar and contradictory to be included as an element in a systems assessment of the family dynamics and of symptoms. A systems model would instead attribute those four symptoms–as well as any others–to being the outcome of the "the frightening dynamics of the divorce process" and to "an array of parental behaviors." According to systems theory, the triangulating process is the root of the "frightening dynamics," and of the dysfunctional behaviors of the parental subsystem. Systems theory defines the triangulating as the process by which the child is co-opted by an aligned/alienating parent into forming a cross-generational coalition against the other parent. And yes, I unequivocally concur with Johnston that this triangulating process likely commenced long before the parents decided to separate: I have yet to recall an alienated parent–and I have worked with several hundred–who did not express the following similar sentiments: "I saw the alienation coming long before we separated. My spouse and my children were always ganging up on me, excluding me, keeping secrets from me, putting me down, ignoring my input, rejecting my parenting ideas, etc."

In Johnston's AC model, then, the alienated child's vulnerability to the subsequent alienation cannot, according to systems theory, be attributed to the intrapsychic concept of being "temperamentally vulnerable" but rather must be a direct result of the family's predivorce history of triangulation. And indisputably, this triangulating required the active co-opting by the aligned/alienating parent. The family's "frightening dynamics" and "array of parental behaviors" cultivated a seed for the alienation, and in this seed is also included the budding alienating maneuvers of the alienating parent, which thusly accounts for all three criteria in Gardner's PAS model. Indeed, Johnston acknowledges the triangulating process as a factor in the development of an alienation when she states:

> Common features of these cases include a history of intense marital conflict, often from the time the child was very young, wherein the child was triangulated or where the child replaced the rejected parent as the central object of a spouse's affection; a separation that was experienced as inordinately humiliating by the aligned parent; and subsequent divorce conflict and litigation that, can be fueled by professionals and extended kin. (p. 6)

So how did the triangulation occur? Would Johnston maintain that children triangulate themselves? Not likely! The triangulation requires the active initiation on the part of the aligned/alienating parent. Johnston's description of how the child becomes susceptible to the alienation in the AC model is

therefore not only inconsistent with systems theory; it actually requires that there be an aligned parent who actively engages in alienating maneuvers.

Johnston's critique of the PAS model is further flawed by another significant deviation from systems theory: namely that her explanation for the formation of an alienation places emphasis on the "there and then" history of the family instead of on their "here and now" experiences with each other. This emphasis is at extreme odds with the philosophical underpinnings of systemic theory, which accounts for symptom formation, instead, on the dysfunctional interactional patterns occurring **in the present**. So it seems quite peculiar that Johnston reverts to history for an explanation of the alienation rather than focusing on the current interactional patterns between the child and the aligned parent, with whom the child is living. Johnston herself criticized the PAS supporters for their failure to consider all the dynamics in the family systems as factors in creating an alienation when she stated that they "would be better served by a more specific description of the child's behavior in the context of his family" (p. 2). So which context is more relevant and impactful, the present here and now experiences or the past there and then memories? Systemic therapists would unquestionably respond with the present here and now experiences. Once again, one must reach the conclusion that the aligned/alienating parent is actively participating in, encouraging, and maintaining the alienation.

As I stated in the introduction, it is important to address the complementary role of the alienated parent in the family system and how she/he contributed to the development of the alienation, participation in which systems theory asserts must have occurred. I wish to be perfectly very clear: when I affirm that the alienated parent played a role in the family dynamics, I am referring to the relationship with the other parent; I am not insinuating that she/he did anything in interaction with the child to justify the child's antagonism and rejection. Most professionals who have been involved in the detection and/or treatment of an alienation, including Gardner, Johnston, and Kelly, noted that alienated parents often display a passivity, from the time when they were still living with the family. This passivity resulted in their underinvolvement and their spouse's overinvolvement with the children and which simultaneously sanctioned the empowerment of their spouse as primary decision maker for their children. For example, virtually every alienated parent expressed to me that they very often "surrendered" to their former partner in marital/parental disputes because it was too hard to fight or that they are conflict adverse or because they did not wish to expose their children to the hostilities. Alienated parents acknowledged having incredulously acquiesced to their former partner's demands that they not pick up and hold their baby and that their family of origin could not see the children. And quite a few alienated parents shared with me that they declined to have their former partner arrested after she/he had absconded with their child(ren) to another country or across America, instead choosing not to subject their children to such a traumatic event. In the end, it was more likely that the alienating parent succeeded in having the alienated parent arrested at one time or another and sometimes multiple times as a result of making erroneous allegations of domestic violence and/or of sexual child abuse. When I engage in treatment with the PAS family, my work with the parental subsystem involves redistributing the power imbalance that typically exists between the alienating and alienated parents but which is often being exacerbated by the professionals in the larger

social systems who have become co-opted by the alienating parent.

It is interesting, however, that Johnston (2001) deems the alienated parent to be generally healthier than the alienating parent. She explained it this way:

> Common personality predispositions of the aligned parent include narcissistic vulnerabilities that escalate under threat and present as paranoid and borderline dynamics. Such parents may not be consciously spiteful and vindictive but nevertheless behave in emotionally abusive ways that damage the child's relationship with the other parent. They often harbor intense, abiding distrust of the rejected parent, hold convictions that the other parent is at best irrelevant and at worst a pernicious or dangerous influence on the child, and believe that he or she has never loved or cared about the child. Consequently they see the child as urgently in need of their protection from the rejected parent. On the other hand, typical personality predispositions of the rejected parent are associated with a range of parenting limitations that do not, however, rise to the level of abuse and neglect. These may include passivity and withdrawal in the face of conflict, a tendency to be self-centered and immature, to have diminished empathy and limited parenting skills, and/or to be overly critical, demanding, and counter-rejecting in response to the child's provocative and obnoxious behavior. (p. 6)

It is a mystery to me how Johnston's above characterizations of the aligned parent support her argument that the aligned parent is innocent of fostering the alienation. Johnston seems to imply that when the alienating maneuvers of the aligned parent occur on an unconscious level, it makes the alienation more palatable. Well, it certainly makes the aligned parent **less** treatable. But I cannot see how this exonerates her/him. If a mugger impulsively, rather than premeditatively, stabs to death her/his victim, the outcome is equally disastrous for the victim.

I would like to elaborate on Johnston's assertion that the aforementioned systems exacerbate the alienation–a contention that cannot be overstated. Indeed, one of the points of this book is that the PAS would have little momentum were it not for the support which the alienator obtains from the professionals in these systems. Power struggles are common in families but do not evolve into such a disparity as it does in situations of the PAS unless powerful outside authorities align with the alienator. It is my contention that when the professionals in the mental health, child protection, law enforcement and judicial systems embolden the alienator, the alienator is able to maintain a significant advantage and upper hand over the targeted parent. The victimization of the alienated parent arises, then, from the overwhelming confluence of power and authority of the co-opted professionals in support of the alienator which accounts for the disempowerment of the alienated parent. The victimization could not result from the alienator's efforts if unaided. This is the basis for my argument for the multiprofessional systems which intervene in the family to work collaboratively with the family therapist by affording a level playing field between the alienated and alienating parents. When this is the backdrop for the therapy, I have generally been effective in reversing and eliminating the PAS.

Johnston (2001) grossly misrepresents Gardner's work by asserting that the making of false allegations of abuse by the alienating parent is a necessary component for the PAS to be diagnosed (p. 1). Although making such allegations is frequently a maneuver employed by the alienating parent, Gardner by no means claimed that it must occur for the PAS to be diagnosed. As the reader will discover from the experiences of the professionals interviewed in this book and from

my clinical practice, making false allegations of abuse–and particularly that of sex abuse– is frequently employed as an alienating maneuver because it almost certainly guarantees that visits between the targeted parent and the child will be suspended during the CPS investigation.

I must make an important point to the women's groups which oppose recognizing parental alienation as a syndrome: it is an exploitation and misuse of the PAS to employ it as a defense against domestic violence or sex abuse. This is a total misread and misapplication of Gardner. Just because there are those in the abusive population who attempt to do so, does not discredit its appropriate label as a syndrome. That would be as irrational as blaming Benjamin Franklin for every electrical fire to befall humanity just because he had harnessed its application.

All this being said, I fail to comprehend how a systems therapy approach, which is the only modality I have been using to treat these families for the past 17 years, is incompatible with assessing as a syndrome the family's transactional pattern of an alienation. As with any other syndrome in the *DSM-IV,* the family arrives with the member who is labeled as the identified patient and whom the members perceive as having an intrapsychic condition at the core of the dysfunction. And as with any other family myth that is presented to me, I provide a reframe which offers to the family an interactional or systemic interpretation of their presenting problem.

I am persuaded by my own clinical observations during 40 years of practice as to the very real existence of the PAS. Throughout these years, I had countless times observed in all too many heartbreaking cases the replication of Gardner's eight symptoms in the children along with the co-existing alienation-maintaining maneuvers of the alienating parent. Indeed, before I became aware of this syndrome, I had frequently misinterpreted situations in which children expressed an inexplicable hatred for a parent. In my early years of practice, I failed to employ an appropriate curiosity about how a child developed what appeared to be an abhorrence for such a significant, cherished, and intimate relationship. Like all too many therapists today, I mistakenly assumed that, beneath the surface, there must be repressed memories of abusive experiences with that parent. Given the increasing dialogue and revelations in the recent literature about the PAS, there can be no justification, however, for a professional in current times to accept carte blanche the child's stated loathing of a parent. Nor should the verbalizations and explanations of only one parent be accepted as the complete reality for what is occurring in the family.

Robert Hiltzik, Esq., is a litigation and matrimonial attorney who has been in practice for more than 22 years. He is a former partner in the law firm of Raoul Felder, and Partners, LLC. He is currently in private practice in Jericho, N. Y. He represents clients in Nassau and Suffolk Counties as well as in the five boroughs of New York City. He specializes in family law, including divorce litigation and child custody. I have known him professionally for two years and have shared many cases with him during that time period. I would be understating it to say that he is one of the most passionate, dedicated, principled, and knowledgeable attorneys with whom I have had the pleasure to collaborate—especially on some of the most severe cases of PAS. It would not be unusual to find him preparing for a trial with his client at 1:00 a.m. or on a Sunday afternoon or responding to client questions through emails at all hours. Often I have found him emailing me at midnight with a question about the PAS that would be of help to one of his clients.

Mr. Hiltzik was interviewed for this book on 12/29/2010. (A video recording and written comments are in the possession of the author.) Throughout his years of practice, he has routinely dealt with cases of parental alienation, which he characterized as "an alienating parent's objective to sever the relationship between the other parent and their child." He elaborated that: "PAS is used as a weapon, a tool utilized by a parent whose primary objective is to make the other parent miserable." He is particularly troubled about parental alienation because of its ensuing harm not only to the alienated parent but more importantly to the children. His experience and anecdotal evidence indicate that "alienation is prevalent in most cases of divorce to some degree because it is a natural reaction to a divorce proceeding." He estimated that 25 percent of his cases are seriously problematical for alienation, meaning that there has been a major rupture to the relationship between the alienated parent and the child. I believe that the explanation as to why Mr. Hiltzik does not experience a higher rate of severe alienation on his cases—a rate that more approaches the previously stated norm—is because of the efforts he invests in reaching out to collaborate with the other side when he smells a whiff of the alienation and also because he counsels his own clients against engaging in any alienating behaviors.

Evie Zarkadas, Esq., has been practicing as an attorney for more than 20 years. Nearly all her current practice is as an Attorney for the Children, and her office is in Centereach, New York. She earned a BS degree in genetics, an MA degree in computer science and energy science, and a JD degree. She sits on the ethics committee of Suffolk County Bar Association. Ms. Zarkadas and I have collaborated for the past two years on several mutual cases involving visitation, custody, and alienation issues, and she, too, has impressed me with her exceptional qualities. She is a highly committed, highly energetic, and a highly persevering lawyer for the child. When she is assigned a case, she not only interviews the child, she interviews the child with each parent, each parent separately, and the parents together. She contacts every adult involved in her client's life–all for the purpose of making the most informed and meaningful recommendations to the court. She utilizes the information she has collected about her client in hopes of brokering an amicable settlement between the parents.

Ms. Zarkadas was interviewed for this book on 1/7/2011. (A video recording and written comments are in the possession of the author.) She explained her thinking and her approach as follows, "Outside of the divorce, the parents are generally normal people who truly love their children. It is the divorce that is abnormal. It is a disease of the moment called divorce." I asked Ms. Zarkadas if she has experienced parental alienation in her practice and, if so, how she would describe it. Ms. Zarkadas confirmed that she frequently encounters it, and she defined it as, "an attempt by the custodial parent to erase the other parent from the child's life" and she described having witnessed its devastating consequences to children.

> The nature of the beast, divorce, is a euphemism for "we go to war." Divorcing spouses will use any weaponry, and the children are the most accessible weaponry. They become weapons of mass destruction by the party who exercises the most control over the child. And the parent with this control is usually the mother, who has been the primary caretaker. Human misery is evolving from this.

Ms. Zarkadas described this human misery to encompass severely acting-out, defiant children who are likely to develop serious psychological disturbances.

Ms. Zarkadas clarified she believes that the explanation as to why she has experienced the mother to be the principal alienator is because of the "opportunity" that is afforded the mother by typically having been the primary caretaker and because she is the parent who usually retains residential custody. As I stated in the introduction, I agree with Ms. Zarkadas's explanation that it is "opportunity" which accounts for the greater frequency of the mother being the alienator.

Dr. Burkhard confirmed that the PAS can be a severe problem and appears often in high conflict divorce cases. Given the agency's extensive treatment of abused and neglected children, she and Dr. Kelly are in the unique position to observe "a very different dynamic with a group of children who are engaged in irrational visit refusal." She expressed her concerns about what she observes during therapy sessions between these children and their targeted parent. According to Dr. Burkhard, "This group of children exhibits extraordinarily rude and disrespectful behaviors as opposed to the behaviors of the children with documented histories of abuse or maltreatment, who generally tolerate visits and may even seek a relationship with their parent."

Dr. Burkhard described the behaviors of the group of children demonstrating visit refusal as having "such an atypical type of pattern." She articulated her assessment of these children as follows, "They are playing a role with a script. They have a very specific script, and they walk out on stage for their lawyers, for the judge, and for the evaluators." Dr. Burkhard confirmed that the script is sometimes furnished by and performed for an alienating parent.

Dr. Kelly reported to me in her interview that she has no doubt about the existence of the PAS. She related that she became acutely aware of it after her years of treating truly abused and neglected children, who still sought to have relationships with their parents. She, too, was struck by "a starkly different dynamic in children from high conflict divorce cases than those in the abused group of children." She stated the following about PAS children in reference to their visitation refusal, "The refusal response is generally disproportionate to what has occurred in the past." Dr. Kelly expressed that the child's behavior is a response to a process, which she described:

> Negative statements and ideas about the targeted or absent parent are reinforced. At times, this may initially be an inadvertent process. Children in a divorce learn to balance their report to one parent about the good times with the other parent in order to spare the parent's feelings. For example, a child may state, "I had a good time at the zoo with dad but then he wouldn't give me dinner." In reality, the child may have eaten at the zoo and didn't want a meal at dad's house. Mom may overreact to the statement that the child was not fed at dad's house with overconcern and attention to the child, establishing a pattern of rewarding negative statements about dad.

The differing dynamics between these two groups of children–those who had been truly abused and those who exhibit an irrational visit refusal–led me to the inescapable conclusion that the PAS does exist. Having worked for 24 years with a foster care population, children who were removed from their homes due to neglect or abuse, I observed how they still zealously craved contact with their parents. It simply defies logic that children in a divorce situation could reject a parent with whom they had had a wonderfully loving relationship prior to the divorce proceedings.

Robert Previto, Esq., has been an attorney in New York for 17 years, and he practices primarily as a matrimonial attorney. He sits on the 18B panels for both Family and Su-

preme Court in Suffolk County, New York. His office is in Huntington Station, New York. I contacted Mr. Previto for an interview upon recognizing his exceptional concern and efforts which he had demonstrated in representing his client in an alienation case for which I subsequently provided co-parent counseling.

Mr. Previto was interviewed for this book on 4/19/2011. (An audio recording and written comments are in possession of the author.) He stated that he has experienced some degree of alienation in most of his matrimonial cases. He pointed out that if parents were able to communicate rationally, they would be seeing a mediator and not litigating custody. He explained, "The children become pawns. I see it again and again and again. When the parents get to the stage of litigation, they are at a stage where it is very difficult dealing with each other. This is the springboard for the contentious litigation." Mr. Previto defined parental alienation as occurring when "the custodial parent frustrates the other parent's rights to the child. The words, acts, and deeds of the custodial parent is to cut the child's affections for and contact with the other parent." According to Mr. Previto, the alienation card gets played because, "Children are used as a source of information and the go-between." Mr. Previto further indicated that the child is selfishly used by the alienating parent: "If you don't want to see the other parent yourself, you can accomplish that by getting the kids not see the other parent."

Mr. Previto asserted that alienating parents will create a situation in which they erroneously justify the withholding of visits if child support falls into arrears. The tactic they invoke is a method for calculating child support called "imputation of salary," which he declared to be frequently unjust and punitive and often abused. He asserted that it affords the custodial parent unprecedented and unwarranted power by allowing them to allege–sometimes with very little verifiable evidence–that the noncustodial parent is "willfully earning less than what he is capable of." He declared that he has had several cases in which his client was assessed an egregious child support payment based on unverifiable and weak imputed statements by his former partner. He asserted that, although there is a very strict burden of proof to establish this, the proof which is accepted is at the discretion of the judge, who can be biased. Mr. Previto exclaimed:

> There is a real opportunity here to abuse the system and relegate the noncustodial parent to an extreme disadvantage. The judge should not have the right to base these rulings solely on the credibility of a witness. That's not enough to prove that a party is earning more money than he or she claims. And when child support obligations fall into arrears, it is used as an excuse for alienation to withhold the visits.

Susan Saltz, Esq., has been a practicing attorney in New York State since 1983, and her office is in Huntington, New York. She is another dedicated and compassionate Attorney for the Children with whom I have collaborated on a very difficult custody and visitation case, which has been ongoing for almost three years. She has always been receptive to my input and many times sought out my professional assessment of the family dynamics on this case. She also represents parties in divorce proceedings. Ms. Saltz was interviewed for this book on 5/4/2011. (An audio recording and written comments are in the possession of the author.) She estimates that she experiences alienation on at least one-third of her cases, and she defined it as "one parent turning the children against the other parent deliberately or negligently by their behavior and by words." Ms. Saltz continued:

People going through divorce are so angry that they don't realize what they are doing. When they go through divorce they do things they would never do under other circumstances. Their anger just makes them blind to what they are doing, and that includes engaging in alienation.

Ms. Saltz cited examples on her case load in which the alienating parent will allow the children to overhear their conversations which they are having with friends or family about their other parent, and they say the most awful things about that parent. "The children almost always hear the conversations," Ms. Saltz exclaimed.

Susan A. DeNatale, Esq., was admitted to practice law in New York State in 1999. She was employed at the Suffolk County Attorney's Office from 1998–2004, where she worked in the Family Court Bureau prosecuting child abuse and neglect matters. In 2001, she was transferred to the State and Federal Torts Bureau, and in May, 2004, she began her private practice, focusing primarily in the area of Family Law. She accepts appointments as the Attorney for the Children as well as representing litigants. A large portion of her practice is dedicated to appellate work. I have shared a number of cases with Ms. DeNatale during the past several years, and I found her to be highly committed to representing her clients. Ms. DeNatale submitted written answers to questions as her practice responsibilities did not permit a face-to-face interview. She responded to the question as to whether she has encountered parental alienation in her practice, "I do believe I have confronted alienation in both matrimonial and family court custody matters," and she defined it as "a parent's attempt to portray the other parent in less than favorable light in order that the child will report to the court and attorneys that they prefer the alienating parent." She further punctuated the point that ascertaining the motivations of the alienating parent is important although not easily determined: "I am not sure that this is done in all circumstances with intent to alienate; it may be done because of a parent's irrational fear that they will lose custody or out of some other emotion." Ms. DeNatale cited a hypothetical situation which nonetheless exemplifies what she frequently encounters:

Daddy is not paying his child support, and mommy is working and paying for everything. Little boy comes home from a visit with dad with an expensive new toy. Mommy, under her breath, says, "If daddy paid child-support, mommy could buy you presents too." Child then feels guilty about having the gift and feels bad about his father. In this scenario, which is very typical, I do not believe the mother's statement comes from a place where she intended to alienate but rather from frustration and anger. Mother's anger is legitimate. Her expression of the anger is misplaced. Perhaps a telephone call to father to discuss the need for child support rather than a new videogame system would be a better way for mother to approach the problem.

Ms. DeNatale made a very important point about the importance of determining the motivations underneath the alienating behavior. As the reader will discover in later chapters, the mental health professionals, researchers, and forensic evaluators who were interviewed for the book all confirmed that a critical component of treatment is identifying such motivations so that the alienating parent's concerns and fears can be resolved in therapy.

Ms. DeNatale further articulated a common dilemma also cited by her colleagues: the difficulty in assessing for the presence of alienation in a particular case. She affirmed, "Not all cases that involve alienation are so blatant that they can be easily labeled." In

further agreement with many of her colleagues, she declared that the nature of divorce brings out the worst in the litigants along with a "certain naturally occurring rivalry between the parents to curry favor with their children and be the most wanted and most loved parent."

Dorothy A. Courten, Esq., currently practices primarily Matrimonial and Family Law, and her office is in Hauppauge, New York. She has been an attorney since 1988, initially working for the Legal Aid Society as an investigator in the criminal division and subsequently as a public defender before going into private practice. In addition to her current practice, Ms. Courten offers a pro bono consultation to battered spouses who are clients of Victims Information Bureau Services (VIBES). I sought out Ms. Courten for an interview after learning about her from my clients who had benefited from her pro bono consultation. Ms. Courten is exactly the kind of attorney whom an abused person would want in her/his corner. At the conclusion of spending just a few hours with her for this interview, I felt as if I had known her for a lifetime, and I believe the feeling was mutual. She is accessible, reassuring, unpretentious, and eager to learn from other professionals while simultaneously impressing with her understanding of the law, her unassuming professional confidence, and her motivation to defend her clients passionately. She was interviewed for this book on 5/27/2011. (An audio recording is in the possession of the author along with written approval of the interview.)

Ms. Courten defines alienation as "a manipulation of the children by one parent against the other parent. It is the twisting of a little mind." She asserted that the goal of the parent who engages in such behaviors is to sever the relationship between the other parent and their child. She judges alienation to be a "gigantic problem" particularly because of its very deleterious effects on children. In her practice, Ms. Courten has experienced that it is the father who predominantly engages in the process of alienation. She deems that "monetary motivation" is often the basis for father alienation on the cases she has confronted. She stated, "The fathers engage in the alienation because they do not wish to put money in the pocket of their former partner. They don't trust their former partner to use the money appropriately for the needs of their children." According to Ms. Courten, if they can obtain custody by severing the relationship between their child and the mother, they thereby resolve their monetary mistrust issues. She further expressed that most men generally do not pursue divorce unless they have another woman waiting in the wings, and they thus have a desire for the families to blend and to provide financially to the maximum for their blended family. On the other hand, according to Ms. Courten, alienating mothers can be motivated out of revenge, just plain hurt, or feeling neglected. Out of these motivations, according to Ms. Courten, they will express to the fathers, "You can't see the kids. You're not coming over. You can't come to the school function." When these mothers are successful in obstructing the father's involvement with their children, they will then advise the children, "Your father is really bad. Look how your father has abandoned you." Although determining the ratio between alienating mothers and alienating fathers is not the purpose of this book, Ms. Courten's anecdotal experience with alienation seems to provide credibility to revised thinking that the ratio between men and women who engage in an alienation is much closer to 50–50 than was originally believed.

Because of the tremendous emotional turmoil which divorcees are undergoing, Ms. Courten insists that each of her clients be in therapy. She attests to the positive results she

has experienced from this requirement: "If you can address in therapy the underlying motivations for the alienation, then some of the really bad behaviors of trying to turn the kids against their other parent will get better."

Francine H. Moss, Esq., has been practicing Matrimonial and Family Law for 32 years. Her office is in Ronkonkoma, New York. She has served as a Law Guardian, now renamed as Attorney for the Children for 17 of those years, and her practice is currently approximately 50–50 between the two roles. Before obtaining her JD degree, she majored in sociology in college and in graduate school. Ms. Moss and I have shared a number of cases during the past few years in her role as representing children. She, too, is a highly dedicated and energetic representative of her minor clients, and she extends herself for her clients by reaching out to the parents in an attempt to encourage them to subvert their hostility for each other to their love for their children and thereby proceed in the best interests of their children.

Ms. Moss was interviewed for this book on 5/12/11. (An audio recording and written comments are in possession of the author.) When asked about her experience with alienation, she confirmed that it has been quite prevalent in her practice over the years, describing it as follows: "The hallmark of alienation is the child's inexplicable resistance to maintaining a relationship with one of her/his parents." She confirmed that this resistance is at the behest of the other parent, whom she described as follows, "The alienator will take everyone down with her/him if possible." Ms. Moss clarified this to mean that the alienator is intent on achieving her/his goal of severing the relationship between the other parent and their child and is unperturbed as to who gets in her/his way, even if it includes their child. She characterized the alienator as follows, "These parents are very self-absorbed, and it's very difficult to get them to see the position of the other parent. It's hard to get them to prioritize for someone other than themselves. It's the children whom you think they should be able to do that for, but I'm not so sure." The determination of alienating parents, according to Ms. Moss, "creates a difficult if not an impossible situation for their children to want to see the alienated parent. For these children, it's like a salmon swimming upstream. Because when you live with the alienator in the household, there will be consequences for any expression of desire to see the other parent."

Joshua Hecht, Esq. is a practicing matrimonial attorney in Hauppauge, New York. He is the only attorney with whom I have had no prior professional experiences. I contacted him cold and was very glad that I did so. He was interviewed for this book on 5/13/2011. (A video recording and written comments are in the author's possession.) Mr. Hecht impressed me as being evenhanded, dedicated, and very knowledgeable. He practices almost exclusively in the area of Matrimonial and Family Law, having been admitted to practice in 2006. Prior to founding a separate practice in 2010, he was associated with two different law firms. Although he differentiated himself as a fathers' rights attorney, he clarified for me during our interview that he views himself more as a practitioner whose goal is to truly bring gender neutrality to the courtroom. He expressed concern with how, in his view, fathers and husbands often fall prey to false allegations of domestic violence placing them at a distinct disadvantage in the matrimonial proceeding, particularly with respect to the issue of custody. He noted, for example:

A husband and father can quickly find himself ordered to stay away from the marital home where he had always played an integral role in caring for and raising the parties' children, based upon the wife's obtaining a Temporary Order of Protection as a result of her filing a Family Offense Petition, wherein the husband wasn't even present to provide his side of the story. Without notice and following a sheriff's knock on the door, a husband may have just minutes to leave his home. All of a sudden he is out of his house and away from his children, with his wife dictating his every move with their children. Having never run afoul of the law, this gentleman could easily find himself embroiled in a divorce proceeding, a Family Court proceeding, and, based upon the nature of the allegations and how they were reported, perhaps a criminal proceeding.

According to Mr. Hecht, as a natural consequence, the wife is often presented with an opportunity to gain an underhanded tactical advantage in the ensuing divorce proceeding, particularly with respect to the issue of custody. Mr. Hecht concluded, "The wife becomes the de facto custodial parent, and this affords them a tremendous amount of leverage."

Mr. Hecht's practice is dedicated to representing both husbands and wives. However, his experience has led him to the conclusion that, while the courts purport to be gender neutral, such is not always the case.

When I asked Mr. Hecht to define parental alienation, he characterized it as:

The poisoning of the child's mind against the other parent either, whether consciously or unconsciously, intentionally or unintentionally, the ultimate effect of which is to drive a wedge between the child and the other parent. Parental alienation could simply involve withholding parenting time or visitation, or, for instance, a parent using his or her financially superior position to drive a wedge between the child and the other parent, or perhaps interposing the child in the finances.

In Mr. Hecht's experience, it is perpetuated by fathers as well as by mothers, and he estimated that 20 percent to 25 percent of his divorce cases with children involve some degree of parental alienation although he did preface that with the following comment:

> The degree of alienation can be rather mild, such as in situations where a father would use his financially superior position to lavish gifts upon the children and curry favor with them at the mother's expense. Consequently, he becomes "the Disney dad," for example, by taking the children on expensive trips, and the mother simply doesn't have the resources or financial wherewithal to compete. All of a sudden, it drives a wedge between the mother and the children even though it may not have been the father's intent to do so.

Paul E. Levitt, Esq., is an attorney who practices in Melville, New York but now no longer handles Matrimonial Law. He had been the matrimonial attorney who represented the father, Stephen Young, in the landmark case, *Young v. Young* (1987, 1995) in which the Appellate Division overturned the trial court ruling handed down from Supreme Court which had denied the father's petition for custody. The Appellate Division rendered a judgment in favor of the alienated father and then applied the remedy of transferring the custody of his four very young children to him. Although Mr. Levitt had been practicing matrimonial law for only a few years when he began the Young case in 1987, he relinquished practice as a matrimonial attorney shortly after the Young case was finally resolved. Mr. Levitt was interviewed for this book on 6/2/11. (An audio recording and written comments are in the possession of the author.) He stated, "I had too many sleepless nights from practicing this kind of law. I was concerned about the effects on children of high conflict divorce, and I wasn't happy."

When I asked Mr. Levitt how frequently he encountered parental alienation in divorce cases he stated, "As a matrimonial attorney, I used to see it too many times. It's the difficulty of representing someone going through an emotional state. You are dealing with people who are at their worst. And sometimes these parents are so impulse-driven that they can't control what they say and do." The consequential behavior from this emotional state very often produces the process of alienation for which Mr. Levitt offered the following definition, "Alienation is the weapon of choice. The alienating parent knows what buttons to push. And they know how to get what they want." According to Mr. Levitt, "The ammunition that fires the weapon of alienation is sometimes fallacious, stinging, and devastating allegations of sex abuse. Other times, it takes on less insideous forms of PAS. He provided some examples of how this weapon is fired. The monetary parent, for example, may play financial war games by hiding income for the purpose of lowering child support and maintenance payments. In order to level the playing field, the nonmonetary parent may use the children by withholding them and turning them against the other parent. Regarding the Young case, Mr. Levitt conveyed:

> The alienating mother inflicted an indoctrinating process on the children by telling them what she wanted them to say. They were manipulated by her to admit to horrendous sex abuse acts, such as being sodomized with a stick, which morphed into a branch, etc. There were always escalating embellishments which are incredibly detrimental to children should they begin to believe what they have been forced to repeat.

It was the frequency of such using and abusing of the children in an unnecessary war between the parents that kept Mr. Levitt awake at night.

What follows in the subsequent eight chapters is a differential definition of each of the eight symptoms which Gardner identified as being indicative of the PAS. In order to bring to life for the reader the distinguishing characteristics and the effects of these symptoms, I will be portraying examples of 56 children in 32 families taken from the PAS sagas in my practice—sagas that represent the syndrome at various stages of its progression. Fifty children and their families are from my practice during the years from 2006 to 2011. The remaining six children and their families were in treatment sometime during the years from 1995 to 2006. Eight of the 32 targeted/alienated parents of nine children are mothers.

A subsequent chapter provides treatment summaries of 16 of the families, and these summaries demonstrate how the PAS can be reversed and frequently squelched by using a structural family therapy modality; but the summaries further indicate that treatment is swifter and more successful when the larger social systems guaranteed a level playing field between the alienating and alienated parents. On the other hand, when professionals in those systems aligned with the alienating parent, the therapeutic process was frequently protracted and less efficacious in reversing the PAS, if at all.

The last focus of the book suggests changes to the mental health, child protection, law enforcement, and judicial systems so as to interrupt and reverse the alienation progression. My suggestions took into consideration the ideas and experiences of those who were interviewed for this book.

Chapter 2

THE CAMPAIGN OF DENIGRATION

An Eternity of Midsummer Nightmares

Everett (2006) declared that all families have "themes" (pp. 230–231) which are shared mutually by all of its members. Themes lend cohesiveness to family identity and form the basis for normative collective and individual member behavior. For example, one family theme may be "We are our brother's keeper." In a family guided by this theme, the parents will encourage the children to pursue careers in public service, religion, the helping professions, or other magnanimous pursuits.

Themes become myths when they are fundamentally specious, have malevolent goals, and maintain dysfunctional family functioning. Examples of myths would be: "All men cheat." "All women are gold diggers." "Only the family can be counted on." "The world is a dangerous place." The consequence of such myths undermines the child's ability to trust in object relations. Myths may be attributed to individual family members, such as occurs in the scapegoating of a child. An example of child scapegoating is, "We would have no problems if little Johnnie would only stop playing with matches." Myths are readily accepted by individual family members in part due to how "normal" they are perceived because a precedent had been set by the acceptance of family themes.

The campaign of denigration is an example of the construction of family myths which are used for the purpose of turning a child against a previously loved and loving parent. Although it may originate on an unintentional and unconscious level, it frequently progresses into a conscious scapegoating of the targeted parent by the alienating parent with the goal of severing the relationships between the targeted parent and the children. The probable progression is the single most important rationale for early intervention. The child is programmed to believe that her/his other parent is worthless, selfish, unloving, malevolent, undeserving, and dangerous, and so on. The effective result is that the children become convinced they will be happier, healthier, and better adjusted if their targeted parent is eradicated from their lives. Alienators have rejected their former partners and seduce their children into introjecting their feelings and executing their maltreatment of their other parent. Seduced children develop a disingenuous loathing of their targeted parent as a result of the alienator's brainwashing. According to Gardner (1998) these children

23

"speak of the alienated parent with every vilification and profanity in their vocabulary—without embarrassment or guilt. . . . In many cases, the elaborations are ludicrous, and even preposterous, thereby providing the clue to their speciousness" (p. 77). PAS children acquire—sometimes overnight—a spontaneous and incomprehensible amnesia when it comes to preserving any memories of their targeted parent's prior participation in their life. Gardner (1998) continued, "It is as if there has been a total obliteration of that segment of the child's brain in which were embedded memories of the life with his (her) father prior to the father's departure" (p. 79). I would modify this statement to indicate that fathers in equal percentages to mothers engage in an alienation, and this is the position that Gardner adopted towards the end of his career.

Baker (2007) assessed that the alienating parent employs five primary manipulation techniques to facilitate the campaign of vilification. Paraphrasing her, they are:

1. expressing persistent and merciless denigration of the target parent's character in order to minimize her/his importance;
2. creating the notion that the target parent is detrimental to the child and thusly must be feared;
3. questioning the target parent's love for their child in order to destroy the psychological bond between the child and the target parent;
4. withdrawal of love by the alienating parent from a child who acknowledges positive feelings and regard for the target parent; and
5. obliterating the target parent from the emotional and physical life of the child (pp. 63–81).

My esteemed colleagues whom I interviewed provided many examples indicative of the campaign of denigration which they experience regularly in their respective practices. Dr. Havlicek described a young child who exclaimed to him "I want to see my father dead. I want to bite his arm until he bleeds to death." When Dr. Havlicek inquired of the child as to what the father could have done to evoke such feelings, no examples were provided. This same child then concocted an inflammatory fairytale which was then exclaimed to the mother upon her arrival for pick-up after the therapy session concluded with the father. "My father attacked me!" the child exclaimed. Stating that it did not happen, Dr. Havlicek was nonetheless unable to disabuse the child of this. The mother inflamed her child's fantasy, however, when she expressed, "My child did not lie. It's just my child's point of view." Dr. Havlicek conveyed to me the gravity of the mother's rejoinder when he declared, "This is the basis for the development of psychoses. The child is learning to manipulate reality due to enmeshment with the alienating parent."

Dr. Burkhard related how alienating parents frequently model for their children an irrational fear of the other parent. This may be conveyed as much through body language or nonverbal communication as by direct verbal communication. She explained:

In our office, a visit with the targeted parent is going to be safe. Children with a known history of maltreatment are able to discriminate that our office is a safe place to meet with the parent. Children who are alienated may be encouraged or reinforced to display irrational fear or anxiety responses as if they are going to be molested, beaten, or verbally or physically assaulted with the therapist present in the room.

However, despite the obvious safety, Dr. Burkhard and her staff frequently see children cringing in the waiting room and being soothed by the favored parent in anticipation of the visit with their targeted parent. Dr. Burkhard expressed:

After observing what the alienating parent is modeling, it would be unrealistic to expect that the child would act otherwise. The children are really in a no-win situation, as they cannot please both parents; but because they live with the favored parent, they will likely follow that parent's lead. If the mother is acting fearful, then the kids will do likewise. Would you really expect the child to say, "Mom cut it out. It's perfectly safe here. I want to go see Daddy." That's not likely to happen. And this happens even in cases where there has been no documentation or evidence of any abuse by the targeted parent.

In working with these families, the favored or alienating parents may model noncompliance for their children, and Dr. Burkhard expressed this as follows:

The favored or alienating parent provides spurious explanations for being unable to keep the visit: the child has an activity that unexpectedly arose an hour before the planned visit; the child must study for a test or complete a school project for the next day; the visit interferes with religious instruction or tutoring, etc., as if the parent had been unaware of these issues when she scheduled the session time. Many times, the alienating parent has declined in front of the child my suggestions

to foster a relationship with the other parent. I often hear, "She doesn't have to do that. She can't do this or that."

Ms. Zarkadas cited cases of alienation from her practice, one being a latency age child whose parents had had a bitter divorce. The child expressed to her, "I don't want to see my father anymore." According to Ms. Zarkadas, the mother supported this behavior by sanctioning her child's feelings and resistance. Another latency age client exclaimed to her in reference to the targeted father, "I'm afraid of him. He yells. I have to do my homework his way. He's a loser, he's disgusting. I don't have to talk to him. And my mom says I don't have to." According to Ms. Zarkadas, this last comment revealed it all and comports with the mother's ongoing pattern of behaviors to sever the relationship between the father and their child. She affirmed that it was clear to her that a child this young was taking cues from the mother, who was sanctioning the noncompliance with the agreement for phone calls and for the visits. In another case, she stated that a preteen child announced to her, "I'm very angry at my daddy. He's never on time. He's always tired. He wouldn't buy me a tutor." Ms. Zarkadas was particularly curious about this last expression and asked the preteen to explain its meaning. The only explanation she received was that the comment had been expressed by the maternal grandmother. Another latency age client exclaimed to her, "My father's a jerk; a philanderer; he cheated all over the place on my mom." Ms. Zarkadas confirmed that when these children are asked for specific incidents that would explain why they characterize their targeted parent so negatively, they are unable provide such examples, and they offer no credible explanations that are commensurate with their visit refusal and expressed enmity.

When Ms. Zarkadas confronts cases of alienation, she evokes her role as "counselor" and attempts to get parents to broker a settlement regarding custody and visitation. She stated that she is frequently successful in facilitating a resolution by calling the parents to her office for a "discussion." She is not afraid to use their authority to broker a settlement. She relies on a psychological principle that is the basis for my therapy: bringing parties face-to-face has the potential to resolve differences.

Mr. Hiltzik stated that alienating behaviors can be subtle but nonetheless devastating and humiliating to the targeted parent. He cited as an example one of his cases of an interfaith marriage in which the alienating mother, who is Christian, sent the child to her Jewish father flouting a cross around her neck–although the parents had agreed to raise her in the Jewish faith; this was a particularly pointed humiliation because it occurred immediately after visits resumed after a year of visit refusal. He cited other examples in which the children will call their alienated parent by their first name or, in situations where the alienated parent is the father, the children will request permission to use their mother's maiden name. According to Mr. Hiltzik, the alienated parents he has represented always have difficulty obtaining their children's medical and educational records and are generally excluded from their children's extracurricular activities. Even more humiliating, he frequently has to defend his clients against multiple false allegations of sexual and/or physical abuse, and this devastating humiliation to his clients is exacerbated because these allegations generally result in the suspension of visits with the children while the CPS investigation runs its course.

Mr. Previto expressed his amazement at some of the derogatory comments related to him by many of his clients that they are labeled by the custodial parent in front of the children. These labels included: "whore" or a "slut" and "Mommy left us." He has also heard comments from the alienated father that his estranged wife communicates to the children that he is not supporting them when he actually is.

Ms. Saltz described one of her cases in which she represented three siblings, one in the mid-teens, one preteen, and one latency age:

> The preteen child walked into my office for the first time, and even before any introductions could be made, the child announced, "I hate my father. I just don't want to see him. I don't know what I'm doing here, and that's all I'm going to say." The latency age child hid under a coat and would not even acknowledge me. The teenager required to "see the papers their parents filed against each other" before deciding with whom to live. Now how does a child know about papers? In this case, the mother had basically told the children everything negative there is to know about their father, including his affair. In fact, she was pushing the children to visit with their father at his girlfriend's house so that they could see her in the flesh and know that their father was cheating. Now how are these kids not going to be screwed up?

Ms. Saltz related that she inquired of the preteen for a reason to justify the feelings about the father, and the child responded, "Well, he had an affair." She counseled the children that this was between their parents, and she described what happened next, "I attempted to draw out the preteen child about anything the father might have done to the children, but I did not get any response to this question." Ms. Saltz continued:

I think one of the terribly alienating maneuvers occurs when the children are shown legal papers. People will do all kinds of horrible, terrible things to each other during divorce, but you surely don't want the children to see that. Kids will accept that what occurs between the parents is between them, but only if they are not poisoned by one of the parents. Children don't need to hear these things, such as an affair. It has long-term negative effects on the children.

In another case cited by Ms. Saltz, she represents the mother of a latency age child who is in the custody of the father with the mother having supervised visits. The mother arranged for a party for her child's communion after having obtained the approval of the supervising resource to provide the acquired supervision on that day. The party was scheduled for one week away, and the father had yet to give consent, even though the invitations had long been out, and relatives of both sides had been invited and RSVP'd their attendance. Ms. Saltz commented, "You tell me what's going on here? The mother wants to do something for their child, and the father is refusing to talk to her about it. I believe that he is trying to alienate the child from her mother."

Ms. Saltz recognizes the heavy burden that has been placed with her to protect the welfare of her minor clients. One way she attempts to accomplish this is by relieving them of the painful ramifications of feeling caught between their parents and having to choose sides. She uses her role to counsel them away from taking a position on where they want to live. She informs them that they have three options and not just the two obvious choices of picking mom or dad. She will advise them that they can simply state they do not want to choose, which is a perfectly acceptable position for them to take.

Ms. Moss cited a number of her cases in which there was an alienation. In one case, her latency age client was so enmeshed with the mother that the child refused to visit the father. The child stated to Ms. Moss, "I hate him. He's mean. He's mean to my mom and he never calls and he never writes." The child was unable to cite any specific instances to back up these feelings. Ms. Moss wondered why her client was so upset about the father's lack of contact if there was so much hatred for him. Ms. Moss questioned the authenticity of the child's feelings for the father upon having revealed too much knowledge of an explosive incident that had occurred between the parents and for which her client could not possibly have had so much first-hand knowledge. "It seemed like it was greatly embellished," according to Ms. Moss. In another case, her client was a child in the mid-teens who would pass the alienated mother in the hallway of the school, where the mother was employed, and not give her the recognition of even a "hello." When her mother went to observe her child's games, she was ignored. In yet another of Ms. Moss's cases, a child in the late teens, who was estranged from the father, switched her last name to her mother's maiden name.

As with Ms. Zarkadas, Ms. Moss takes very seriously her role as "counselor" and thereby invests extraordinary efforts to work with the parents of her clients in hopes of brokering a settlement which not only reflects her clients' wishes but also serves their best interests. Ms. Moss is forceful in speaking with her minor client, seeks an explanation whenever there exists the refusal to have a relationship with the noncustodial parent, and explains to her clients that it is unlikely that a judge will order that there be no visits. Her antenna for alienation goes up when she receives responses in which "the situation described doesn't seem to be a good enough explanation for refusal to have a relationship with the parent. The reason given is just out of proportion to the feelings of antipathy." When this occurs, Ms. Moss recognizes she has a tough road to hoe. Ms. Moss will talk to the parents as well in an attempt to minimize the conflict and hostility. She reminds them that children are not necessarily accurate reporters and that if they are telling tales about one home, they are most likely telling tales about the other as well. According to Ms. Moss, "Children often play one parent off against the other." She also acknowledged experiencing a very common phenomenon with PAS children when she stated, "There are rewards for telling the parents what they want to hear."

Mr. Hecht cited a number of cases where, to his own consternation and frustration, it was his clients who were culpable, though he notes that a parent may engage in alienating behavior without even realizing it, for example, when a mother states, "We can't do X because your father won't pay for it." According to Mr. Hecht, such comments, particularly when repeated with regularity, "drive a wedge between the child and the other parent." In one of his own cases, his client had her small children write letters to their father about things they needed him to pay for. The judge admonished his client as to the adverse effects of her behavior on her children, but the judge's admonition simply did not register or resonate with his client.

Dr. Baker described a typical alienating behavior which obstructs the visits between the other parent and their children when she commented on her experience that the alienating parent is "conveniently waiting in the driveway of the targeted parent's house with the car engine running to pick up the kids in case the slightest thing goes wrong."

In my own practice, I experience on a recurring basis the precise behaviors which my colleagues describe as routinely occurring in their respective practices. I shall shortly portray these tragic sagas. I encourage the reader to note the similarity in the children's themes, expressions, attitudes, and performances, as if they had all attended the same theatrical retreat in order to ascertain how to best enact their roles in the family drama. And I encourage the reader to further note the similarities of expressions and behaviors of each alienating parent with every other and with their children. The resemblance of each child to every other child and each alienating parent to every other parent is indicative of a syndrome.

But if the predicable, virtually identical attitudes, declarations, and deeds of the children and the alienating parent provide empirical evidence for the objective observer to reach the conclusion that the syndrome is present, we must be careful not to rush to judgment in interpreting the **motivations** of the parent who fosters an alienation; we can only initially observe and describe their alienating behaviors. Until we discover exactly who is the individual presenting before us with her/his idiosyncratic feelings, beliefs, and attitudes, we must resist stereotyping with maligning characteristics and pathologizing diagnoses. A grouping of parents is comprised of individuals whose similarities cannot be prejudged to extend beyond the title of "parent" and of the consensus which we, as a culture, have reached about what it means to be a parent. Motivations to engage in a programming vary markedly from overprotectiveness to naiveté to insecurity to fear of losing the love of one's children to mistrust due to the culmination of an uncivil marriage to anxiety due to the anticipated loss of one's social and economic status, and yes, to revenge, for some. And then there are those who facilitate an alienation because they had learned from their family of origin that emotional cut-off is the customary way of handling (or more likely mishandling) disagreements. This is exactly what my sister and I learned from our family of origin history when my paternal grandfather and grandmother severed their relationships with their siblings in response to insignificant disagreements–the origins of which had long been forgotten and is exactly the theme depicted in the short story, "The Lottery." So when my mother and my maternal grandmother engaged in the PAS, it appeared to my father to be normal behavior precisely because he had been acculturated by his parents to perceive ruptures in family relationships as normal family development.

I am therefore advocating that the mental health professional not prejudge, vilify, or marginalize the alienator but instead attempt to ascertain the motivations for the alienation. Ascertaining the motivations of and then conveying empathy for the alienator will enable the therapist to join with her/ him, who then feels understood by the therapist. Joining is an essential preliminary step to the subsequent challenging process in which the therapist will engage with the family members in order to facilitate the family's restructuring.

The following are my case examples which are illustrative of the symptom called "denigration of the targeted parent." But because the eight symptoms can overlap, the examples cited may be illustrative of any of the other seven. For example, "borrowed scenarios" will also be present when the comments indicate a cognitive development beyond the actual age of the child; "reflexive support of the alienating parent" is also present when the child's words indicate a coalition; "extension of the deprecation to the extended family of the alienated parent" is present when these formerly loved relatives are rejected, and so on. Each symptom, however, has a dedicated chapter for an in-depth discussion.

A boy in early puberty who had not visited with his father in seven months asserted

to me that he did not believe that his anesthesiologist father was competent to treat him when he is ill. He exclaimed, "He does not know what to do when I get sick, but my mom does." (I can stipulate that his mother had no medical background.) On one occasion, upon falling ill under his father's care before the visit refusal commenced, the boy immediately sent a text to his mother about the situation, and she raced to her sick son's bed to rescue him from his physician father. At other times, the boy labeled his father, "a liar," "stupid," "mean," and "off his rocker." He accused his father of being "fake" when his father expressed to him how much he loves him and misses him. Even after his father reminded him of everything he had done for him, given him, and participated in with him, the boy continued to insist that his father's feelings for him are "fake." He failed to cite any examples of the epithets he had labeled his father.

In another case, an alienated father was alleged to have an "anger management problem," by his preteen daughter who had not seen him in several years because her mother had absconded with her to Canada. During the sessions, the girl frequently exclaimed to him, "You are not a good father." At other times she uttered in response to his limit setting, "Nobody's talking to you. I don't have to listen to your crap." When her father requested that she do her chores in a timely fashion, she snapped, "I'll take as much time as I want to, so just get used to it." When her college professor father attempted to encourage her to pursue her studies more diligently, she derogatorily responded, "I know you are just the encyclopedia of knowledge." At other times, she engaged in dismissive gestures such as rolling her eyes, pointing in his face, and looking away while he was talking to her. There were also a number of instances in which she punched her father in the face and struck him in various parts of his body. She frequently labeled him a "liar," a "disturbed person," an "abuser," and "a jerk."

In the case of a boy in puberty who had not visited with his pediatrician father in almost a year, he demeaned him by calling him a "quack" but could not explain in what way. When I commented that it did not appear that he held his father's occupation in high regard, he responded that he is not sure if his job is important. In fact, he frequently called his father, "stupid," "mean," "a liar," "crazy," and "passive-aggressive." The boy was unable to cite any specific examples that would justify these characterizations, and he further could not define "passive-aggressive." He stated that his father has a problem "managing his anger." He, too, described his father as being "fake" when he expressed his love for him.

A preteen girl refused all visits and all contact with her mother for a year after having had an extended phone call with her farther, who coincidentally arrived to take her to his parents' home where he was living. Just like that, the girl decided to erase her mother from her memory and life. Her much younger brother did not accede to the brainwashing and remained meaningfully involved with both of his parents. In the initial therapy session, the girl arrived sobbing as if the sky were falling because the judge had ordered the therapy sessions with her mother, and she exclaimed "I told my lawyer that I did not want to have any contact with you." She declared that she was fearful of her mother in anticipation that she could become physically aggressive with her. (As if this would actually occur in the office of the court appointed therapist!) Her mother did nothing in the session to realize the girl's prophesy. She was, instead, supportive and empathetic of her daughter and persuasively expressed her love for her and conveyed to her the emptiness she had endured due to

their estrangement. In response to her mother's vulnerability and outpouring of emotions, the girl uttered, "You're being fake. You're lying. You're only being nice because she's here." Even when the mother sobbed regarding the state of their relationship, the girl exclaimed, "Your tears are phony. You're putting on an act." In anticipation that her mother might attempt to hug her, the girl exclaimed, "Don't you dare come near me. I order you not to touch me." She further called her mother, "fuckin' nuts" and "mean." When I asked the girl for examples that would justify her panic about being in her mother's presence, she was unable to cite any that were commensurate with her expressed fear. She alleged that her mother had an "anger control issue," but she was unable to cite any instances in which her mother had become angry with her other than the typical parental requests to do homework and chores, to keep her room clean, and not to pick on her younger brother. When I pressed her to cite the verbally abusive language which she had accused her mother of using, she stated, "I can't remember any; it was such a long time ago."

The mother of a young latency-age boy was obstructing visits with his father due to spurious allegations that he had an "anger management problem." In sessions, the boy regularly called his father "crazy" and "mean." He stated that his mother and aunt, with whom he lived, regularly told him that his father does not love him; they encouraged him to hang up the phone on his father whenever he called; and they refused admittance of his father into their home when he arrived for the visits. The effects of the poisoning on this little boy resulted in his defiance of his father. In the therapy sessions, the boy frequently exclaimed to his father, "My auntie says you are not the boss of me." He proceeded to justify his defiance by exclaiming, "I don't have to listen to you. It's because you're a baby; you're boring; everything with you is junk. I'll be happy if you don't pick me up anymore." He added, "Mommy doesn't listen to you either." At other times, he called his father "a liar" as a result of hearing his mother repetitively contradict his father in his presence. He frequently told his father, "Keep your big mouth shut," and he attempted to overtalk his father whenever he did not like what his father had to say. At other times, he exclaimed to him, "You have a big problem" after which he then punched his father in the stomach. He was unable to cite any specific examples of his father's behavior which warranted this barrage of epithets. The father reported to me that the Rabbi of his synagogue had one time confronted his son about his son's maltreatment of him which the Rabbi had witnessed. His son responded to the Rabbi, "Well my mommy and my auntie disrespect him." The boy exhibited anxiety because his mother yelled at him whenever he asked to call his father, thereby confirming that his expressed animosity for his father was specious. All this brainwashing conveyed to the boy that his father is only incidentally significant to him, as reflected in the boy's comment to his father, "I don't have to visit if I don't want to. I have my rights."

The brainwashing by the boy's alienating mother and aunt is evident: children this young are not capable of expressing themselves with this terminology, and they clearly lack an understanding of these concepts. I have not known the rights conveyed by the Constitution to its citizens to be on a grade school syllabus.

I was providing therapeutic visits to a father and his two teen-age sons whom he had not seen in 13 months after they precipitously stopped visiting, coincidently when their mother had applied for an increase in child support on the basis that there was "a change in circumstance." The boys entered the first therapy session, and in a manner like that of a dragon spitting fire, the older boy proclaimed to his father, "You are a psycho!" He then turned to me and exclaimed, "You need to understand all the reasons why we hate him so much!" But such citations were not offered—either for the father's alleged mental instability or for the boys' expressed hatred. When his father offered apologies for these nonspecific accusations, the boy pronounced, "Your apologies are phony. They don't seem sincere." The boy was unable to indicate how he had arrived at the interpretation that the apologies were not genuine and were nonetheless echoed by his brother, who was also unable to provide citations. The boys repeatedly expressed that they had no desire to see their father. The younger son admitted to having called his father, "a fucking bastard." The father's "crime" that warranted this explicative was that he had bought him a pair of sneakers for having improved a failing grade. The younger boy called his father a "liar" and suggested that he forget about having them in his life. But when I asked the boy my routine question in PAS cases as to whether he could imagine his father not being at his high school graduation, he became maudlin and teary-eyed and did not answer. This reaction is clearly indicative of the speciousness of his supposed hatred for his father.

I was providing therapeutic visits for a latency age boy and his father who was alleged to have an "anger management issue," in a situation where there had been no visits for five months. Arriving under the influence of his alienating mother, he announced, "I hate him, I hate him, I hate him. I don't want to see him." Throughout the first several sessions, the boy repeatedly ranted against his father with these words. He called his father, "crazy, lazy, and a liar." When his father asked him why he expressed those sentiments, he responded, "You don't treat me with love, so I don't treat you with love." He was unable to explain the connection. (A latency age child is not capable of this level of abstract thinking.) During the first several sessions, the boy hit, kicked, spit at, and stuck his tongue out at his father. When his father asked him why he did not speak with him on the previous day when he had called him, the boy replied, "The babysitter stated that I am not allowed to talk to strangers." The sitter was indisputably executing the dictate of the boy's alienating mother. The boy was unable to cite any justifications for his alleged statements of hatred towards his father.

I was providing therapeutic visits for two children, one preteen and one teen, and their father whom they had not seen in five months. He was alleged to have an "anger management problem." In the sessions, the younger child frequently demonstrated no restraint in expressing to the father a tirade of hurtful comments such as, "I hate you," and "Go to hell!" When the father attempted to provide discipline, the child exclaimed, "My mom said you are not the boss of me." The older child cursed him on a regular basis. One of the "nicer" comments was, "What is your problem? Are you sick in the fucking head?" They teased him about his efforts to improve his parenting skills by reading a number of books on the subject. Instead of recognizing his effort to become a better parent, they chided him for essentially not having been born with parenting knowledge. Outside of the therapy session, the older child left abusive and threatening messages on his phone. Many therapy sessions were quite stressful in that I felt like I was coaching the father about how to deal with children who demonstrated no respect for him and were invested in degrading him at every opportunity. He frequently sobbed to me in pain about how his children relentlessly barraged him with these hurtful indictments and

denigrations. The children offered no credible explanations for their enmity for him other than to cite a totally fabricated history of having physically abused them; this history was never substantiated with examples. Because they had been brainwashed by their alienating mother to believe this, both children accused their father of being "a phony" whenever he expressed his love for them and how much he misses them. Their mother, also, had alleged to me about such an abuse history but was unable to provide any credible evidence to support her claims. The fabricated emotional abuse is only half the story. The younger child frequently became physically abusive of him—one time deliberately punching him in the genitals.

A very young adult regularly regurgitated the epithets he had heard his father spew at his mother by calling her "bitch," "cunt," "fatso," "white trash," "a piece of shit," and "demented." He had witnessed his father physically abusing her, and he replicated this treatment. The abuse consisted of attempts at choking her, slapping her in the head with a book, and kicking her in the stomach. She was so much at risk by remaining in the marital residence that she fled to a relative's home. She since had no contact with her son for more than eight months as he made no efforts to repair their relationship or apologize to her at the very minimum. In fact, ever since divorce proceedings were initiated, the only interaction between the mother and son was of the abusive nature just described. The father had previously announced to the mother that he would do everything in his power to destroy the relationship between her and their son if she pursued the divorce.

I was requested by the attorney for a preteen boy to provide family therapy for him and his father, who was alleged to have an "anger management problem." (Does the reader notice a pattern in these cases?) The mother was attempting to win the boy to her side in a very nasty custody proceeding. Although the boy and his father were living the same home, he had refused to acknowledge his father's existence or go near him as if the father were a leper. During the therapy sessions, it was like pulling teeth to get the boy to talk to his father. Typically, he gave him the silent treatment, which was most humiliating and disempowering. Mimicking the epithets he had heard his mother spew at and about his father, the few words which he would utter to his father was to call him: "white trash," "a psycho," and "a piece of shit." The boy would not even extend to his father the courtesy of a "hello" when passing him in the hallway of their home. This father was also accused by his son of being "fake" when he expressed his pain regarding the state of their relationship.

A boy in his puberty stage had been brainwashed by his mother to believe that his father—alleged to have an "anger management problem" and also a drinking problem—had abandoned him while he was serving as a Navy Seal. The mother intercepted the father's mail, email, telephone calls, and gifts and concealed from the boy all of these contacts. She instead unremittingly "reminded" him of his father's lack of interest in him. The boy expressed in session, "My life stinks because my father does not care about me," and his mother did nothing to disabuse him of this myth by enlightening him about all of his father's countless efforts to remain in touch with him. The boy exclaimed, "My father does not want to be around me. I don't believe him when he told me he loved me." He added, "If he came back now I would tell him to get lost. I never want to see my father again. He always disappoints me and makes promises he does not keep. He's a liar and a phony." When I asked the boy for examples of how his father disappoints him, he was unable to cite any examples

other than the myth that his father had made no efforts to contact him during his deployment. Under the auspices of the mother's "counseling," the boy alleged that the father had been physically abusive to him before his deployment. But no examples were cited. Throughout all of her son's laments of heartache, this alienating mother was unmoved by his pain—all the time concealing his father's extraordinary efforts to contact him.

The mother had deceived me as well—until the father sought me out during one of his leaves and documented for me all of his efforts to remain in touch with his son. Upon meeting the father, I was impressed with his commitment to his son. I subsequently supervised a number of visits during which time the boy and his father were loving and affectionate with each other. The father was appropriate with him, and the boy enthusiastically responded. Yet once under his mother's control after his father's redeployment, the boy again vilified him. He further never called his father to thank him for his birthday presents delivered during one of the therapy sessions, and he did not call him on Father's Day either. But such consideration from a child this age would need to be encouraged by his mother.

I received a referral for family therapy from the lawyer of a multisibling group ranging in age from latency to late adolescence, all of the children having expressed to him their hatred for their father in remarkably similar terminology but failed to provide any credible justifications. There had been no visits for more than eight months, and the lawyer suspected alienation. When I met with the children and asked for the rationale for their feelings, they were unable to provide credible and reasonable examples that were commensurate with their overwhelming enmity for him. They expressed that he "abandoned" them even though he had explained to them before separating from their mother that he and their mother were getting divorced but that he would remain involved with them. Nevertheless, the children insisted that their father had rejected and abandoned them. The oldest child in her late teens lamented, "I'm tired of feeling thrown away like garbage by him." She was unable to provide any examples of how her father makes her feel this way. Her preteen brother stated, "We are coming to determine if our father deserves a relationship with us." He was unable to provide any examples to explain his reticence about visiting with his father. (As stated by my colleagues, the expression of feelings and beliefs in the person of the "we" or "us" indicates an enmeshment with the alienating parent in that the children have introjected their alienating parent's feelings for their other parent.)

An alienated father of preteen children, who are discussed in this book and who had refused all contact with him for eight months, played for me several audio recordings of being defamed by his former wife in front of his children. In the recordings, his former wife was heard shrieking at him, "You're a mental case. You're hated. You're immature. You're crazy. You have always been worthless to me and to the boys. You're cruel and mean. That's why I divorced you, and that's why your children refuse to see you." Their children were heard in the background mimicking their mother's words as they screeched at him: "Daddy, stop coming to pick us up for visits. We don't want to see you. Mom already told you that." A number of alienated parents have played similar audio recordings for me in which they are being verbally abused by the alienating parent in front of their children with their children frequently chiming in. They had been advised by their attorneys to make such recordings whenever they have contact with the alienating parent

in order to have evidence to defend against false accusations of domestic violence–a common alienating maneuver.

A father of two girls, one in puberty and one preteen who are also discussed in this book, shared with me a common lament of alienated parents–that his daughters call him by his first name and further asked to change their last name to their mother's maiden name. The girls often teased him about his bald spots. The father recalled one particularly painful incident in which he had given his younger daughter a necklace for her birthday and had inscribed, "Love Poppa." The girl made it a point to advise him that she kept it only because she had been able to sand off the inscription or else she would have thrown the necklace in the garbage.

Another alienated father of two children discussed in this book, one preteen and one in adolescence, stated to me that his former wife yelled at him in front of their children whenever he called to discuss them or confirm visits; she humiliated him with demeaning labels such as "worthless" and "incompetent;" always criticized what he did during the visits; and attempted to orchestrate how he spent the time with their children. She repeatedly coached the children to express to their father her issues about how he organized his home and activities when they visited. These alienating behaviors conveyed to the children that their father is not competent to plan their activities or to care for them adequately, and this is exactly what the children came to believe; they repeated verbatim their mother's complaints, and they mocked their father in the identical angry and dismissive tone used by the mother. The mother used any excuse to withhold the visits. She frequently took him back to court falsely alleging that he had been verbally abusive to the children and requesting that his visits be terminated. The court eventually dismissed all those petitions, but only after great cost to the father in terms of finances and lost time with his children–more than a year when I had been assigned by the court to provide therapeutic visits.

Another father of three preteen boys discussed in this book reported to me the "feedback" with which his brainwashed preteen son berated him subsequent to a therapy session in which I had recommended a parenting book on discipline. The next time the boy visited him, he excoriated his father when he exclaimed, "Your training manual made me feel like a dog." In fact, his alienating mother modeled disrespect not only of the father but of me: during one session in which the father was talking with his three sons about their defiance of him, the youngest boy sent his mother a text message about his unhappiness with the discussion, and she promptly arrived at my doorstep demanding that the father immediately terminate the session. (The world of texting has become an indispensable aid to alienating parents as it allows for instant communication between them and their children. Many a therapy session or visit was disrupted when the alienating parent rushes to the "rescue" of their children after receiving a "distressing" message.) This was not the first such incident of the crashing of my therapy session; unfortunately I suspect it will not be the last.

A father of two children, one preteen and one in adolescence, who were visiting with him only sporadically during a period of years due to their mother's manipulation of them, had contacted me for co-parenting counseling and family therapy in the hopes of reversing their estrangement. After several therapy sessions with the group and with various subgroups, the relationships between the father and his children as well as between the parents had improved and visiting increased. But all was lost upon the father's request for additional visitation time beyond

the customary one night a week and every other weekend. At that point, the mother unilaterally terminated the therapy because she feared that any reduction in her time with the children would result in a reduction in the child support. The children quickly followed their mother's lead by again breaking off contact with their father, and it has not been reinstated as of the writing of this book. This family's organizational patterns had been established during the marriage when the mother failed to support the father's authority with their children and thus made him out to be "the bad guy." Indeed, in one family session, the mother had labeled the father in front of the children as being "fanatical," "autocratic," and "insensitive."

An alienated mother of a boy in his late teens had no contact with her son for many years except those times when the boy and his father had a physical altercation. The painful alienation saga of this family began when the boy was a toddler after which time the mother left the father, taking the boy with her, due to a history of having been physically and verbally abused by the father–behavior which the boy had witnessed. The verbal abuse included "fucking cunt, bitch, white-trash, and psychopath." The mother permitted the father unfettered visits with their son, but she soon began to notice that her son's behavior towards her upon return from the visits was becoming extremely defiant, disrespectful, and even aggressive. The same behaviors were soon transferred to the boy's teachers. Indeed in his latency stage, he had become physically abusive to his mother. Verbal abuse had begun even earlier, and included all of the above epithets and more. He was becoming his father by the way he treated her. On one occasion, the boy attempted to choke her with a scarf but eventually backed off before the deed was accomplished. She was rapidly losing control over her son, and he was becoming a lost soul. Despite multiple interventions from CPS, law guardian counseling, psychotherapy, and parent coordination throughout the years and throughout the boy's adolescence, no one except for the mother recognized the PAS. And surely no one understood how she ultimately had no option but to relinquish custody of her son in order to protect her safety and possibly her life. Now, in the present day, completely alienated from his mother, the young man is a walking advertisement for the detrimental results of a violent upbringing and of the introjected fabrications uttered to him by his alienating father that "your mother threw you away."

A latency age girl had had no contact with her father for a year resulting from the alienating maneuvers of the girl's mother, who had knowingly filed against the father several fallacious allegations of sex abuse–all of which were eventually deemed to be unfounded. I was assigned to provide therapeutic visits between the girl and her father at which time the alienation was just in its nascent stages. In the sessions, the girl expressed to her father how much she loved him, how much she had missed him, and how much she enjoyed spending time with him. She would not leave her father's side, and she continually hugged and kissed him. Upon seeing this interaction, I recommended that the father's normal visitation be immediately restored. This recommendation very much displeased the mother, and she became the instrument to sever their relationship now that her CPS ally was no longer prohibiting the visits. She "plotted" with the girl to reject her father: when he arrived for visits, she refused to go with him. She stood in the doorway to her home and exclaimed, "I don't want to go with you, daddy. I hate you, daddy. I'm afraid of you. You're mean. I'm mad at you daddy." Whenever the father called her for his daily phone

contact, the girl refused to talk to him– whose mother could be heard in the background coaching her to be rude to him and to terminate the conversation after a few seconds. One would not have believed that this loving and affectionate girl from just a short time earlier had become so rude, defiant, distant, and resistant in relation to her father.

A toddler whose parents share joint legal custody and who split residential custody 50–50 returned after being with the father and inexplicably began to call the mother by her first name. When the mother directed the child to call her "mommy," the child announced to her, "My daddy says you are not my mommy. My daddy told me I have a new mommy. My daddy said that he lives with my new mommy. He said I have to call her 'mommy,' and I have to call you by your name." On another occasion, the child told the mother, "Daddy says you're a cunt." And yet another time, the child stated that the father had declared to her, "Your mommy is a bad mommy so I'm going to keep you for myself." The child's defiance of the mother gradually escalated with each return to her after being with the father.

The parents of two latency age boys contacted me for therapy due to the children's defiance of their mother and because they were demonstrating temper tantrums and aggressive behaviors towards each other. I met with the entire family, and I soon concluded that the father was engaging in a campaign of denigration against the mother due to his resentment and anger that she had initiated a divorce proceeding. The father accused the mother in front of these young boys of cheating on him and told them, "Your mommy is breaking up the family because she doesn't love daddy anymore. She loves someone else." At other times he told the children, "Mommy is making daddy cry. Mommy and her friend will make daddy go away." Although these children were too young to understand the concept of an affair, the effectiveness of their father's deprecation of the mother was evident when the older boy expressed, "Daddy says mommy has a boyfriend and that makes her a bad mommy. The boyfriend does not like my daddy and wants him to disappear." The father told the children that their mother loves her boyfriend more than she loves them. The younger boy exclaimed to his mother in another session, "Daddy said you're mean and selfish." The father manipulated the children to confront their mother about her refusal to attend his extended family's annual reunion with them. The younger boy asked his mother, "Why don't you like my grandma and grandpa? Daddy says you're not going because you don't like his family." The father repeatedly gave the mother the finger in front of the children—a sign of which they became precociously aware. I spoke to the mother two years subsequent to the treatment and after the divorce was finalized. She stated that her former husband has not relinquished his alienating behaviors although his contact with his children is minimal because he chooses not to take full advantage of his visitation. The mother stated that the children are still caught in the middle, and they continue to demonstrate defiant behaviors towards her. Her older son, for example, had become angry with her because his father had told him he cannot afford to buy him a Wii because, "Mommy takes all my money." The boy regularly demonstrated anger for his mother by defying her supervision.

The four prior cases exemplify how insidiously and surreptitiously the alienation process commences, and it should be an early warning sign to the targeted parent, to the mental health professional, to CPS, and to the judicial system that alienation is better addressed sooner than later. The horrendous outcome for the boy in the first of the previous four cases is an omen of what occurs—

and may yet occur to the children discussed in the subsequent three cases—when the PAS is unrecognized and unchallenged. This is precisely indicative of the rationale for this book: awareness and early intervention.

Forty-nine children of the 56 discussed in this book explicitly exclaimed to their alienated parent in some form, "I don't have to listen to you. I don't have to answer you." Many also demonstrated this sentiment in their defiant behaviors.

The denigration of targeted parents takes many forms, and another example of this occurs when they are not apprised of their children's medical and educational developments, extracurricular activities, and social experiences. The interviews from my colleagues in the mental health and legal professions confirmed that they, too, have experienced a general pattern that alienated parents are not kept in the loop regarding any aspect of their children's' lives. Indeed, due to the extraordinarily manipulative behaviors of alienating parents, alienated parents are routinely and effectively excluded from receiving any information about their children. They must overcome major hurdles in the rare situations when they are able to acquire such information. Several alienated parents had to incur legal expenses in order to obtain a court order directing the alienating parent to share this information with them. Others endured the humiliation of having to provide proof of joint custody to the school authorities and medical providers before they were privileged with this information. Targeted parents have to beg to receive their children's report cards, yearbooks, and school pictures although often they are the ones who had paid for the pictures and yearbook. Alienated parents are routinely excluded from participating in medical decisions and appointments affecting their children. Indeed, another common alienating maneuver which deprives the targeted parent of contact time with her/his children occurs when the alienating parent schedules these exclusionary medical appointments and activities during the targeted parent's visiting times. The alienation is deepened when it then appears to their children that their targeted parent is uninterested in them because of failure to be in attendance. It is a major failure by mental health, medical, and educational professionals when they operate as if a child had been conceived as a result of the Immaculate Conception and they consequently neglect to collaborate with the non-residential parent. As validated by my esteemed mental health colleagues, this occurrence is all too often the norm and not the exception.

The denigration of the targeted parent takes other forms such as when their children are forbidden to keep pictures of them in their home, not even in their bedrooms. Numerous targeted parents have lamented to me that this situation is akin to their children wiping them from their memories. It is disheartening to hear the laments of alienated parents who have sobbed that their children are prohibited from keeping gifts and cards from them and are often not informed that such items have been received. They never know if their gifts and cards go unappreciated or are actually intercepted as they rarely receive verification of receipt from their children. One targeted parent related having left Christmas presents for the children with their other parent's relatives because all contact with them had been thwarted for almost a year. Yet another delivered Christmas presents to the children in my office in April of the following year, and still another delivered Christmas presents on Father's Day of the following year. Nor do targeted parents receive gifts from their children—not even a card or a phone call for their birthdays or for Mother's Day/Father's Day. Another targeted parent related an ago-

nizingly hurtful episode of having been hospitalized on Christmas Day, and the other parent refused to bring their children for a cheer-up visit and to exchange gifts. Indeed 29 of the 32 alienated parents discussed in this book lamented to me that their phones calls, text messages, and emails to their children were not returned. As with a previously cited case, it is common that PAS children address their targeted parent by her/his first name, frequently referring to them in the third person, and, in cases of targeted fathers, have requested to change their last name to that of their mother's maiden name. Of the 32 targeted/alienated parents discussed in this book, 30 reported having been consistently excluded from and not being informed about most of the above. Alienated parents feel like personas non grata.

One alienated father of a preteen boy discussed in this book was not informed that his son's soccer league had been changed. The father discovered the change only after he embarrassingly appeared at a game in which he expected to see him playing. This was particularly disappointing for the father because, observing his son at his games, was his only connection to him during the eight months in which his estranged wife had failed to comply with his visitation. The boy, himself, explicitly compounded his father's humiliation when he expressed to him that he was not welcome at his games. He entirely ignored his father when he did appear, and he further degraded him by describing his appearance as an example of how "he stalks me." When the mother of a previously discussed girl in her early teens appeared to watch her games, she was ignored completely by her daughter, who would walk a circuitous route around the playing field in order to avoid having any contact whatsoever with her. At other times, she left nasty messages for her mother that she is not to show up at her games or practices. When this mother appeared with flowers to present to her daughter in recognition of her singing performance in the church choir, the girl took a circuitous route out of the church in order to avoid having to accept the flowers. This mother was uninvited for more than a year to all of her daughter's baseball games, cheerleading tournaments, recitals, and school functions. So were the maternal grandparents. During this entire time, the father excluded the mother from learning about and being involved in the girl's educational and medical life. She was not informed when her daughter began to menstruate, and, even though the mother had joint custody with the father, the pediatrician refused to discuss her child with her because he, too, had been poisoned by the father to believe that the mother had a history of abusing the girl–a history of which the girl, of course, confirmed.

The mother of a previously discussed young child was excoriated by her former husband because she had planned a vacation during their child's preschool class trip to the zoo. The problem was not the mother's alleged insensitivity to her child's yearning to go on the trip; the problem was that the father did not apprise her of the trip until the night before, although he had long been informed of the mother's vacation plans. He then told his child, "Mommy doesn't care what you want." Despite having joint custody, the father failed to apprise the mother of every other activity in which he had enrolled the child–including religious instruction, sports activities, and Sunday school. When the mother did not attend the child's activities, the father announced to their child that the mother was unloving and uncaring.

The father of a latency age boy discussed in this book was routinely excluded from decisions which his estranged wife unilaterally made about his school placement, and

she specifically scheduled his medical appointments at times when she knew that he would be working. In order to obtain any medical information about his son, this father frequently had to incur legal fees and lose time from work by involving the court or his son's lawyer in order to compel the mother to provide him with this information. The boy reported to his father in one of the therapy sessions that he will not be able to share his yearbook with him because his mother will not allow him to bring it to the therapy sessions or to their visits. Of course, this yearbook was paid for by the father. On another occasion, the mother was willing to go to the extreme of removing the boy from the soccer field because his father had appeared to watch him play on a day that was not his regularly scheduled visitation. In order to avoid any embarrassment and disappointment to his son, the father left. When this father would inquire of his son about his day at school, the boy conveniently suffered an amnesia spell, generally replying, "I don't remember." Nevertheless, the boy had a remarkably sharp memory for citing the scores of every Knick game which had been played during the week. At other times, when his father inquired as to his soccer schedule, the boy humiliated him by responding, "It's none of your business. You don't need to know this. You asked me this one hundred times. You are like a broken record. You are on a need-to-know basis, and this does not qualify." Eventually, the boy revealed the source of his degrading remarks: he let the cat out of the bag by stating, "I guess my mom thinks it's none of your business."

Another alienated father of two girls previously discussed in this book reported to me that, although he was their soccer coach, they refused to hug him or kiss him or talk to him other than in his official capacity as their coach. The father reported another very common incident in PAS situations in which he was shamefully minimized and humiliated at his younger daughter's bat mitzvah. Although he had paid for the entire affair, he was not accorded recognition or appreciation by being granted the customary candle and nor were his parents. His former wife's family completely ignored him. The girl never thanked him for the bat mitzvah, and he and his parents were not invited to the post ceremony party. Another father of a child discussed in this book reported similar insults and humiliation at his daughter's bat mitzvah, all of which he paid for fully. He was not thanked for the affair, and, in fact, he was told by his daughter that the bat mitzvah was a "dud." In recognition that the PAS is an equal opportunity syndrome, several alienated parents reported to me similar happenings at their children's communions and confirmations; they were not accorded any recognition during the service and were not invited to the post-service celebration despite their hefty financial contribution to the affair.

Another targeted father of children discussed in this book reported to me about the repetitive exclusion by his former wife from every aspect of the emotional, educational, medical, and social lives of his children. He described a particularly painful incident in which he learned of his daughter's recital from the school web site. He arrived at the performance with flowers for her, and his daughter had noted his appearance from afar. Nevertheless, after the recital, she left with her mother without acknowledging him or approaching him so that she may receive the flowers. Indeed, the father reported that his daughter does not grant him the recognition of even a "hello" if she is in her mother's presence.

Eight alienated parents of 11 children had been excluded from and disagreed with the conclusion of their children's psychiatric evaluations which recommended the prescribing

of psychotropic medications. Four of the children were diagnosed with ADHD based on input from only the alienating parent, and the children were prescribed stimulants, which the alienated parent deemed to be a rush to judgment because the diagnosis was based on only a partial picture of the child's life. The remaining seven children were diagnosed with bipolar disorder, one child was as young as 10 years old, and none of the alienated parents had been interviewed by the psychiatrists. The children were nonetheless prescribed psychotropic medications, none of which had a palliative effect because the environment remained a "bipolar environment" caused by the PAS. Had the neurologists and psychiatrists in these cases interviewed the alienated parents, they would have discovered how the poisoning by the children's alienating parents had caused their unraveling, like what occurs to the rope in a tug-of-war. I strongly suspect that the anxiety and depression due to the effects of the PAS accounted for the ADHD and bipolar look-alike symptoms. Even more discouragingly, several of these alienated parents informed me that when they attempted contact with their child's neurologist or psychiatrist to discuss their child's diagnosis and treatment, they were refused any discussion. The medical providers were seduced by the alienating parents into believing that the alienated parents had physically abused their children. The accuracy of each child's diagnosis, of course, was called into question when none of the medications proved palliative. And not surprising to me or to the alienated parents of three of the children was that when they took their children off the psychotropic medications upon a transfer in custody, the three children began to function well within normal limits in all areas. (*All's Well That Ends Well,* for these children at least.)

Several alienated parents, including those

who are medical providers, reported that their former spouses had attempted to have a stipulation written into their divorce agreement that they are to be denied access to their children's medical developments. Another alienated father of previously discussed children reported that he was not informed in a timely manner that his children had been in a serious car accident. He was notified well after their discharge from the hospital, thereby conveying to his children that he did not care enough about them to visit them while they had been hospitalized. Another father of a child discussed in this book reported to me that his former wife does not keep him apprised of his daughter's medical appointments and that she was placed on a strong prescription allergy medication without his knowledge or approval. In some cases, the children discussed here were permitted to move out of state, and the nonresidential parents were kept in the virtual dark about their children. All of these fathers had joint custody of their children, but it seemed that their rights were nonetheless trampled upon.

In one particularly heartbreaking case that was atrociously and inexcusably mishandled by the mental health community, a preteen child had experienced several psychiatric hospitalizations, and the father discovered this only after he received a bill for the co-payment. This was exasperating for the father, who had not been contacted by any of the treatment providers; the mental health community made an assessment of and developed a treatment plan for the child based on a one-sided exploration of the causes of the child's acting-out behaviors and emotional disturbances. The mother's reporting, confirmed by the brainwashed child, attributed the symptoms exclusively to a manufactured history of physical abuse at the hands of the father. Had he been interviewed, he could have clarified the reality of

this fictitious abuse history. He further would have made the credible argument that the significant dynamics influencing his child were the actual aggressive actions occurring in the mother's home, where this child had been witnessing domestic violence, among other negative influences. The father would have further punctuated that the detrimental effects on his child resulted from the PAS, and he would have convincingly argued that his influence over his child had been negligible during the prior several years when his contact had been negligible. It goes without saying that an improper diagnosis cannot produce effective treatment.

Even more disconcerting are those situations in which alienated parents never ascertain information about their children's health because it is the alienator who carries the medical insurance. In these situations, alienated parents do not receive the explanation of payment from the insurance provider or a request for the co-payment.

I contacted the individual therapist of a previously discussed latency-age boy to whom the mother brought after firing me because I could not be seduced into the PAS process. Without having ever spoken to the father, she labeled him "an abuser." Although she had been presumably hired to help the boy conquer his alleged anger for and fear of his father, the therapist found no rationale for contacting the father to involve him in the therapy or to elicit his perspective. It was only after I implored her to meet with him that she agreed to do so. After a twenty-minute interview with him, she assessed him to be a "borderline personality disorder." This is a severe diagnosis and deserves more respect than a twenty-minute interview to assess for it: forensic evaluators administer several hours of written testing before they are confident at arriving at this diagnosis. Furthermore, the individual therapist made no attempt to contact me in my

capacity as being her patient's family therapist, who continued to see the boy in session
with his father. To add insult to injury, the
therapist joined with the mother's lawyer in
submitting supporting "documentation" for
the mother's petition for sole custody, the
basis of the documentation being the boy's
corroboration in the mother's presence of
her mythical history of the father's abuse of
the child. The boy subsequently revealed to
me and to his father that his individual therapist had declared to him, "Mothers are
more special than fathers." I am not a therapist who relies solely on client self-reporting
so I would require corroboration from another reliable source before I would attribute
the comment to the boy's individual therapist. But I was concerned that he had been
inculcated with this suggestion from some
significant adult in his life as it is not a
thought that was commensurate with the
cognitive development of a latency-age
child. This suggestion was indisputably
implanted and was contributing to his negative perception of the father/son relationship. One wonders what damage is being
done to this boy's self-esteem when the parent with whom he must identify is so disparaged. My conclusion was validated when the
boy subsequently exclaimed to his father and
to me, "You should be with your mommy
because you came out of her tummy." The
legitimate focus of the child's individual therapy should have been to help him develop
an appreciation for the value and importance of both parents to his growth and
development.

In the case of another previously discussed latency-age boy, he, too, was in treatment with an individual therapist while I was
simultaneously providing family therapy for
him and his father. I received a similar attitude from this therapist as I had from the
previously discussed therapist. She was completely uninterested in the father's version of

the family's history and accepted verbatim
the fantastic abuse allegations made by the
mother–which of course had been verified
by her brainwashed son. The therapist was
treating the boy for posttraumatic stress disorder, thereby validating her little patient's
misconceptions about his father. She additionally humiliated the father in front of his
son by telling him that the reason his father
must be in therapy is because he was in trouble with the court for having abused him.
There were absolutely no incidents of abuse
in this case.

The failure of the mental health profession in this regard was further exemplified
when the mother attempted to locate another therapist for her son after this individual
therapist was prohibited by the court from
treating him. Each therapist whom the mother contacted, three in all, initiated treatment
with the boy without contacting the father. It
was only when he received the explanations
of benefits from his insurance company that
he became aware of the treatment–even
though his divorce order specifically stipulated that the mother must keep him apprised of all medical care. The father contacted each of these therapists, and none of
them was aware of parental alienation. None
of them was willing to make any accommo-
dations to his work schedule in order to
involve him in the therapy. The father managed to have each of them terminate treatment on the basis that family therapy and
not individual therapy had been mandated
in his divorce agreement. Despite this, the
mother again sought out yet another therapist who was willing to treat her son without
including the father, and she attempted to
conceal the new therapist from the father by
changing their son's address with the father's
insurance company so that the explanation
of benefits would then be sent to her.

The ultimate form of humiliation and disempowerment suffered by the targeted par-

ent occurs when the alienating parent employs the classic maneuver of thwarting visits entirely. Suspension of visits goes to the heart of how the process of the PAS is culminated. As stated in the introduction, access to the child by the alienating parent, coupled with lack of access by the alienated parent, is the environment that initiates, sustains, and achieves the goal of severing the relationship between the targeted parent and the children. Targeted parents not only lose the opportunity to enjoy and bond with their children; they lose the opportunity to counter the malicious and fabricated brainwashing. It has been my experience in my treatment of perhaps two hundred alienated children that many of their alienating parents will employ extraordinary measures to circumvent the law in order to disrupt, sabotage, or totally prevent the visits between the other parent and their children.

In the case of an alienating mother of a previously discussed latency-age boy–a case which I cite because it so perfectly exemplifies the objective of the PAS process–she unabashedly revealed her alienating intentions to me in the first session when she exclaimed, "I would like and hope for nothing more than for the father to disappear out of my son's life. I wish he would run his SUV over a cliff and die. I have told him he will never see his son again." Most alienators are not so blatant and transparent about their feelings and intentions, which are generally kept covert. They reveal only veiled intentions as reflected in their ineffective "efforts" to motivate their children to comply with the visits and to maintain a meaningful relationship with their other parent. They convey impotency while simultaneously insisting that they undertake extraordinary efforts to achieve compliance. In actuality, the alleged encouragement covertly conveys to the child an implicit **choice** about whether to participate in visits. These alienating parents do not

demand compliance with the visits; they never impose a consequence for failure to comply; rather, they frequently grant a reward for noncompliance. And it is truly a pity that even the most experienced professional is deceived time and again by these severe alienators, who are so convincing in conveying their "superhuman" efforts to encourage their "resistant" children to maintain a relationship with their targeted parent.

The following is a tiny sample of comments expressed by the alienating parents of the children discussed in this book–comments which are indicative of the alienator's "diligent efforts" to support and encourage the relationship with the targeted parent: "Perhaps you should go on the visit." "Maybe she won't be so selfish with you this time." "I think he learned his lesson and will be nicer to you." "Maybe his girlfriend won't be there to boss you around, and he will pay more attention to you." "Are you sure you don't want to go?" "Do you want to go with him?" "What goes wrong at your mother's that you would not want to go with her?" "I don't know why you would not want to go." "I believe he has discovered how to act in your presence." "Perhaps he is benefiting from the anger management classes." In addition to conveying that the child has a choice about attending the visit, these comments imply a veiled implication that there is a problem or a safety issue at the targeted parent's home. Just imagine giving children a choice about attending school! Would a parent actually say to her/his child, "Would you like to go to school today?" Imagine conveying to children the covert message that school is not important: "Maybe they will teach you something today if you go." Several alienating parents revealed a superficial helplessness with regards to getting their children to go on the visits. The following are typical comments which were expressed to me: "I do not know how to get the children to go." "It puts too much pressure on me to force them to go." When I asked these parents what they would do if their children refused to attend school or medical appointments, they all responded quite affirmatively, "I would make them go."

It is so baffling to me that alienators recognize the necessity for their children to acquire learning experiences from their teachers, medical providers, and even sports coaches while simultaneously being unable to appreciate the necessity for the learning experiences provided by the other parent. Out of this ignorance arises the failure to use their authority to require that their children maintain a relationship with their other parent.

A number of alienating parents of children discussed in this book walked the fine line between appearing to support the visits between their children and the targeted parent while simultaneously facilitating the alienation. They accomplished this ploy by feigning encouragement for the visits in remarks which concurrently conveyed to their children the message that their targeted parent was the source of the family's ills. The following are examples of what was expressed to their children: "You need to go, or I'll be in trouble with the judge." "You must go, or I could go to jail." "If you don't go, I will have to pay a huge fine." "If you don't go, I will lose custody." "Fool them by keeping the visits for now; once the court case is closed, you won't have to go." "If you don't go, the judge will say that it's my fault." "If you don't go, the judge will accuse me of alienation." "Why don't you keep the visits to show the judge you are not alienated."

The reader should not be surprised by the responses that the children subsequently declared with great hostility to their targeted parent. The following are sample remarks: "You keep saying we're alienated. We are not alienated." "You blame our mother/

father for the alienation. She/he did no such thing." "You have alienated yourself." "If you send our mother/father to jail, we will never, ever talk to you again." "If you make her/him pay this fine, you're taking food out of our mouths." "It makes us very, very mad to keep hearing you say we're alienated when we are not alienated. If anything, it's these comments which make us alienated."

Some of the alienating parents discussed in this book conveyed their genuine, if not misguided, belief that they needed to protect their children from their other parent, who was somewhat inept at child rearing. Others disclosed their fear of losing a connection to their children, who were filling the void of an empty marriage. Yet others justified alienating behaviors by their raison d'être as having been the primary caretaker of the children throughout the marriage while the other parent had been only minimally involved–if involved at all–with their children's care. Thus downplaying the targeted parent's history with their children, they conveyed to me their sincere belief that their children would not experience a great loss if the relationship with the other parent was minimal or even nonexistent. Others were not so "genuine" in their concern for their children, and their motivations were not so magnanimous. These alienating parents uttered the following sentiments to me about the other parent: "He expressed no interest in the children; he did not want children." "She surprisingly did not bond with our children." "She never did her motherly duties such as cooking, laundry, and shopping for them." "I thought he wanted children. "He showed no interest in them. He did not bond with his children." "He showed no interest in the children except when impressing other parents." "She never saw anything positive in our children. Can a mother really love her children if she only picks on their negatives?" "You're missing the big picture if you think she is really concerned about the children." "She is a very good actress; she knows how to fool the therapist into believing that she really cares about the children. I see she has fooled you." I am sure the reader is not oblivious to the not-so-veiled implication of the last comment indicating that the therapist had been deceived by the alienated parent or that the therapist is naïve.

The alienator's hypercritical support for the visits–particularly that of these latter alienators–would be comical were the PAS not so tragic. Of the 32 alienating parents discussed in this book, 29 proclaimed to me they desired that their children have a relationship with the other parent. However, there was the "**if only**" caveat. Of the remaining three, I did not receive the "if only" response for the following reasons: one was deceased when I became involved in the case; another was residing in another country at the time of the alienation; one was openly blatant about the resolve to sever the relationship between the other parent and their child.

When visits are effectuated, the children often receive a double message from their alienating parent at the time of transition. Again implying that the targeted parent is dangerous and incompetent, several alienating parents of children discussed in this book conveyed reassurances to them such as, "If you need me, I will come get you." "You have your cell phone if you need me." Another alienating parent stated to me that she unequivocally conveys to her sons that she believes that their father wants to be involved with them, but she then quickly contradicted herself when she added, "I can't say for sure that this is true." Conveying even further confusion, she commented, "I don't think they actually despise their father; it's just really dreadful when they visit with him. They don't feel protected and loved." The use of oxymoron messages is a very

commonly used alienating maneuver. When I hear such ambivalence, I am skeptical of the professed commitment of support for the relationship between the other parent and their children.

With all the PAS cases from my practice either included in or omitted from this book, the laments are deafening from targeted parents that their time with their children is curtailed, disrupted, controlled, and thwarted by the alienating parent. It has been my experience that many alienating parents generally give their children grief should they enjoy the time with their targeted parent. Alienating parents ascertain their children's feelings by interrogating them upon their return home, and this interrogation has the effects of not only turning the children into pseudo-CIA agents in their targeted parent's home but also of orchestrating an extremely negative experience with the visit. Our advanced state of technology has further afforded the alienator ingenious methods to sabotage the visits. A commonly reported pattern is that the alienator engages in clandestine contacts with their children via the cell phone and through e-mails. The ostensibly innocent premises for these contacts are to reassure the children that their alienating parent is thinking about them and to convey concern about them. In actuality, alienating parents are checking up on the targeted parent, who is presumed to be placing their children at risk or is being insensitive to their wishes and needs. These contacts affirm for the children that a plea for a needed rescue is an easy "techno-means" away. Having been co-opted by their alienating parent and recognizing that the alienating parent's continued love is conditional upon causing grief to their targeted parent, PAS children typically engage in disruptive and disrespectful behaviors immediately after having communicated with their alienating parent. Although PAS children were initially seduced by the alienator into doing their bidding, they will augment the humiliation and maltreatment of their targeted parent with their own contributions. For example, they frequently initiate the communications with their alienating parent so as to portray a horrific time during the visit. The alienator expects these communications, and these children have learned that they will suffer the consequences for failure to comply. The lengthy communications between the children and the alienating parents further rob targeted parents of quality time with their children.

Alienated parents have reported to me that they are astonished by the resourcefulness which their former partner employs to obstruct the visits. Alienators frequently refuse to allow the visits–despite court orders–and targeted parents may or may not be given a lame excuse as to why the children are unable to attend. Alienators will avail themselves of any opportunity that falls into their lap to accomplish their goal of complete alienation. For example, the work schedule of a targeted father of a multisibling group of previously discussed children was changed over his protest so that his scheduled weekend to work occurred when he had his visits with his children. His former wife refused to switch the weekends and provided him with the explanation, "I chose to do this. You can't stop me." He had to incur the expense of returning to the court to have the weekends switched by court order.

An alienating mother of children who were permitted to move one hundred fifty miles away from the father failed to keep two-thirds of the visits which the divorce order had stipulated as a condition for approving the move. It was always an ordeal for the father to have the children on Father's Day, on holidays, and for extended summer visits. The following are some of the excuses the alienating mother offered as a rationale for her "inability" to keep the visits: "The roads are wet, my tires are bald, I have no gas money, someone has homework, someone has a test, the traffic is heavy, someone is sick, someone died, someone has a play date, someone must attend a party, my cell phone is not working, your child support check was a day late, the children don't feel like going, the children arose too late to go," etc. The mother additionally portrayed the visits to the children as punitive because she would cancel a visit as a form of punishment–or as an excuse–if they had misbehaved. This further conveyed to the children that the visits are optional rather than required. When the children requested to call their father, they suffered the penalty of incurring her opprobrium. Eventually, the children stopped asking to see their father or even to call him.

Sabotage of the visits takes many forms. I have heard it repetitively from children and from their targeted parent that they are made to feel guilty by their alienating parent when they do visit with their targeted parent. One typical example of this is reflected in the following statement conveyed to me by an alienated father of previously discussed children, "My former wife runs a guilt trip on the children whenever they visit; her going away message to them is, 'I will be lonely without you.' This cannot make for a pleasant visit." One teenage boy reported the following in a session regarding the emotional burden he carries for his mother as a result of visiting with his father: "I feel so bad when I leave mom because she gets so depressed." Other children, ranging in age from latency to adolescence, revealed that they feel obligated to call home multiple times during visits so as to reassure their residential parent that they miss her/him. Many of these children were under orders to text home regarding every discussion and activity they have with their targeted parent during the visits and in the therapy sessions, thereby indicating that their targeted parent and the therapist cannot be trusted to be appropriate with them. Most targeted parents rarely have their right of first refusal honored if the alienating parent is not available to the children. The babysitter is generally perceived by the alienator to be the preferred choice. A previously discussed latency age child gave me the following response to my inquiry about how the reinstated visits were going with the child's targeted father: "Well, my mom says that the visits are too much for me. And if I come home too late, then I can't kiss my auntie good night because she will be asleep, and she feels bad when this happens." Is it any wonder that this young child was assessed by the pediatrician to experience anxiety after returning from visits with the father? But, of course, the pediatrician–having declined to speak with the father as a result of the unfounded child abuse charges–made the erroneous assumption that something inappropriate must have occurred while in the father's care.

Another alienated father expressed that he could never count on his visits being kept with his previously discussed multisibling group of children, and he had to return to court multiple times to enforce compliance with his visitation. His former wife always intercepted the children on his weekday visits, and she had frequently disappeared with them on his weekends. He received e-mails from his children excoriating him for insisting that they keep their visit with him instead of allowing them to attend a play date. (The e-mails were written in sophisticated language that was well beyond his children's cognitive development, and this is indicative of the symptom called "borrowed scenarios.") On the rare occasions when they did visit, they conveyed to him that they resented being with him, and they were rude to him and to his extended family. They often

did not say one word to him during an entire weekend visit, but they took lengthy phone calls from their mother. Subsequent to the calls, they increased their provocation.

The divorced parents of previously discussed siblings entered co-parenting counseling with me, and it soon became apparent that the mother was doing everything in her power to sever the relationships between the children and their father. This mother allowed the children to believe that visiting their father was at their discretion. She expressed it this way to them, "It's your choice. You don't have to go." She further guaranteed that her children would make the "correct" decision about the visits by scheduling exciting activities during the father's visitation time. This incentive had the purpose of making the children feel deprived because they would miss out on something better if they kept the visits. She continually dropped the children off hours late for the visits, called them on the cell phone multiple times throughout the visit (here we go again), encouraged them to return home if they had a disagreement with their father, criticized everything their father did with them, labeled him with many demeaning characterizations such as "tyrannical" and "calculating," and interrogated them when they returned home about what had transpired during the visit. If she objected to something, she immediately contacted the father to chastise him. She made the children feel guilty about the visits by declaring to them, "I miss you when you are with your father." (This really does seem to be a common refrain from the alienating parent as they send their children off to the visit.) Her interference with the father's visits were so extreme that even a member of her family expressed in a session that she should enjoy being off-duty when the children are with their father but that her micromanaging of the visits negates that. Thirty-one children discussed in this book expressed that their alienating parents made them feel guilty about keeping the visits.

When a father of a previously discussed preteen boy asked him how he is so certain that his mother supports their relationship, he offered as "proof" the following remark, "She doesn't care one way or the other about my relationship with you." Another alienated father of previously discussed children described to me an occurrence that was remarkably analogous to others which I have repeatedly heard in PAS cases: his children had sent a text to their mother alerting her to their location at a concert. The maternal aunt coincidentally appeared and whisked them away. The aunt proclaimed to the father, "When will you realize that they don't want to be around you? Why do you think they alerted me to your location?" The aunt had caused such a commotion that the police were summoned. Had the father not presented his court order specifying his visitation time, the police would surely have allowed the children to remain with their aunt and might have arrested him. (It is strongly advised that targeted parents keep their order for visitation on their possession at the time of every visit.) This father concluded that his children visit with him only because the judge had threatened their mother with severe penalties if she did not comply with the visits. He expressed his dismay regarding the alienation when he stated, "My children have absorbed all the enmity and resentment of their mother into themselves. Legal remedy had taken too long."

A previously discussed latency age boy became exceedingly anxious as the end of every visit approached. This was because he suffered reprisals if he returned home a mere five minutes late, as if he were responsible for this. (Now here is a real incentive to visit.) In the therapy sessions, he was vigilant about knowing exactly when the therapy session

was to end because he feared that he would be in trouble with his mother if he was late returning to her. The same situation applied to another previously discussed latency age boy who became anxious as the end of the therapy session with his father approached, and he insisted upon playing it exceedingly safe by running out my office door five minutes prematurely to the waiting arms of his mother. He had been conditioned by her to expect an angry response whenever he did not exit promptly.

Another alienated father of previously discussed children lamented that when he arrived to pick up his children for visits, the transition never went smoothly. He was frequently kept waiting half an hour or more before often being informed by his former wife that the children would not be going with him. She referred to his apartment as "squalid" and not suitable for **her** children. If he had arrived for the visits while his children were playing outside, their mother would warn them to run and hide anywhere in order to escape him. The father expressed to me regarding this experience, "The look on my children's faces was of pure terror." Another previously discussed father expressed an analogous experience. If his children were playing outside of their home when he passed by, hoping for a glimpse and a chance to say hello, the children were quickly scurried into the home by their mother. Both fathers were made to feel like the local pedophile.

Another father of a previously discussed sibling group described a commonly occurring tale in PAS cases: he went to court for many, many years attempting to enforce his visitation rights. His former wife had been running continual interference with his relationships with his children during the entire time, and he missed virtually every Christmas, every birthday (his and his children's) and every Father's Day. The visits were so sporadic that he recalled multiple occasions when he had given his kids their Christmas presents six months later. When visits did take place, his children were questioned upon return home, as if they were in the Inquisition, regarding what had occurred during the visit; as a result, they became anxious as the end of each visit approached in anticipation of what was to come. The father was frequently called by their mother within minutes after the drop-off to hear complaints. He expressed to me, "I was amazed at how quickly she was able to manipulate the children into giving up this information. If she disapproved of something that had occurred, she punished my kids." Now that's a real incentive for the visits! The father described to me the difficulties he encountered at transition time beginning with the toddler stage: his wife had so agitated the children against him that they became terrorized when he picked them up, at which point their mother agitated them further by screaming, "How sick you are to emotionally abuse your children like this." His children's panic-stricken reaction to him made him feel like a kidnapper. (Make your selection, pedophile or kidnapper?) When the father called the police to enforce his visitation, they would not support him in carrying off hysterically crying toddlers. The father provided the police with his court order for visitation, but this made no impact. When the children reached the latency stage, their mother anointed them with the power to decide whether to visit. She was quite self-assured that they would make the "correct" decision and not counter her transparent preference. She frequently scheduled activities, play dates, parties, and medical appointments during the father's visitation time, and he was denied the option to participate. He was never compensated for his lost time. The children accepted nonstop calls from their mother during the few visits which did

occur. (Was the invention of cell phones an apocalypse in the hands of the alienating parent?) But to the contrary, the children never accepted his phone calls, did not call him on Father's Day or his birthday, and failed to initiate any other contact with him. The ultimate humiliation occurred when the mother petitioned for and received sole custody by alleging him to be an "uninvolved father." She served him with the subpoena for this court action on Father's Day.

The father of previously discussed preteen children reported to me that his estranged wife thwarted visits for more than seven months. She repeatedly failed to open the door to him and frequently kept him waiting outside for extended periods of time even in snow, in rain, in exceedingly cold temperatures, and in windstorms after which time she informed him that the children would not be attending the visit. Several fathers described identical painful situations in which their former partner refused to open the door to them for the scheduled visit, pretending not to be home, while their children were simultaneously observed making faces at them in the window. Some alienated parents reported that their children hung signs in the window expressing a variety of humiliating remarks, and the following is just a sampling: "I checked my schedule, and you are not on it." "Go away." "It's not your scheduled time to visit." "I do not want to see you." "I have not decided if I want to see you yet." "I have something more interesting to do." Several alienated parents described the humiliation of seeing their former partners drive away with their children in tow after they had been kept waiting an inordinate time for the children to be sent out to them. Compounding the humiliation, the children were observed to be laughing and sneering at them as they drove past. Indeed, 29 of the 32 alienated parents discussed in this book had to climb all sorts of barriers to pursue their visits. The remaining three cases were accounted for as follows: two alienated parents were living in the home with their children, and visits with one alienated parent and his child could not occur because his former partner had fled with their child to another continent. And this is an excellent segue into the next alienating maneuver.

Alienating parents are a flight risk—with their children in tow. The following are examples of what some of the alienated parents discussed in this book have endured to recover their children. One father incurred expenses of nearly $200,000 and had to enlist the aid of the court in The Hague to bring his child back from Europe where the mother had fled with the child. This father lost almost five months in his child's formative years. Another father incurred expenses of nearly $250,000 and lost multiple years in the lives of his children because his estranged wife had fled with them to another continent. Three fathers of six previously discussed children each had to incur extraordinary legal expenses to the point of bankruptcy to have their former wives ordered to return from having fled with their children across the country, where they had taken up residency.

Okay, I have heard the contention from professionals, not just from lay people, that alienation is not present when the children are visiting with their targeted parent. These naysayers postulate that visitation is an oxymoron to an alienation. We should not rush to judgment in reaching this conclusion: the interactions that occur between PAS children and their targeted parent during the visits must be assessed before arriving at such a determination. The following accountings expose the shocking maltreatment that targeted parents discussed in this book have endured from their children. The abuse and maltreatment was often so intolerable that the visits often had to be terminated prema-

turely. This is a double-bind for targeted parents because they are subsequently accused by the alienating parent for not taking full advantage of their visits and because their children are "counseled" to interpret the early termination as an indication that their targeted parent is indeed not interested in them. Twenty-seven alienated parents of 49 children complained of oppositional, disrespectful, and sometimes aggressive behaviors during the visits. Eighteen of the 49 children were physically abusive to 18 of their targeted parents, five being targeted mothers and 13 being targeted fathers. Because men—who comprise the majority of the targeted parents discussed in this book—do not readily acknowledge being abused, I suspect that the figure regarding the physically abused parent is underreported. Each of the five attacked mothers had required medical attention but declined to seek such care because she did not wish to implicate her child(ren.) The three mothers who were not physically assaulted were mothers of very young children, but these children were verbally abusive to them by uttering their father's malicious epithets, and they frequently defied their mother's supervision. Twelve alienated fathers acknowledged having been physically attacked by their former partners, and many of the attacks were witnessed by their children. (What does the reader think these children are learning about authority and the likelihood that they will transfer the aggression and maltreatment to other authority figures?)

Examples of the children's oppositional behaviors and maltreatment included: (1) verbal and nonverbal expressions of hatred, derision, and rejection; (2) manufacturing of false accusations that the targeted parent exposed them to sexual materials or were sexually inappropriate with them; (3) physical attacks; (4) destruction of their personal property; and (5) refusal to accept their discipline and limits.

The following are examples of the maltreatment which were cited to me by the targeted parents discussed in this book:

A father related that he had sent his preteen daughter to her room as a punishment for her defiance of him. She promptly returned, stating that she was not going to accept his punishment. When he subsequently received her cell phone bill—which he continued to pay voluntarily—he noticed that she placed a call to her mother at the exact moment when she had been sent to her room. A preteen girl in another case repetitively assaulted her father by spitting at him, kicking him in the groin, throwing water at him, punching him, and pulling his hair. She damaged his expensive business iPod in a fit of rage, and she was completely unapologetic for these behaviors. When her father punished her by withholding an electronic game, her mother placated her in front of the father by offering to replace the game with an even more expensive one. A latency-age boy on another case frequently hit, kicked, spit at, and stuck his tongue out at his father. Another unrelated latency-age boy punched his father in the stomach, spit at him, kicked him, and made threatening hand gestures in his face. A preteen child threw a book at the targeted mother while driving in the car and kicked the mother's driving leg. Along with the physical attacks came a sequence of verbally abusive epithets which all included the F-word. In another case, a girl in her late teens punched her father in his face in a crowded public facility. And to remind the reader, two unrelated boys, one in his early twenties and the other a boy in his late teens, physically attacked their respective mothers just as they witnessed their fathers having done so during the course of the marriage.

In another case, a father had contacted me ostensibly to help renew the relationship between his former wife and their young adult daughter who had six months earlier left her mother's home, moved in with his extended family, and refused all contact with her mother since that time. When she was living with her mother, she physically abused her on several occasions. The father was enabling his daughter's estrangement from her mother by financially supporting her in his relative's home despite his verbalizations to the contrary that he was "distraught" over the severed relationship between the two of them. He expressed that he supported their reconciliation—but **only if** his ex-wife would cease her incessant criticisms of their daughter. He then spewed out a barrage of deprecating epithets against his former wife, which I later discovered he liberally shared with their daughter. He labeled her "a whore," "a mental case," "a druggie," and "a narcissist." Despite his professed request of me to facilitate a reunification, it was obvious that he was actually fostering an alienation between the two. In a subsequent session with the mother and daughter, the girl viciously exclaimed to her mother, "**We** would not be upset if you dropped dead tomorrow. We don't give a crap about you." She expressed these words with an insensitivity so sharp that it could have cut an iceberg. She acknowledged that she was speaking for both her father and for herself. Her use of the word, "**we**," confirmed her enmeshment with her father and of the family's history of triangulation. The mother's "crime" for meriting this rebuke had been the sensible limits she had attempted to impose on the girl throughout her childhood but which were generally overruled by her father. In the session, when the mother attempted to correct the girl's distortions of the family's history, the girl rolled her eyes, shot her mother a look of utter contempt, and then looked away with disinterest. She assumed the role of the puppet of her ventriloquist alienating father when she spewed the identical epithets at her mother which her father had beforehand expressed to me.

In the case of a previously discussed latency age boy, the alienating mother called just prior to the first therapy session to express that he did not wish to attend, and she requested that I cancel the therapy session. I refused, and I implored her to use her parenting skills to convince him to participate. When they arrived, he was "performing" for her; he screeched that he did not want to see his father and that he was afraid of him. The mother announced to me in front of him, "I told you he did not want to come." This statement empowered the boy to escalate his tantrum in opposition to the visit. He thrashed about the hallway and refused to enter the office. The mother's poisoning of this boy against his father set the tone for the session, which was horrific and painful for the boy, for the father, and for the therapist. He repeatedly exclaimed to his father, "I don't have to be here if I don't want to." He physically attacked his loving father by kicking, punching, and spitting at him. There was only one explanation for the boy's maltreatment of his father: he was standing on his mother's shoulders.

An alienated mother contracted with me to help her repair the relationship with her adult daughter, and she related the following family history about how the PAS had achieved its goal of severing their relationship. The children were very young when her nightmare began: her husband locked her out of the family home upon returning from a marriage counseling session. Because he had a history of physically abusing her, the police strongly encouraged her to go elsewhere. She was never again to reside in the marital residence. Because legal proceedings grind so slowly, the alienating father was afforded the time he needed to successfully brainwash the girl against her mother, although her much younger brother escaped

the process. The girl was eight years old when her mother was expelled from the home, and the next time there was any meaningful contact between the two, the girl was in her early 20s. The alienating father had intercepted the mother's phone calls, cards, letters, and gifts which she sent to her daughter in the subsequent years. He convinced the girl that her mother had abandoned her, and she reported this to her attorney and to the forensic evaluator who was assigned during the ensuing contentious custody proceeding. Although the forensic evaluator concluded that an alienation was present in this case, she nevertheless recommended that the alienating father receive custody of the girl on the premise that the alienation had reached "the point of no return." In between the time of the mother's expulsion from the family home and the renewed contact with her daughter, there were two excruciatingly painful incidents which had occurred between them. The first incident transpired when the girl was in her early teens: she was screaming on her mother's front lawn all the epithets that she had heard her father label her. These epithets included, "whore, insane, egotistical, and worthless." The next contact occurred when the girl was in her late teens: she again unexpectedly popped into her mother's home and punched her so severely in the chest that she was black and blue from shoulder to shoulder. The mother's "crime" for being the recipient of this abuse was that she had pursued legal remedy to enforce the payment of child support arrears for her son. As a consequence of the mounting arrears, the judge ordered the father's incarceration, and the girl was determined to punish her mother for this situation.

In none of the above situations did the alienating parents admonish or punish their children for the disrespectful and abusive treatment displayed towards their targeted parents. Some children were even rewarded with privileges and material items. Indeed, every alienating parent of the abusive children justified the maltreatment due to spurious allegations of sexual, physical, or domestic abuse and to anger management issues.

Mr. Hiltzik stated that many courts labor under the misperception that if visits are occurring, then there is no alienation. He could not disagree more. He asserted:

> Even if the kids visit, they are incredibly disrespectful and really take advantage of the alienated parent. It is a complete lack of respect, a lot of manipulation going on. I think it is clearly alienation any time the custodial parent fails to comply with case law that requires them to foster a loving relationship between the other parent and their children. Frequently these children will engage in highly provocative behaviors during the visits with their alienated parent.

Mr. Hiltzik cited cases in which the children refused to interact with their alienated parent, even to the point of not even saying "hello" and "goodbye." He often hears complaints from his clients, generally the alienated father, in which alienating parents convince the children that it is "a chore" for them to visit with their fathers. The alienating parent conveys the following message to the children, "You **HAVE** to go see your father this weekend. If you don't go I will be in big trouble with the court. I do everything I can do to make them visit. But I just can't get them to go." According to Mr. Hiltzik, this kind of behavior does not comply with the previously mentioned case law. He affirmed, "This is a form of alienation."

Dr. Kelly described having heard alienating parents sob to their children about the visits, "I know it is terrible for you to spend time with her, but if you don't go, I'll be in so much trouble." In characterizing the effects of such comments, Dr. Kelly stated, "The child has to act in conflict to what he knows to be accurate and real in order to keep the peace."

I am in agreement with the concerns raised by Dr. Kelly and previously by Dr. Havlicek: the effects of the denial of reality can lead to serious psychological issues, including psychoses.

Ms. DeNatale cited from her practice examples of the denigration of the targeted parent by the alienating parent as follows:

> I have seen parents show and read court documents to children, speak badly in the presence of the child about the other parent, unnecessarily call the police on a parent, contact child protective services, contact school officials regarding the other parent, go to the school to meet with school officials regarding the other parent, and tell their children that their other parent is not paying for support.

Ms. DeNatale deemed the last behavior to be very common and all the behaviors to be quite detrimental to the children.

Mr. Previto described numerous incidents in which there is the thwarting of visits with the alienated parent by the custodial parent. He, too, commented to me how he frequently hears from the opposing attorney that her/his client, the custodial parent, is unable to get the child to visit. He expressed it this way, "The excuse is always that they can't get the kids to go to the other parent. Well, if you can get the kids to go to school and get them to go to the doctor, you can get them to see the other parent." He also maintains the belief that if the custodial parent is unable to foster a meaningful relationship between the children and their other parent, then they are probably not competent to retain custody.

Ms. Saltz criticized the current system: "I

think sometimes we give kids way too much power in this area. But I do know at least one judge who affirms that the kids are not going to drive the visitation bus." She concurred with this when she declared, "I do not believe that kids are entitled to make a decision about visits on their own." Nevertheless, she recognized that there may not be resolute and consistent support for her position. She further addressed the difficulty in enforcing visits with adverse older children when she commented:

"Is visitation an area where children should have a say so? Not for eight or 10 or 12-year-olds. But when you're dealing with children 14 and older, some judges will say that a 14-year-old can refuse. It used to be up until the age of 18 that judges would take the position that they do what we tell them to do. But people nowadays want to be friends with their kids."

Nevertheless, Ms. Saltz does not accept visit refusal by older children without a challenge to them. She fully enacts her role to counsel:

"I always try to get children at least to agree to therapeutic visitation when they have refused all visits. I encourage them to tell their mom or their dad about how they are feeling and to do it in a safe environment with somebody who is trained to help them to do that. Sometimes I convince them to agree."

Nevertheless, Ms. Saltz acknowledges that with the children who are truly victims of alienation, it is virtually impossible to get them to agree voluntarily to attend therapy with the alienated parent.

The reader will be learning much more from Ms. Courten, Ms. DeNatale, Mr. Hecht, Mr. Hiltzik, Mr. Levitt, Ms. Moss, Mr.

Previto, Ms. Saltz, Mr. Steinberger, and Ms. Zarkadas in the chapter discussing judicial recommendations.

It is important to impress upon the reader that the abusive behaviors and the hurtful verbal and nonverbal messages of PAS children do not reflect their genuine feelings for their targeted parent. These children have, to the contrary, repressed their loving feelings for their targeted parent. There is no gene for parental rejection. During my 24 years working with children in foster care, I became an expert on appreciating the child's yearning for connection to her/his biological parents. Despite having endured abuse and/or neglect severe enough to warrant removal from their home, virtually all these children were passionate for contact with their biological parents. And the day a child "graduated" from the foster care system, she/he, in overwhelming percentages, sought out the biological parent(s.) Indeed, I have concluded—based on 40 years experience working professionally with children and families—that the instinct to maintain a relationship with a parent is superseded only by the instinct for survival and the instinct to protect one's young. Only the unrelenting programming by the alienating parent can account for the rejecting and hurtful expressions and deeds which these children demonstrate towards their previously loved and loving parent. Children become experts on their parents just as parents are experts on them. Children study their parents and interpret their wishes, which are conveyed to them both verbally and nonverbally. As children mature and develop their cognitive abilities, emotionally healthy children learn to discriminate for themselves what is valuable information as opposed to unhelpful information which their parents have imparted to them. This process culminates with the maturity and independence of adulthood. The minor PAS child, however, becomes an indiscriminate mirror of the alienating parent, first reflecting that parent's malevolent perceptions of the targeted parent and then acting out the abusive and rejecting behaviors towards the targeted parent based on those introjected characterizations, which are compounded by their own contributions. These children are so convincing about their feelings because they express their hostility with such passion and conviction. It is therefore often impossible for me to convince some targeted parents that their children's feelings and behaviors are not their own but are entirely the result of the indoctrination and encouragement by their alienating parent.

Most of these targeted parents have responded with their incredulity in some version of the following remark, "Well, I have been thoroughly duped."

Without therapeutic and judicial intervention, the PAS process will continue unabated, and the repulsive images of the alienated parent have the potential to become permanently etched in the child's mind, thereby becoming characterological and quite frequently irreversible. This, then, becomes a loss not only for the alienated parent but for the alienated child as well. For the alienated parent, it is a loss of a relationship. But for the alienated child, it is also a loss of self.

Chapter 3

WEAK, FRIVOLOUS, AND ABSURD RATIONALIZATIONS FOR THE DEPRECATION

These words are razors to my wounded heart.
—Shakespeare, *Titus Andronicus*

This symptom reflects the distortion of family events or "the enshrining of revisionist history" by the alienating parent and the PAS child about the targeted parent in order to portray that parent in the worst possible light. PAS children remain armed with a laundry list of vague injustices, deceptions, and disappointments which were allegedly inflicted upon them by their targeted parent. These children exploit the opportunity to reiterate their complaints ad nauseam when they respond with their inventory of grievances to nearly every question asked of them about their relationship with their targeted parent. When they are requested, however, to provide specific incidences or explicit examples which support their accusations, they are unable to document credible, significant, or factual examples. To the contrary, these children utter nothing more explicit than vague comments such as "she/he lies;" "she/he is embarrassing," "she/he is annoying," and so on. Sometimes these children will say, "She/he is abusive," but they will be unable to cite specific incidences to support the claims. These children, nevertheless, have the potential to create havoc for their target-

ed parent when they fabricate fantastic, ludicrous, and exaggerated accusations to justify their deprecation, such as child abuse allegations. What these children can specifically articulate is the nastiness of their alienating parent as well as that parent's corroboration of their misperceptions of the targeted parent. The PAS thus catapults to life because of the repetitive exploitation of deceit, untruths, and hyperbole.

Few would dispute that parenting is a process of trial and error. As such, it is expected that trivial offenses and mistakes will be committed throughout this learning curve. When targeted parents commit such "transgressions," however, their children's responses of vilification are utterly out of proportion to the mistakes. This transpires as a result of the poisoning by the alienating parent coupled with the embellishment of the child's own contributions. This process occurs as follows: when the child is co-opted by their alienating parent, a coalition develops between them, and they collude (either consciously or unconsciously) to co-create fantastic tales designed to justify the deprecation and rejection of the targeted parent.

Their complementary interactions maintain a symbiotic bond between them, and the symbiotic bond in turn permits them to sustain each other, inflame each other, and encourage each other to culminate the process of the PAS–which is the dissolution of the relationship between the targeted parent and the child.

The power and energy resulting from the symbiotic relationship between the alienating parent and the PAS child is akin to the cumulative force of a snowball having reached the completion of the descent which began at the summit of Mount Everest. The symbiotic relationship engenders a fire and fury for the targeted parent which spins equally out of control as did the snowball. If the reader takes umbrage at this dramatic portrayal of the PAS, I request that judgment be held in abeyance until absorbing the horrifically painful PAS tales which follow in the subsequent chapters.

Targeted parents are blamed by each participant in the symbiotic relationship for everything that goes wrong in their children's lives, and they receive no credit for their support, help, nurturing, or their enormous sacrifices. The PAS child and symbiotic partner imaginatively invent issue after issue for which to criticize the targeted parent. These issues are either fantastically embellished with barely any relevance to reality or are entirely fabricated. Examples of the hyperbole which I have heard from these children and from the alienating parent include: failure to feed their children; causing their children to miss their practices, games and other extracurricular interests; planning boring activities and vacations; interfering with their children's social lives and peer relationships; preventing their children from "vital" communications with the residential parent during the visit; asking "meddlesome" questions about their children's education, health, and social activities; attempting to

buy their children's affections with clothing, electronic toys, sports equipment, and so on.

But these are relatively mild, nuisance complaints as compared to the more egregious fabrications which the alienated parent must not just dispute but must defend against–frequently at great legal expense. These latter charges have life-altering implications because they allege criminal activity and/or child abuse. Many alienated parents have enlisted my help and the help of defense attorneys to discredit charges that they had exposed their children to pornography and child pornography or that they had behaved with their children in a sexually inappropriate manner or that they had physically abused their children.

Dr. Burkhard related in our interview some of the frivolous and some of the outrageous rationalizations given to justify visit refusal which she has heard from PAS children in her practice. One child cited the following as a justification for her visit refusal: "If he would only stop going on the Internet or talking on the phone, I would be happy to be there." Other comments she has heard were: "He beats me but I can't remember when, but it happens all the time. It happens so much I can't think of a single time." Dr. Burkhard stated she has heard children allege: "He never cared about me. I never want to see him again." But when she asks for specific details of these allegations, she confirmed that the children have a hard time providing the specifics. She elucidated on her experiences with children who exhibit visit refusal with a parent: "With alienation, I get a lot of emotional language but no concrete content."

Dr. Kelly confirmed that she repeatedly hears preposterous rationalizations from these children for visit refusal, and I cite merely one example: the child uttered to her in all seriousness that his father insisted that he become a Yankee fan and forsake his allegiance to the Mets.

Ms. Zarkadas stated in her interview that these children are unable to provide specific examples of the "horrific" behaviors of which they accuse their alienated parent. She is convinced that the visit refusal of these children is sanctioned by the residential parent who conveys to the child covert messages, if not explicitly overt, such as "I guess he loves you, but his girlfriend comes first. He means well, but he can't seem to do what you want." Ms. Zarkadas characterized such indoctrinations this way, "Nebulous statements are thrown out there in front of the child for the purpose of turning the child against the other parent." She stated that another indication of alienation occurs when these children make derogatory comments about their targeted parent that reflect an understanding well beyond their cognitive abilities and for which they could not possibly have had firsthand knowledge. Such comments are not only indicative of frivolous rationalizations but also of the symptom of "borrowed scenarios," to be discussed in a subsequent chapter.

Ms. Moss shared the story that one of her teenage clients offered as a frivolous rationalization for never seeing her father again was that she was disappointed in the expensive sweet sixteen party he had made for her. She also cited the case of a very bright and verbal three-year-old who was nevertheless not so precocious that Ms. Moss could believe that the things coming out of her mouth were legitimately her thoughts and feelings. For example, the girl stated, "I can't be with my mother because she has a black boyfriend, and I can't stay over at my mom's house because the man is not supposed to be my dad."

The following are case examples from my practice which exemplify the wide range of fabricated allegations and myths which alienated parents have had to endure and to defend against.

A mild-mannered targeted father was informed by his previously discussed pre-teen child that the reason for visit refusal was that he had been embarrassing when he had asked the cashier in a large supermarket to speak with a manager. The child was unable to specify exactly how the father was embarrassing and failed to provide any specifics about the "embarrassing" discussion between the father and the cashier. The child followed this frivolous rationalization with the accusation that the father then refused to provide any lunch after returning home with the groceries because the child had expressed having been embarrassed. Another targeted father related to me that his previously discussed teenager justified why it was acceptable to defy his supervision: "My mom said that your punishments don't fit the crime so I do not have to abide by them for that reason." On subsequent visits, the child's defiance of the father escalated, becoming increasingly provocative and thereby making it impossible to have enjoyable visits. The father was convinced that the mother was scheming with their child to devise a strategy to make him conclude that it was too stressful to pursue their relationship. In another very typical comment that PAS children express, the child stated to the father, "My mom told me that if you loved me, you would allow me to see my friends instead of visiting you." This father was also typically accused of not feeding his children when they visited and not paying child support but instead buying himself expensive clothing with the money designated for child support. These allegations were patently untrue.

Forty-nine of the 56 children discussed in this book were ensnared by their alienating parent into the financial conflicts with the other parent by telling them that their targeted parent is either "taking them to the cleaners" and "causing them to go bankrupt;" that the targeted parent does not support them or is delinquent in child support payments; or fails to pay for all their required needs and is, instead, diverting these funds to support her/his need for "toys." Such messages were expressed as: "He didn't do his fatherly duties by paying for camp or braces." "He said he was not responsible for my graduation party." "I won't expect you to pay for my cell phone. That was not a stipulation in the child support award." "Why is it okay to give only four child-support checks in a year and a half?" "You know that you don't want your children. You just want to avoid child support." "You should have bought me that iPad out of the goodness of your heart after mom couldn't afford her share." "I read in the papers how you are trying to avoid child support."

The mother of a latency age boy attempted to brainwash him into believing that his father does not love him because she has to fight in court to get his father to pay child support in a timely manner as well as for the "extras" that the child requires. She told the boy that his father does not visit more frequently, instead electing to work overtime so "he can buy himself nice stuff." She was nonetheless aware that the father needed the extra income precisely because he does meet his child support and maintenance obligations as well as paying for all the extras. In a particularly malevolent alienating maneuver, the mother prepared the boy to expect his father yet knowing that the father had rescheduled the visit due to a mandated work commitment. She encouraged the boy to anticipate his father's arrival, and she eventually announced to him, "Your daddy forgot about you." In the subsequent therapy session, the boy exclaimed to his father, "You forgot about me. You left me standing by the window all day waiting for you to come for me."

Another alienating mother of previously discussed children told them that their father

was permitting them to remain in a boiling hot house during a 90+ heat wave by refusing to repair the central air conditioner, which had broken down. The facts belied the mother's accounting; the truth was that the father had sent a repairman, but the mother turned him away. She did not want the existing air conditioning unit repaired; she wanted it replaced as she was to acquire the family home in the divorce settlement. This alienating mother created the myth that the father was unconcerned about his children's well-being and comfort although she finally relented hours later and permitted the repair. But many years later, his children still believe the fairy tale that their father was so uncaring about them that he was prepared to tolerate them spending the entire hot and humid summer without air conditioning only to save a few pennies on a repair bill.

The eight targeted mothers who were discussed in this book were also the recipients of a barrage of frivolous rationalizations from their children either to justify visit refusal or to deprecate and defy them. The following are some comments that their children belligerently uttered to them in and out of the sessions: "You tricked me when you bought me that iPod. You didn't do it out of love. You only got me that so that I would see you." "You never get the house clean. Why would someone want to visit you in a dirty house?" "Your dress has wrinkles. We don't want to be seen in public with you." "Look at the way you look! None of my friends' mothers look the way you do." "Your hairstyle is ugly. It's so old fashioned. I'm embarrassed to be seen with you." "You embarrassed me because you spilled soda on your blouse at the movies. I can't trust that you won't be careless again. So forget about the next visit." "You're old. You're not young and hip." "Your boyfriend is more important than your children." "You deserved to be hit because you're a nag." "You aren't my mommy anymore. My daddy said he lives with my new mommy." "My daddy says he can't buy me a Barbie doll for my birthday because you stole all his money." "My daddy says you abandoned me." "You threw me away." "What kind of mother would turn her back on her children?" "You fornicated with animals. That's why **WE** had to divorce you." "You never had time for me. You were always talking to your friends on the phone." "You were always on the computer. You forgot about me." "You didn't do your motherly duties by cooking for us or doing our laundry." (The word "wifely" might easily have replaced "motherly" because these latter comments were generally followed-up with the children's explicit harangue of their mother with marital complaints–which had been covertly conveyed in these comments.)

When the targeted parent is the mother, she is blamed for the lower standard of living that is usually the inevitable result of separation and divorce. Many times they must return to their family of origin as they do not have the means to support their families in a separate home. Such was the situation with several of the targeted mothers discussed in the book. The following are some comments with which their children harangued them: "You are not normal. You have to live with your parents." "Aren't you ashamed of yourself for having to live with auntie?" "Why can't you keep a man and have a normal married life like dad does?

Being accused of abandoning their children for failure to attend their activities, medical appointments, or school events is another common frivolous rationalization of which the targeted parent is accused. Very frequently, the alienating parent had orchestrated the non-participation by either moving away or making fallacious child and/or domestic abuse claims which generally lead to suspension of all contact. Most frequently the alienating parent directly thwarts the

contact. A huge number of the children discussed in this book were convinced by their alienating parent that their targeted parent had indeed abandoned them. In this situation, the alienator twisted the marital decision to separate to convince their children of abandonment by the targeted parent. Even in situations in which visits were occurring, the alienator created the illusion of abandonment by distorting events that had occurred on the visits. Twenty-four targeted fathers and six targeted mothers of previously discussed children recounted incidents of having been accused of abandoning their children. Examples of these "abandonment" incidents are provided.

A previously discussed sibling group and their mother had independently described to me in remarkably similar terminology an event in which the father had allegedly "abandoned" the children at a crowded movie theatre. They described how he had entrusted his preteen children to the care of the counter girl while he "disappeared" for almost an hour. In actuality, the father left for a few moments only to avail himself of the men's facilities. He accurately anticipated that he would be accused of leaving his children in an unsafe situation. This was offered as an explanation as to why the children subsequently refused to visit with him for almost a year. Another previously discussed father reported to me that he was accused of abandoning his children by leaving them alone in an amusement park for extended periods when, in actuality, he, too had availed himself of the men's facilities and returned within moments. These children also expressed in all seriousness that this "abandonment" incident was enough justification for expunging their father from their lives. A latency-age child who was discussed in this book had been watching the *Sleeping Beauty* movie with her father, and she announced to him, "The prince will not come back for her. He's going to abandon her." All children in a large sibling group ranging in age from latency to adolescence uttered, "Our father walked out on us." Another unrelated latency age child expressed, "My father left me."

The mother of a previously discussed latency age boy repeatedly conveyed to him that his father does not come to his games because he does not love him. In actuality, the mother failed to provide the father with the information about his sports activities. The boy was so angry with his father for missing his games that he mimicked his mother's criticisms in one therapeutic session by exclaiming, "Daddy is never sorry for missing my games. He is never sorry for anything. He always has to be right." After this, the boy embellished with his own contributions when he exclaimed to his father, "You always have to make trouble. Why don't you just forget you ever had a son?" He was unable to cite any examples of these accusations or even what the concepts meant.

Questioning the targeted parents' love for their children always warrants special attention, as reflected in the following comments: "You lie about your concern for your children. You give your children doubts that you love them." "He does not act like he loves me very much." "I don't believe him when he says that he love me." "She's faking by pretending to care about me." "Your daddy doesn't love you. That is why he doesn't visit you." In fact, there is frequently a double bind for the targeted parent because they are accused of having been unaffectionate and unloving to their children prior to the initiation of the campaign of denigration. Nevertheless, in the initial therapy sessions, most of these children cautioned their targeted parent not to come near them or attempt any physical contact. Forty-one of the 56 children initially demonstrated extreme resis-

tance to any displays of affection with their targeted parent, and 30 of the 41 went into hysterics when their targeted parent attempted to overrule their objections by hugging them. Twenty-six alienating parents lectured and/or "enlightened" the targeted parent in the co-parenting sessions or outside of the sessions about how to establish a meaningful relationship with their children and how to manage their anger. Thirty-eight children were informed by their alienating parent in a therapy session that they were not safe in the care of their alienated parent. If that could be stated in the presence of a therapist, one can only imagine what is said outside of the therapy. And, in fact, the continual communications during visits between the children and the alienating parent is a covert message that the targeted parent is to be feared and cannot be trusted to keep them safe.

The following are examples of some of the more bizarre and implausible justifications that PAS children have expressed to me as rationalization for their visit refusal.

A previously discussed teenage boy in all seriousness justified his visit refusal with his father for almost a year because of the "miserable, awful, and boring" times he had "endured" when on vacations with his father. What were these awful vacations? They consisted of a teen cruise to the Caribbean and a trip to Alaska. Not believable? He persisted in his ludicrous justifications when he alleged that, even though his father took him to the finest restaurants, on camping trips which he had requested, and to amusement parks, the only thing he ever enjoyed with his father was a one-time bike ride! And finally, he added with intense conviction that he hated the trip to the planetarium which he had attended with his father several years previously. The fallaciousness of this last rationalization was manifest because there had been no disruption in their relationship during a period of many years subsequent to the trip. Is the boy suggesting that it took him years to get in touch with his anger? The boy was so solemn in his speech when he offered these frivolous rationalizations, which were supported by the flatness of affect, that he would likely convince a lie detector expert, assuming that the expert was unfamiliar with the PAS. When I asked the boy to clarify the discrepancy between his assertions of misery and that he can be seen laughing and smiling in pictures and in videos of these vacations and trips, he offered no such clarification.

In another case, a previously discussed boy in his puberty offered the following as justification for his visit refusal, "He always makes promises never to do things again. He states that he won't do anything bad again, but he keeps doing it over and over. There were always problems with him. There was no peace." When I asked the boy for specific examples of these indictments, he replied, "I can't think of any, but my sister knows. She'll tell you." I did address the above comments with the preteen girl, and she also was unable to provide any specific examples despite her brother's assertion. As validation, however, of a programming, the girl conveyed remarkably similar criticisms of their father when she exclaimed in a separate session, "He refuses to stop doing the same stuff. Every time we forgive him, he does it again. We keep giving him chances, and somehow he just makes a mess of things. We always forgive him, and he uses us. He makes us feel unwanted." This girl sounded more like a jilted lover (a.k.a. the jilted mother) than does a daughter. One wonders, therefore, if the girl's repetitive use of the words "we" and "us" refers not to her brother but rather to her mother.

Another previously discussed teenage boy offered as justification for his visit refusal and for his deprecation of his father that he hated the model train shows he had attended with his father—despite the fact that he

enthusiastically participated with his father in the exhibition of his father's train collection. Subsequent to one show, he beseeched his father to build him his own colossal train display in his basement, and his father happily complied with this request.

The mother of two children previously discussed in this book cheerfully "enlightened" them about their father's disinterest in and love for them when she led them to believe that he had dumped them during his visitation time because his new family was more important to him. What she did not tell them was that the father had requested to have the children for an extra few days to attend a concert on the last day, but the mother refused his request. And this developed after the father had already purchased the concert tickets for his children!

In the case of the mother who had been physically abused by her young adult son, he offered the following explanation for the abuse, "You deserve to be hit because you nag. Because you talk too much." He alleged that his mother did not spend enough time with him when he was younger. The boy could not be disabused of these beliefs even though his mother reminded him about how very much involved she had been in all his activities, medical care, and his education. The boy himself was unable to cite any specifics of how she had neglected him. What he was able to cite, however, were the vicious verbal attacks he had heard his alienating father spew at her.

A previously discussed latency age boy justified his vilification of his father by exclaiming that, when the father had been living at home, he did not insist that he brush his teeth or wash his face. This boy is the first and only child of the thousands whom I treated who became enraged with a parent for NOT insisting about this. He further exclaimed, "I hate my father because he broke into our home." He was unable to explain how a person breaks into one's own home.

An alienated father of children previously discussed sobbed to me many times in exasperation and in pain over the maltreatment and disrespect he receives from his children. He shared with me a particularly heartless phone call with his teenage daughter in which she accused him of wanting "to sodomize her stepbrother and then cut him into little pieces." The girl's brother, stepbrother, and her mother could be heard laughing in the background.

A previously discussed latency aged boy further bemoaned that his father had stolen a hundred dollars from his piggy bank "before he abandoned me." This was absolutely untrue and had actually been staged by his alienating mother to portray his father in the most reprehensible light.

Two previously discussed siblings in their early teens justified their one-year visit refusal with their father with the following reasons: "The sleeping arrangements were no good; the mattresses were too soft; the mattresses were too hard; the sheets were too cold; the food was yucky or too hot or too cold; activities were uninteresting, etc." The children had not raised any of these issues with their father, but they became issues after their mother began to make them so.

A previously discussed latency-aged girl expressed to her father in a therapy session, "My mom says the swimming pool that you take me to is dangerous for me." She added that her mother told her that her father would be "neglectful" if he failed to put sunscreen on her. Her mother further cautioned her about her father in that she must make sure that he watches her closely when she rides her bike and she must insist about not being with any of his friends unless the mother had approved of them. It is evident that the poisonous programming of this girl by her alienating mother is designed to make her believe that her father is dangerous and

untrustworthy. In an individual session with me, the father related to me that, while he was still living with his wife, she frequently humiliated him in front of their young daughter by accusing him of homosexuality. Imagine that!

The reality testing and judgment of PAS children is undermined when they are brainwashed to perceive their targeted parent to be evil and surreptitious because she/he spends money on them. (Does the reader perceive a double-bind for targeted parents because they are simultaneously vilified as a result of the myth that they not supporting their children?) The following are examples which were expressed in and out of sessions:

A previously discussed girl in her early teens deprecated her mother because she had a "bad habit" of buying her expensive electronic games as a means to defuse arguments they had. She chided her mother, "You thought that being a good mother was buying me things. You lied to me that you buy me things out of love; you only bought me things so that I would agree to see you. You just wanted to make me feel bad about not seeing you." A preteen boy offered in all seriousness the following preposterous rationalization for his deprecation of his father: "I hated the expensive Adidas sneakers which you bought me." He amplified his remark by stating, "You think you can buy me with gifts. You just can't buy somebody to make things all better." He acknowledged that his mother had conveyed these notions to him.

I have heard comments such as the last two repetitively from the many children cited in this book, and this is further indication that PAS children are indistinguishable from each other. These comments include: "You don't treat me like a daughter if you think buying me a dinner will make everything right between us." "You can't build a relationship over dinner." "My father tries to bribe me to visit him by giving me $20, $40,

$50, $100, etc." "He thinks a Barbie doll will make me want to see him." "She buys me clothes to run a guilt trip on me." PAS children have evolved a curious redefinition of terms: they label gifts received from their targeted parents as "bribes." I have been continually re-educated by these children to consider the following as a bribe: dolls, money, sneakers, video games, iPads, cell phones, jewelry, and the list goes on–the purpose of the "bribe" serving to entice children to grant their targeted parent the privilege of having contact with them. Webster's dictionary would have to be totally revised if it were to accommodate to the preposterous characterizations by the PAS child to consider as a "bribe" what their targeted parent buys for them. In all my years of practice, I have yet to encounter a child–other than a PAS child–who considers a present from a parent to be a bribe. When their targeted parents bemoan to me how they are accused by their children of running a guilt trip on them for having spent money on them, my response usually is, "I think you should stop running a guilt trip on them!"

The above examples are indicative of the absurd, frivolous justifications offered by PAS children for the deprecation and rejection of their targeted parent. The following are examples of nebulous rationalizations for visit refusal which PAS children exclaimed to their targeted parent in and out of sessions: "I hate you when you tell me what to do." "I hate all those things you tell me to do which I hate doing." "You were mean to me." "You have such a mean face when you stare at me. You have no idea how intimidating and creepy you would look." "You gawked at me with those eyes when I wouldn't clean my room." "You frightened me to death." "The pants you bought me were too big." "The pants you bought me were too small." "You pointed at me in anger when I did something wrong." "You put your teeth to-gether and foamed at the mouth when you got mad." "He points his finger in a malevolent way." "We can't count on him." "I hate you daddy; but not as much as mommy hates you." "He has an anger management issue." "He is not benefiting from his anger management therapy." "She doesn't act like a family." "He is not exactly father of the year." "He cooked too much." "She didn't cook enough." Each child was requested to cite specific examples of these general remarks, and each failed to do so. But instead of sitting in awkward silence, one child remarked, "Why must you be precise and exact?"

When I receive the above implausible justifications for the deprecation and rejection of the targeted parent, I express my incredulity by sharing my experiences in foster care. I explain how foster children, who had been maltreated and/or abused to the extent of warranting removal from their homes, nevertheless craved a relationship with their biological parents. But the PAS children discussed in this book were unmoved. The following remarks are indicative of the responses I receive to my expressions of incredulity: "Why can't you just believe that he didn't abuse me and that things just arose?" "I can't think of why I hate him, but I know there must be reasons or I would not feel this way." "My father would beat me. I can't think of an example right now. But I know he must have beaten me because my mother said he did." "Isn't it abuse if your father dragged you out of bed for a visit when you didn't want to go?" "She is always making us see family we don't want to see. How could you not get angry about that? Wouldn't you think that's abuse?" "She always found something wrong with me. I can't ever remember hearing a compliment from her. But it was so long ago, I can't give you any specific examples." "Everything I did was wrong to you." "Nothing I did was good enough for you." "You were constantly criticizing me." "Why can't you just accept that he is just a negative person?" "You slapped us around a lot. I was scared of you. But it happened so long ago, I forget the circumstances." "I peed in my pants because of you." "I always got a yucky feeling when I looked at those panties. Why must I have to tell you when that was?"

When I asked these children to explain how their targeted parent presents in the sessions completely different than the person whom they have been describing, I received remarkably similar responses–as if all these children knew each other and had conspired with each other to respond in like fashion. The following are a small sample of their similar responses: "He's fake." "He's acting. It's not the real him." "He has never been like that." "This was one of his rare moods." "She is just like that because you're here. She will change the minute she leaves here." "She can't be trusted to be like this." "His attitude always changes. He's not like this at home." "She's never been like this." "He deserves an Academy award for his acting." "He knows how to fool the therapist."

A frequently employed and effective alienating maneuver in support of the deprecation and rejection of the targeted parent occurs when the alienating parent makes specious allegations of domestic violence–and which are frequently confirmed by their brainwashed children. Our profession should not conclude that such an allegation is true unless speaking with both parents, at the very least. Even more malevolent and devastating are frivolous allegations of child abuse because such allegations frequently result in the immediate suspension of visits during the CPS investigation. It is a particularly pernicious deed when the alienator encourages the children to confirm abuse accusations, especially when they are sexual in nature. The harmful effects to the child cannot be avoided because the child must be convinced that she/he had actually been sexually abused by a parent. Treatment of these children as an adult reveals that they suffer from the same posttraumatic stress disorder as do children who had actually sustained sexual abuse by their parent.

The following are cases from my practice in which alienating parents alleged physical and/or sexual abuse, and they succeeded in convincing their children of this fallacious family history. In many of the cases, the allegations resulted in CPS investigations, during which time all contact between the children and targeted parent was suspended.

In the case of a previously discussed preteen who had refused all visits and all forms of contact with the alienated mother for a more than a year, I initially met with the father, and he alleged that he supports the relationship between the mother and their child, **if only** the mother ceased her physically abusive behaviors to their child and to their younger son, who was not alienated. I asked the father, who was a mandated reporter in his capacity as a teacher, as to why he did not make a CPS report if he was so convinced that his estranged wife had been physically abusive to his children. The father responded that he had attempted several times to do so but that CPS declined to accept any report because the allegations were nonspecific and did not rise to the level for investigation. Nevertheless, the preteen insisted that the targeted mother was guilty of multiple incidences of child abuse, and this history was used this to justify visit refusal for a year. The father could provide no explanation as to why he did not encourage the visits between his estranged wife and their child during this entire time or to attempt to mediate their relationship so as to prevent an alienation.

In the case of a previously discussed preteen girl, whose relationship with her father is currently severed, her mother succeeded in brainwashing her into believing that her father had a long history of domestic violence upon which the mother attempted to obtain several orders of protection. One after another petition was dismissed, but the mother was eventually able to convince one judge of her allegations, and he granted an order of protection. In the co-parenting sessions, the girl repeatedly barraged the father with completely fabricated allegations that he had physically abused her and her sibling along with their mother. In actuality, the girl initially acknowledged having witnessed only one incident of physical confrontation between her parents, and she confirmed that her mother had initiated it by hitting her father in the head with a shoe. The girl nevertheless maintained in all subsequent sessions that her father had a history of abusing the entire family and that her mother had never engaged in any physical abuse of her father whatsoever. The girl used this fabricated history to refuse all contact with her father for more than a year, and the father has sought legal remedy to ameliorate the alienation.

An alienating mother of previously discussed children made several specious allegations that their father had repeatedly exposed them to pornography. In actuality, the mother and the children concocted their elaborate tale based on a single, quite innocent, trivial event that had occurred during a visit with the father in which the ceiling fan blew open the swimsuit edition of *Sports Illustrated* to a page of a girl in a revealing bathing suit. The children scarcely glanced at it, and they quickly became involved in other activities with their father, enjoying the balance of the visit. This was a nonincident for them at the time, and they had actually giggled upon glancing at the magazine on the father's table. The next day, however, when under their mother's influence, the drama commenced. The accusation was made that the father had intentionally exposed them to

observing the act of sexual intercourse. The children suddenly developed a hysteria over what they had viewed. In subsequent separate sessions with me, each child depicted their reaction to this incident using identical terminology: "It was repulsive. It was the most vulgar thing I ever saw. It was terrifying; it was a creepy." When I met with their mother, who could not be characterized as being prudish, she, too, described the incident in the identical terminology as did her children. The resemblance of each description to that of the other descriptions was a further indication that these children were being exposed by their mother to a malicious programming against their father.

The alienating mother of a previously discussed preteen girl modeled for her how to file frivolous domestic violence reports, and the girl was a captive student. She then repeatedly called the police and CPS on her father, making false allegations of child abuse. The father was arrested on a number of occasions. Visits were frequently suspended during the CPS investigations, and the father incurred excessive legal fees to defend himself. As of the writing of this book, this father is still engaged in legal proceedings to prove himself innocent of child abuse allegations. This girl's campaign of disrespect, disobedience, and sometimes aggression caused much anxiety for the father in his anticipation of the visits. He stated to me that he expects that his relationship with his daughter will be permanently scarred out of fear that she at any time can allege inappropriate contact.

Another father of a previously discussed young child had to defend himself against his former wife's allegation–confirmed by a forensic evaluator whom she had hired–that he had viewed child pornography Web sites while she was at work and he was at home caring for their child. He did not have the funds to hire his own expert who might have testified that there are several simple methods to fake the time of the Web site downloads, such as merely changing the time on the computer's clock. He testified under oath that he was innocent of the charge. His inexperienced legal aid attorney did not realize that he could have objected to the admission of the computer into evidence because the other side had not established chain of custody. The result of this legal travesty was that this father not only lost custody; he further lost all visitation and contact with his child because the alienating mother manipulatively used the court ruling to achieve this.

A previously discussed preteen girl who had not visited with her father in a year implied sex abuse to me when she stated, "I can remember a strange feeling when being around my father. Something happened when I was younger. I can't remember anything specific, but there was a pair of panties that made me want to vomit every time I saw them." Her mother previously conveyed to me that she suspected that something inappropriate had happened between her former husband and their daughter, but she was unable to substantiate her speculation with any specific details. CPS declined to accept the mother's report because the allegations were so vague.

In another previously discussed case in which an alienating father had succeeded in severing the relationship between his former wife and their young adult child, he made a CPS report against her alleging that she permitted her paternal uncle to sexually abuse their teenage daughter, further alleging that the uncle had sexually abused her when she had been a child. CPS unfounded the case.

The alienating mother of previously discussed children (who only sporadically visited with their father during a multiyear period) reported the father and his wife to CPS on the allegation that the wife walks around in a revealing nightgown in front of the children. This case was deemed to be unfounded, but visits were suspended during the investigation.

In a case egregiously mishandled by multiple professionals, I began to work with a family consisting of divorced parents and their puberty age daughter. The case was referred by CPS for therapeutic visits between the girl and her father subsequent to a multiyear suspension of visits because of a founded sex abuse case arising from an allegation made by the mother. The mother had previously served notice on the father that she intended to do everything in her power to sever his relationship with their daughter. The allegation was that the father had touched her in a sexual manner while cleaning her as a much younger age child. The father emphatically denied that he had engaged in this activity for his own "sexual gratification." The sex abuse evaluator should have reached that conclusion, having determined that there was no evidence that the girl had been sexually abused or that she was exhibiting any symptomatic behaviors that would have indicated sex abuse. I was provided a copy of the evaluation, which affirmed that the girl's statements, behaviors, and affect were inconsistent with sexual abuse. The evaluation further confirmed that the father had made no threats, imposed no coercion, nor demanded secrecy. The evaluator further concluded that the test scores on the CSBI were inconsistent with the scoring pattern of the sexually abused child. The father voluntarily submitted to and passed two significant evaluations, of which I was provided copies. A polygraph test confirmed that whenever (Mr. X) cleaned his daughter, he did it for hygiene purposes as a father and not for personal sexual gratification. The second evaluation was the Abel screening—a highly reliable test to determine sexual preference. The results indicated that the father's sexual orientation was for adult women, and it ruled out any preoccupation with or fixation on children.

Despite all the evidence to the contrary, the father was adjudicated guilty of having sexually abused his daughter. The finding was made solely on the basis of the mother's testimony that the girl was capable of cleaning herself. There were no other allegations accusing the father of abusing or neglecting his daughter. This symptom-free girl was nonetheless immediately sent to an individual therapist, who initiated a treatment regime for posttraumatic stress disorder. Compounding this travesty, the therapist failed to contact the father even once throughout the girl's multiyear therapy to inquire as to his accounting of the family's events. Nor was the therapist suspicious of the unjustifiable conclusion arrived at by the sex abuse validator. She accepted carte blanche the mother's recounting of the event, and she devoted the girl's therapy to corroborating the myth that her father had sexually abused her. Imagine being so young and being told by a therapist—an esteemed authority—week after week after week for several years that you had been sexually abused by your father! And yet the therapist's treatment notes reflected that she was in receipt of the validator's evaluation which I had received. I am at loss as to understand how the therapist justified her "treatment" of this girl. This entire case was a rush to judgment that resulted from the alienating mother's success in co-opting the professionals in the mental health, CPS, and judicial systems into believing that the father was worthless and dangerous to his daughter. As a result, the girl and her father were deprived of a relationship in the girl's critical formative years, and this is time that cannot be recovered. Shame on those professionals who participated in this travesty!

What follows is further validation that the professionals in the mental health system need to self-reflect and self-police in order to do a better job at assessment and intervention. A court-appointed therapist had preceded me on the case of a previously discussed latency age girl in which the father's visits had been suspended for almost a year after his former wife knowingly reported fallacious sex abuse allegations. All allegations were determined to be unfounded. The court had initially referred the father to the therapist for "anger management" because he "inexplicably" felt anger and contempt for his former wife, although he never threatened her in any way. His anger justifiably developed not only as a result of the consequent damage to his relationship with his daughter but also as a result of the huge legal fees he had incurred in order to defend himself. Being PAS-unaware, the prior therapist interpreted the father's anger—which was never directed at his daughter—to indicate a serious psychological problem rather than being the consequence of the humiliating and despicable circumstances to which he had been subjected. So, even after CPS unfounded every allegation, the therapist recommended to the court that the father's visits with his daughter be reinstated on the condition that it be done gradually and initially with only therapeutic visits—supervised by that therapist, of course. What could possibly have been the rationale for this recommendation? I believe the answer is blatant. Nevertheless, the court abided by the therapist's recommendation. The ongoing therapy with the therapist did not proceed well. The father alleged that the therapist had been biased by his former wife and was seduced into believing that he was guilty of domestic violence and of being inappropriate with their daughter. The father asserted that the therapist criticized his every interaction with his daughter. For example, the father was concerned that his daughter believed that he had abandoned her while his visits had been suspended, and this was exactly what her mother had told her. So the father expressed his love for her, shared how much he had missed her, and conveyed his excitement about the forthcoming restoration of his unfettered visitation. Instead of supporting the father's expressions of reassurance and commitment to his daughter, the therapist criticized him for his "enthusiasm," stating that he "too frequently" expressed to his daughter how much he loved her and looked forward to seeing her again. The therapist conveyed to the father that his expressions of love placed an undue emotional burden on the girl because her mother was simultaneously expressing to her that the visits must be restored slowly, 'very slowly,' very, very slowly; maybe not at all. Indeed, the therapist labeled the father's expressions as "emotional abuse." It seemed to escape the therapist's awareness that it was the girl's mother who had put excessive emotional pressure on her by making her feel that she was betraying her if she desired contact with her father. Talk about blaming the victim!

I am flabbergasted at the therapist's interpretations; any objective, nonseduced therapist would have recognized that it was the mother who was fostering an alienation. I know of no psychological theory or research informed practice which would support the therapist's interpretation of "emotional abuse." And, as a matter of fact, there is no psychological research that supports going slowly on the reinstatement of the visits. Indeed, psychological research supports exactly the reverse. Eventually the father's attorney was able to persuade the court to discharge the therapist, and that is when I was assigned. But if the "treatment" of the case was inexplicable until this point, the therapist's behavior became even more unprofessional: the therapist refused to accept the dismissal and continued to counsel the mother, thereby counteracting my family treatment.

Talk about splitting! The mother failed to commit to my treatment as she had an ally in the prior therapist in the pursuit of her alienation efforts.

By all accounts, the girl was delighted to see her father, hugged him, kissed him, and would not leave his side—all behaviors which the prior therapist acknowledged having observed when providing the therapeutic visits. I recommended that the father's full visitation rights be restored, and the court so ordered.

In the afternoon of the first unsupervised visit, the father called me in a state of panic, stating that his daughter had intentionally groped him in his genitals. He had admonished her before contacting me. I suggested that he ask her from whom she had learned such behavior as a child her age would have to be "educated" to do this. He related back to me that his daughter denied her actions. Suspecting that projection frequently follows denial, I had them come to my office so that I could video a discussion of the incident. I had no doubt that another CPS report was lurking around the corner. In the session, the girl spontaneously revealed the following, "My mommy told me I am to call her right away if my daddy does anything mean or bad to me. My mom told me if anything happens that really hurts me, I must call her immediately; if my father does anything to upset me, I must call her immediately." When asked to define "mean and bad," she responded, "If he touches me in my private parts or makes me touch him in his private parts. I have to call her if anything inappropriate happens." Hmm. I smell a brainwashing. How awful for this child and father.

As I suspected, sadly that evening another CPS report was filed against the father; the girl was subjected to yet another unnecessary vaginal exam, at which time this latest CPS case was immediately deemed to be unfounded. I contacted the girl's lawyer and informed him of the video which I had made of the session, and he arranged to view it with me the next day. But he inexplicably decided to include the prior/unresigned therapist. Based on what the lawyer viewed in the video in conjunction with the feedback he had received from the CPS caseworker, he concluded that no inappropriate sexual activity had occurred between the girl and her father. The prior/unresigned therapist reluctantly concurred but nevertheless suggested the immediate suspension of the father's visits! (If the reader can find a legitimate rationale for the prior/unresigned therapist's recommendation to suspend the visits, please contact me immediately because I cannot fathom what that could have been.) The therapist's stated rationale, however, was that the girl felt emotionally caught between her parents. I facetiously responded to the prior/unresigned therapist by stating, "Maybe we should place the girl in foster care so neither parent is able to talk to her about the visits." (At least that would have had the palliative effect of preventing any further brainwashing!) Responding to my transparent message, the girl's lawyer affirmed, "We have no legal reason to suspend visits."

The reader need not be a therapist to recognize the detrimental poisoning against the father that this alienating mother was instilling in her daughter—and unforgivably with the support of a professional whose job it is to prevent such harm. When one considers how impressionable and vulnerable children are to the influence of a parent—particularly the residential parent—it is quite conceivable that this little girl at some point is capable either of making a false accusation that her father sexually abused her or of misinterpreting healthy father/daughter affection. This is another father/daughter relationship that will likely be permanently marred. The fantastic ideas that this girl's mother is implanting in her about her father is truly an inex-

cusable, destructive brainwashing of her against a loving and dedicated father. In addition to all the lost contact that has occurred between the girl and her father, the additional tragedy is the very real possibility that this girl will come to believe that her father had actually sexually abused her and will be sitting as an adult in a therapist's office being treated for PTSD.

Another egregious example of therapist maltreatment occurred in the case of divorced parents and their daughter in her mid-adolescence. I was assigned to provide therapeutic visits between her and her father, with whom she had not had any contact for more than a decade because of a founded incident of sex abuse that had occurred when she was a toddler. The contact had lasted all of ten seconds, and the father had not initiated it, which I verified by legal documents. The girl completed a course of therapy at the time—whatever kind of therapy would be offered to a toddler in order to remind her weekly of an incident about which she would likely have had no memory. (But this is not the malpractice I am citing here.) Life went on for the girl and her mother to the total exclusion of the father. CPS closed their case a few years later, but the mother refused to permit visits between the father and their daughter. Eventually the father despondently concluded that his former wife would never consent, and he petitioned the court for enforcement of his parental rights. Just subsequent to the father's filing of the petition, the mother coincidentally sought therapy for the girl, now in her teens, to readdress the incident. When I was assigned, the girl had been in individual treatment for several months and was being treated for having been sexually abused by her father. I immediately contacted the individual therapist to coordinate care. The therapist acknowledged having not contacted the father to obtain his account of the incident nor had he obtained verifiable, objective documentation of the incident to learn the actual details. Due to this negligence, the therapist was treating the girl for a sexual abuse incident that had never happened but which was accepted by the therapist as having occurred because "it was verified by the mother." I expressed that the girl's recollection appeared to me to be an implanted memory—a fabricated memory that the father had initiated sexual contact and had done so purposefully. I conveyed that I did not find it credible that a toddler independently retains such a meticulous memory—especially when what was "remembered" did not happen and lasted for seconds. The therapist responded, "But she's revealing a fantasy." Okay, I stipulate that credible practitioners urge against challenging a psychotic fantasy. But the girl is not psychotic, and the fantasy does not have its roots in a psychosis; it has its roots in an implantation. The therapist nevertheless confirmed the plan to continue treating the girl for the purpose of "readying her for her father's apology for having sexually abused her." Why would this therapist be so invested in continuing to perpetrate such a deceit, which is so detrimental to his patient?

In the case of two girls, one in puberty and one pre-teen, the parents had concluded a very nasty divorce proceeding. The mother hired me ostensibly to repair the relationship between her children and their father, whom she alleged to have an anger management problem and a sexually abusive history. She explained to me that her goal for the therapy was to enable the children to express their anger at and fear of their father. She offered the following as justifications for the children's alleged negative feelings for their father, which involved only his relationship with the younger girl: the father peers at her when she is bathing and changing, and he insists that she sleep with him

when she visits. The mother offered no explanation in response to my query as to why the father did this only with the younger girl. Nor could she explain why the father does this overtly, does not conceal it from the older girl, and made no request for secrecy. The mother stated that she had filed multiple reports with CPS and that the father has been indicated for sex abuse. (Her statement that she had filed multiple reports was true. Her statement about the father having been indicated was a complete fabrication.) I spoke to the girl separately, at which time she denied having any feelings of anger for or fear of her father. She adamantly disputed all of her mother's allegations, asserting that nothing sexually inappropriate had occurred between her and her father. She affirmed that she always has complete privacy in the situations about which her mother had described. She asserted that her mother created these issues for her by basing them on events which were exaggerated and misrepresented. Having provided to me details about these completely innocent situations, she then exclaimed, "My mother makes nothing things into a big deal!" I separately interviewed the girl's older sister, who confirmed her younger sister's accounts.

Upon meeting with the father, first individually and then with his daughters, it was evident that he was a loving, dedicated father who interacted appropriately with the girls. It subsequently became evident to me that the mother was engaging in the process of facilitating an alienation, and I then discovered that her ulterior motive for the therapy was to gain support for her sole custody petition, which she had filed before the ink was even dry on the divorce agreement granting joint custody with the father. I met again with the mother in an attempt to reason with her about the detrimental consequences to her daughters if the relationship with a loving father is severed. My efforts were to no avail. She was determined to sabotage the relationships between her daughters and their father, and I was determined to resign as a therapist for this purpose. She continued to file fallacious CPS reports again, and all of them were eventually unfounded, but visits were suspended while the investigations were proceeding. After I resigned (or was fired, depending upon which side of the coin one is viewing), the PAS deepened with the aid of several subsequent PAS-unaware therapists, whose mission it became to rescue the children from their father. In the process of co-opting each therapist, the mother became emboldened in her pursuit to attain the ultimate goal of an alienation–that of severing the relationships between her daughters and their father. Father Time was not on this father's side, and, as of the writing of this book, he is completely alienated from his daughters.

In another case, I contacted a therapist to share my input regarding a previously discussed latency age child. The therapist was assigned after the alienating mother had me removed, alleging to the child's attorney that I was "biased" for having reached an assessment that she was facilitating an alienation. The newly assigned therapist was not a family therapist, working individually with the child for the purported purpose of "readying the child for a relationship with the father." Nevertheless, during a period of six months, the therapist met with the father only once and not even one time with his child. So how does a therapist ready a child for a relationship with a parent who is unknown regarding a relationship that has never been observed? The mother had brainwashed the child into spouting hatred for and visit refusal with the father. The therapist sanctioned the child's visit refusal by failing to invite the father to participate in the sessions. What logical parent–let alone a therapist–in any situation other than divorce, would

deem it appropriate for a child to determine visitation with a parent? What are the legitimate decision-making realms to be granted to a latency age child? Perhaps which pair of jeans to wear, the black or the blue? But certainly nothing more momentous than that. Most of the sessions with the child were conducted in the presence of the mother. The therapist, nonetheless, felt confident in reporting to the court and to the child's attorney that she had concluded that the child is "afraid" of the father and "judges him to be "mean." The therapist acknowledged to me, however, that she never requested the child to cite rationales for the fear or to cite examples of the meanness. Instead, the therapist offered as validation for her assessment that the child's reporting was believable because "the mother had confirmed it."

The above cases represent a tiny fraction of families with an alienation and which are improperly and destructively handled by PAS-unaware mental health professionals, CPS personnel, and judicial personnel. Due to lack of knowledge about parental alienation, their interventions and rulings validated and needlessly perpetuated the progression of the PAS by emboldening the alienator. The mental health therapists allowed themselves to be seduced by the alienator and consequently failed to request the targeted parents' accounting of the family history and dynamics. To proceed in this manner is as preposterous as listening to only one side of a debate and casting a vote for that position. To accept without independent verification the fantastic fabrications and deceptions put forth by the alienator is negligence at best and highly destructive of lives at the worst. By not recognizing how readily children are influenced by the residential parent and by neglecting further exploration of the family history from all family members–particularly from the other parent–these irresponsible professionals accepted as truths the fallacious allegations leveled against the targeted parent. These rescuers were convinced as to the veracity of the alienator's lies upon receiving confirmation from the brainwashed children. How preposterous! And yet the mental health profession recognizes that client/patient self-reporting is highly unreliable and untrustworthy. Acceptable clinical practice requires that the professional hold opinions and assessment in abeyance until information is received from all family members who are available. Obtaining the most inclusive possible picture of the family is the minimum standard of care that the mental health professional must provide, particularly when a child is the identified patient. And to the more significant point: obtaining the most accurate information about the family results from observing the interactions among the members and not from verbal articulations with an individual. It boggles my mind how therapists can initiate a course of treatment of a child for posttraumatic stress disorder before ever having interviewed the targeted parent/alleged perpetrator and without ever obtaining independent verification of the alleged abuse. I consider it malpractice to proceed in this manner.

CPS personnel also have a good deal to account for in the manner in which they handled the above cases. They, as well, all too frequently accepted as veracity the fallacious allegations of the alienating parents, especially when verified by the brainwashed child. CPS must inform itself about how to identify the PAS as well as to recognize it as a form of child abuse. (The reasons that I and those interviewed for this book advocate for the PAS to be considered a form of child abuse will be discussed in later chapter.)

And finally, the judicial system must be held accountable for permitting the PAS to progress by permitting the lingering of visit obstruction with no justifiable reason.

Dr. Havlicek becomes quite concerned about children's well-being when it comes to sex abuse allegations. "There is, relative to the number of claims, a very low incidence of sex abuse in child custody cases; I have had one case in several dozen evaluations," according to the doctor. He provided the context for this development: "Allegations are frequently made when all else fails to get the targeted parent out of the child's life. Because the courts are so sensitive to allegations of molestation, the alleged offending parent is immediately slapped with a restraining order and cannot have any contact with the child. This is a very negative dynamic for the child as well as for the alleged offending parent."

Ms. Moss commented regarding situations when sex abuse is alleged, "The court finds the allegation of sex abuse so shocking, and if true, so detrimental to the child, that it often prohibits contact between the alleged perpetrator and the child, choosing to err on the side of caution." She cited two of her eventually dismissed cases in which the alienating mother had made such allegations. The first case was of a three-year-old who had accused her father of inappropriate sexual contact; but it was later revealed that the mother was rewarding her with food for making the allegations. In another case, the father was accused of fondling his daughter on the visit in front of an entire house full of people–including his in-laws. Even though Ms. Moss won this case on appeal and the charges were thrown out, she asserted that the effects have long-term negative consequences for the father/child relationship in that "their relationship is forever scarred because the father will always be afraid to be alone with his child."

Dr. Kelly is also concerned about the serious damage to children from false sex abuse allegations as she, too, believes, "It confirms damage to the child as if the abuse really happened."

When I asked Ms. Saltz for her opinion regarding the assertion by the alienating parent to go slowly in reinstating the visits with the other parent after a long suspension due to the alienator's false allegations of child abuse/neglect, she compellingly expressed:

They are arguing against giving full rights immediately? I would say that's another way of depriving the children and the alienated parent of getting their relationship on the right track. You can't shoot your parents dead and then request mercy from the court because you are an orphan. The alienator is the one who caused the separation, and then they have the audacity to demand that things proceed at a snail's pace? And even during the abuse and neglect investigation, I never recommend suspension of visits. The visits should be supervised and therapeutic but not suspended because the kids will then start believing in the false allegations. Even if they didn't initially think it happened, they will tell themselves, "Well maybe I'm not remembering it. It must have happened if there are no visits." They still need to have relationship with that parent. I firmly believe that.

Ms. Saltz agreed with many of her colleagues that we have a two-tiered system in which parents of children who were placed in foster care have more rights to their children and to visits than does the alienated parent in divorce proceedings upon becoming the subject of what is generally a frivolously false allegation of abuse.

Mr. Hiltzik also commented in his interview about the delay in justice that ensues when allegations of abuse are made, especially those of sex abuse. He stated the following about this typical, egregious development, "Courts make a big mistake when CPS is involved. Judges become fearful when abuse is alleged. They take it as a sign to shut everything down. You are convicted just by being charged. Frivolous allegations? Of course! The vast majority of cases are unfounded."

Mr. Previto had a similar reaction to situations in which abuse is alleged. He cited one of his cases of two young siblings in which the custodial father was withholding the children from visits with their mother, who was his client. Immediately after Mr. Previto had filed a petition for habeas corpus regarding the violation of the mother's visitation rights, the father alleged that the mother committed horrific sex abuse with the children. "It was clearly a vindictive measure. But once CPS gets into the mix, things get drawn out. It was just awful for the mother. This is an excellent example of abusing the system to alienate the child." To add insult to injury, during the CPS investigation when the visits were suspended, the father told the children, "Your mother doesn't love you. She left us." Commenting on another of the eight symptoms indicative of the PAS, Mr. Previto continued his elaboration of this case by stating, "It's always '**us**.' But the mother always wanted to parent the children." He further confirmed from his professional experiences what Dr. Havlicek had previously asserted as to his experience with sex abuse in custody cases. Mr. Previto exclaimed, "Sex abuse by parents . . . well, it's like going back to the Greek playwrights. It's pretty heinous, but it is a pretty rare occurrence."

Costas Constantatos, M.D., F.A.A.P., pediatrician, who was interviewed on 6/8/11, stated that he encountered three to four unsubstantiated cases of child sexual abuse per month upon physical examination when he had been working three-quarters time in just one hospital emergency room.

Those who were interviewed for this book generally agreed about the level of perniciousness and fallaciousness of sexual abuse allegations and the probability that they have been fabricated in service of the alienation process. I completely concur with my colleagues, who recurrently deal in their respective practices with the awful consequences of such an allegation: namely that it immediately results in the unjustifiable and protracted suspension of visits between the targeted parent and child and has the potential of scarring that relationship for a lifetime–even after the allegation is determined to be bogus. And compounding the harm from the suspension of visits is that the programming by the alienating parent continues in the absence of any forum to counteract it. I have had several cases in which visits were suspended for almost a year because of multiple fallacious allegations.

The sagas of alienation which I just summarized are only the tip of an iceberg for what occurs in high conflict divorce. What is left behind in the wake of its cold and heartless impact is often irreparable damage to the relationship between a child and a parent.

The statistics on the families presented in this book are heartbreaking and eye opening. Of the 32 targeted parents and 56 children presented, 30 parents had to dispel the malicious misperceptions and accusations which 53 of their respective children held about them surrounding the events of the divorce and custody. The alienating parent of these children exposed them to adult material which not only turned them against their targeted parent but which caused them emotional distress. In 27 families with 45 children, the alienating parent alleged physical and/or sexual abuse and/or exposure to pornography. The alienated parents of 37 children were investigated by CPS, frequently multiple times, and only two parents were indicated. In both cases, the allegation was so flimsy that it would likely have been overturned had the parent had the funds to pursue a trial instead of entering a plea bargain. During the ensuing CPS investigation, the visits of most of the targeted parents were suspended, sometimes for three months or more. The larger tragedy in one of the two cases was that the alienating mother used the neglect finding to persuade the judge in her divorce proceeding to allow her to move out-of-state with the children, thereby exacerbating the already estranged relationships between the children and their targeted father. Of course, the brainwashed children conveyed to their attorney that they supported their mother's request to move.

In 18 of the 32 families involving 30 children, the alienating parent alleged domestic violence on fictitious grounds. In 11 cases, orders of protection were granted but all were on highly questionable grounds. In two cases in which the court dismissed the alienator's multiple petitions for an order of protection, the alienator then filed an allegation of animal cruelty, and the ASPCA raided the targeted parents' homes!

In every case in which the targeted parent had been prevented from contact with her/his child due to order an order of protection or due to CPS's suspension of visits, the alienating parent conveyed to the child that the lack of contact was willful on the part of their targeted parent.

When listening to the superficial, specious, and preposterous justifications of PAS children for their degradation of their targeted parent, the evaluator or therapist wonders if she is experiencing the absurdity of the events in Franz Kafka's novel, *The Trial.*

Chapter 4

LACK OF AMBIVALENCE

How sharper than a serpent's tooth is to have a thankless child.
—Shakespeare, *King Lear*

Ambivalence is the condition of simultaneously experiencing contradicting feelings running the gamut from positive to negative, pleasant to unpleasant, pleased to angry, happy to sad, composed to anxious, appreciative to disapproving, and so on. All healthy relationships embrace a degree of ambivalence, and the more meaningful and intimate the relationship so is the likelihood for a greater degree of ambivalence. It follows that a relationship with a spouse will likely engender greater ambivalence than would a relationship with a cousin and that living intimately with family members will likely arouse the full range of feelings, thereby giving rise at various times to ambivalence. It is, however, through the appreciation of the ambivalence which we provoke in fellow family members and which they provoke in us, that we are afforded the opportunity to address the disagreements which underlie these contradictory feelings. And it is the eventual resolution of our disagreements with another family member which engenders the development of an even greater level of intimacy between us.

When a family is functioning within the normal range of feelings and behaviors, the parent/child relationship similarly embraces moments of ambivalence as do the spousal and sibling relationships. PAS families, however, do not function within the normal range of feelings and behaviors. Instead of embracing ambivalence, a staunch certainty of feelings is characteristic of the PAS child, who does not experience ambivalence for either parent, albeit the child stands at the opposite ends of the feelings spectrum with respect to each parent. In other words, PAS children are quite self-assured that they possess unambiguously negative and repulsive feelings for their targeted parent and unambiguously positive and appreciative feelings for their alienating parent. PAS children perceive the alienating parent to be above reproach and the targeted parent to be completely appalling. According to Gardner (2001), "The concept of mixed feelings has no place in PAS children's scheme of things" (p. 153).

When families are functioning in a healthy manner, children are able to identify and appreciate each parent's strengths, attributes, and contributions to them and to the family. Children in well-functioning families are also able to recognize each parent's weaknesses and limitations as well as the areas in which each parent needs to improve and change. PAS children, however, can be predicted to recite a long list of deficits about their targeted parent while minimizing or refuting any positive attribute or redeeming quality of that parent. PAS children are curiously stricken with "amnesia" when it comes to acknowledging and appreciating their targeted parent's lifetime involvement with them. Targeted parents receive no recognition for the time, energy, and emotional and financial support which they had invested and continue to invest in their children. Instead, everything targeted parents utter, accomplish, propose, and offer to their children is viewed with disdain and negativity. The inventory of characteristics is just the reverse for the alienating parent, who is idealized, appears to possess a halo, is perceived as capable of walking on water, and reveals no character flaws whatsoever. PAS children have relinquished any interest in engaging in an objective assessment of each of their parents. On the one hand, they consider their targeted parent to be unadulterated evil. On the other hand, they demonstrate an unshakable reverence for their alienating parent, even when an objective observer would evaluate the alienator to possess insufferable, problematical, and even reprehensible attributes.

Gardner (2001) summarizes this phenomenon as follows: "The vilified parent may have been deeply dedicated to the child's upbringing, and a strong bond may have been created over many years. Yet it seems to evaporate, almost overnight, at the time of the onset of the PAS" (p. 153).

PAS children hold to their convictions staunchly and cannot be disabused of their beliefs even when confronted with strong empirical evidence to the contrary. I have witnessed time after time situations in which the targeted parent produces photos and videos of joyful times which they had shared

with their children, and yet many of these children do not alter their negative perceptions and distorted memories. When asked how they account for the joyful times depicted in the photos and videos, these children respond that they either feigned happiness or were otherwise bribed or threatened by their targeted parent to appear happy.

Dr. Burkhard described how these children behave when they arrive in her office. She stated that the children come with an attitude of "knowing it all." She continued:

> There's a great deal of black-and-white thinking. There is tremendous polarization between the parents. That is, as per the children, the problems are always the targeted parent's fault. It's his fault that they cannot have a dress or that they cannot join a soccer team because there is no money. Everything the targeted parent does is terrible. There is no room for human error. Making mistakes and asking for forgiveness are unheard of. Every little thing he does is a catastrophe. The favored parent, on the other hand, makes no mistakes. The favored parent is viewed as just about perfect.

Reflecting on the atypical nature of this thinking, Dr. Burkhard commented, "This is very unusual, particularly when dealing with a teenager. What teenager thinks any parent is perfect? And the other parent is particularly satanic. There is a complete lack of ambivalence."

Dr. Burkhard noted the very observations that I have seen repeatedly in my practice; PAS children fail to credit their targeted parents with any meaningful prior involvement in their lives: they never attended a soccer game; they did not coach a baseball team; they never made their birthday party; they never threw a ball with them; they forgot to give them praise for a good report card; they never took them to a movie or to a dinner or to the park, and so on. In severe cases, they disputed having a good time as seen in the videos and pictures of them and of their alienated parent. Dr. Burkhard describes this as, "cognitive distortion." And cognitive distortion leads to an undermining of cognitive maturation, frequently to emotional disturbances, and quite often to dysfunctional peer relationships.

I can certainly appreciate the reader's probable incredulity regarding this discussion about these children's blindness to reality. Despite my protracted experience with the PAS, I have been astounded at times by the fantastic rationalizations, the refutation of truth, the blindness to reality, and the adherence to a polarized world view which characterize PAS children. It is as if one has traveled to the twilight zone when entering the world of PAS children. I concur that it is atypical to embrace such inflexible and extreme negative judgments about a parent and such a perfunctory acceptance and validation of the other. It requires tremendous energy and imagination on the part of these children to be able to refute and to deceive themselves as to how each of their parents actually presents. Nevertheless, the depiction of the PAS child has not been overstated.

The following are case examples from my practice of children who exhibited this symptom.

Previously discussed siblings, who had moved hundreds of miles away, regularly "advised" their father that he was wasting his time traveling to see them. They exclaimed to him that he had nothing to offer them and that he was of no value to them. They frequently expressed to him in and out of session that they would not be upset if he dropped out of their lives. They exclaimed to him, "If you come to see us, we won't be home; and if we're home, we won't open the door; and if you don't leave our property, we

will have you arrested." During other sessions, the children proclaimed to him that he was "totally worthless" because he does not provide child support. Despite producing canceled checks of his child support, they could not be disabused of their beliefs because their alienating mother continued to inculcate them with misinformation, and his limited access to them mitigated against his ability to defend himself against these false accusations. Nothing he did for them was seen in a positive light; and nothing selfish and irresponsible that their mother did could debunk their perception of her as Mother Theresa–not her screaming and cursing at them, not her hitting them, not her allowing her extended family to verbally abuse them, not her failing to show interest in their education, not her showing more interest in her social life than in them, and so on. The children insisted that their mother and stepfather fulfilled their every need and desire and that their father never supported them.

In the case of the two previously discussed teenage brothers, they verbalized their unambiguous loathing of everything their father did while simultaneously expressing their unambiguous acceptance of everything their mother did. Both children insisted that they could not remember even one enjoyable experience they had with their father despite multiple vacations, cruises, and day trips. (Oh, there was that bike ride as a toddler which one of the boys enjoyed.) In one therapy session, the father confronted them with the discrepancy between their statements and their joyful appearances in videos and pictures. They were unable to provide an explanation to resolve the discrepancy. Their father further requested an explanation for their last-second decision not to attend a recent camping vacation with him despite their enthusiasm in preparing for it. The younger boy had been so delighted with the father's purchase of clothes and camping equipment for him that, after returning home with these items, he put on the clothing, set up a campground in his father's backyard with the newly purchased equipment, and pretended the trip had already begun. However, after receiving a phone call from their mother, they refused to go on the trip and exclaimed to their father that they were feigning excitement. In a therapy session, the father asked his sons to explain their astonishing last minute refusal, and the younger boy responded, "I was just pretending to enjoy the camping equipment. I never wanted to go in the first place. It's time you realize that there is **nothing** we enjoy doing with you so you might as well forget about us." He provided no further explanation. Although the boys crucified their father for his every trivial oversight, such as once forgetting to bring home dental floss, they simultaneously excused their mother for having filed multiple petitions requesting an order of protection based on bogus abuse charges–charges which they knew to be bogus and about which they knew their mother had perjured herself. The children characterized these transgressions to be "insignificant mistakes."

Other children who were discussed in this book demonstrated typical polarized patterns of behavior in that they universally exonerated their alienating parent from the most egregious/aggressive behaviors against their targeted parent while crucifying their targeted parent for merely defending themselves. Indeed, a number of these children absolved their alienating parent for committing perjury for a variety of reasons "or for" concealing marital assets "or for" having affairs "or for" having their targeted parent arrested "or for" physically abusing their targeted parent. The "or for" was always excused no matter how reprehensible. And they simultaneously crucified their targeted parent for minor "transgressions" such as not sitting next to their alienating parent at their

games, failing to send the alienating parent a birthday card, arriving two minutes late for a visit, arriving two minutes early for a visit, chewing gum in public, and so on. I think the reader understands the point.

A previously discussed teenager who had lived most of her life with her mother and from whom she had been inseparable but from whom she was now alienated for more than a year, declared in therapy sessions that her mother never came to any of her games, medical appointments, or to school conference; never once did anything special with her; and never "hung out with me like my dad always does." It was as if the majority of her life with her mother had become a blank slate, wiped clean with one stroke of an eraser. She had no memory of the shopping trips, the special vacations, cheering on the sidelines during games, the school trips, the hair stylings, the manicures, and so on. In all seriousness and with a completely straight face, the girl denied having even one memory of a positive experience with her mother; nor could she cite even one positive attribute about her mother. She declared that her father's house is "normal" but that her mother's household is totally "abnormal" because they were living in the home of the maternal aunt and uncle and their children. She labeled her alienated mother "psycho" because she has not yet remarried, and she deemed her father to be "emotionally stable" because he had–despite the fact that he was now in the process of divorcing his third wife! She deemed her father to be above reproach, the only parent required to meet all her needs, and can be relied upon to teach "good moral character." Without any concern for her mother's feelings, the girl announced that her father and paternal aunt now comprise her family and that her mother is "unrelated to me." She emphatically expressed that she would have no problem if her mother walked away from her and never looked back as she has nothing to offer her. On the other hand, she indicated that her life would be over if something happened to her father.

A previously discussed preteen boy repeatedly declared that he had no use for his father because his mother fulfilled all his needs. He announced to his father that he would have no regrets moving with his mother across the country–something which she had been contemplating in order to be near her extended family. When the father explained to him that it would likely result in "parentectomy," the boy shrugged his shoulders to indicate his lack of distress. He solemnly asserted that he had no apprehension about the possibility of never again seeing his father because, "All I need is my mother."

A targeted mother heard the following from her preteen child, "My father teaches me everything I need to know in life. I learn nothing from you. He teaches me right from wrong. I am doing fine with dad. You're crazy that you think I am not growing up right. That's why I have no use for you."

A previously discussed preteen girl insisted that her father was "of little importance to me" and that "I could take or leave him." She expressed in a session, "The only good stuff about dad is that he sometimes helps me with my homework." The girl continued to devalue her father's importance to her when she stated, "My father is lazy and takes the easy way out because he does not cook for me but instead orders in Chinese food." The girl surmised that she could live a "very productive and satisfying life" without any participation whatsoever from her father. Her feelings for and assessment of her mother were quite the opposite. She stated, "Except for being somewhat overprotective, my mom makes no mistakes," and the girl normalized her mother's overprotectiveness by declaring that it is "typical of all mothers." The girl continued to extol her mother's vir-

tues by stating, "My mother does everything for us: she makes sure we have clean rooms, cooks for us, does our homework, and teaches us good values." The girl provided further indication of her unambiguously positive feelings for her mother when she then withdrew her apparent criticism that her mother was overprotective: she revised her comment as follows, "Well, that's not exactly valid anymore as she is now letting me have sleepovers with the girls I know from the girl scouts." In conclusion, the girl did not perceive her mother to exhibit any traits which needed correction. On the other hand, she assessed her father to require "extensive therapy" in order to overcome his many shortfalls, including his "anger-management issues." In every weekly therapeutic session, the girl arrived with a long list of grievances against her father which were "coincidentally" identical to those of her mother, such as accusing him of having had abandoned her, when in actuality the mother had moved her fifteen hundred miles away over the father's objections; of not really loving her or wanting custody except to avoid paying child support; and of having "too free a hand." I remember that I commented to the girl in a session that she reminded me of the puppet of her ventriloquist mother because she speaks but her mother's words come out.

When I am assigned to do forensic evaluations to assess for the PAS, I ask each child in separate interviews the standard task of naming three positives and three negatives about each parent. I invariably receive the identical response from these children: a long list of positives and not a single negative about their alienating parent and just the reverse about their targeted parent. In one such evaluation involving three siblings ranging in age from 10 through 15 years, I received the predictably scripted responses from each as follows: "My mom listens to me; she does my homework; she chauffeurs me to all my activities; she's always home for me; she is respectful, caring, and responsible; she teaches me to live a moral life." (PAS children seem to be "obsessed" with establishing that their alienating parent has good moral character.) All three children similarly insisted that they would change nothing about their mother, and life with her was described as: "It's terrific! It's been peachy!" I wonder how many children who have not been subjected to the PAS would assert such perfection in a parent, particularly an adolescent who is characteristically disagreeable. In predictably scripted responses, each of the three children similarly declared that they could not think of a single positive attribute about their father. Each made an identical flippant remark indicating that he does nothing for them and that "life would be fine if I never saw him again." Nevertheless the youngest child became choked up and held back tears in an attempt to convey the father's worthlessness, thereby indicating that the words were a cover for genuinely positive feelings for him. During a subsequent session with him, the children's deprecations were categorically discredited by the facts. The father revealed how thoroughly knowledgeable he was about their lives and activities: he was familiar with the names of all their teachers; he had regularly participated in parent-teacher conferences and was able to discuss each child's performance in every class; he knew about all their friendships; he had conversed with their coaches; he was aware of all the moves each had made on the baseball field; and he was aware of all their extracurricular activities, including a recent judo class in which they had enrolled. It was indisputable that their father had actively participated in their lives prior to having been prohibited by his children and ex-wife from continuing to do so.

I generally ask targeted parents to bring to the therapy sessions photos, videos, and any memorabilia of their involvement with their children. Many of these parents who are discussed in this book were unable to do so as they did not have in their possession any memorabilia: their former spouses had refused to share such items with them, and they had left the marital home with barely the clothes on their back due to the frivolous orders of protection. Those alienated parents who were able to share such items with their children created cognitive dissonance for them because of the difficulty in denying empirical evidence of the happy times and meaningful activities which had been shared together. This is often an effective therapeutic tool—PAS children are awakened to their true feelings by the memories evoked when they travel down memory lane with their alienated parent. This clearly can be accomplished only in a face-to-face session between the alienated parent and child. I cite the effectiveness of this technique in the case of a previously discussed father whose relationships with his children were obstructed for more than a decade. In the therapy session, the father sobbed as he recounted to his children about his involvement with them while he had still been living in the family. His teenage daughter was unmoved. I suggested that the father sit next to her, and soon the girl was sobbing in her father's arms. They declared their love for each other, and the girl acknowledged her desire to resume visits immediately. I become overwhelmed with joy and satisfaction when such developments occur. My therapy provides the environment for PAS children and their alienated parent to experience with each other memories which evoke laughter, giggles, and feelings which run the emotional continuum. Such positive, emotional interactions further provide explicit evidence of the speciousness of these children's expressed negative feelings for their targeted parent.

Chapter 5

THE INDEPENDENT
THINKER PHENOMENON

The lady doth protest too much, me thinks.
—Shakespeare, *Hamlet*

PAS children proclaim uninfluenced ownership of their "horrific" opinions of and feelings for their targeted parent. Moreover, they accept sole responsibility for their abusive, disrespectful and rejecting behaviors towards that parent, adamantly affirming that their alienating parent does not encourage them in the slightest. Imagine, a child accepting absolute culpability for their reprehensible deeds! And surprisingly, these children spontaneously volunteer their declarations of independence without being queried by the therapist or by their targeted parent as to the source of their thoughts, feelings, and deeds. Their voluntary declarations, indeed, are often completely extraneous to what is being discussed. It appears that these children have an insatiable need to impress with their "autonomous" thinking. When listening to the declarations of independence by these children, one is reminded of Shakespeare's expletive: "Me thinks the lady doth protest too much." Gardner (2001) characterized their declarations as follows: "Children who have their own opinions do not have to profess vociferously their opinions with disclaimers about the programmer's input" (p. 164).

What could possibly be the motivations of these children to accept blame for another's deeds? Firstly, they are assuming a protective role with regards to their alienating parent; that is, the alienator cannot be culpable for a programming crime if it were not committed in the first place. Secondly, these children gain brownie points with their alienating parent for executing her/his desires and deeds while simultaneously exonerating her/him from any culpability. Thirdly, these children have learned that it is not safe to challenge their residential parent, upon whom they are so dependent.

As discussed in prior chapters, the alienating parent and the PAS child are enmeshed whereby the actions of each reinforce and encourage the actions of the other. To that end, alienating parents will support their children's denigration and offensive actions by bestowing unjustifiable praise upon them for having "minds of their own," the "courage" to express their feelings and thoughts, and the capacity to follow through with "self-protective" actions. In service to the charade of independence, alienating parents affirm that they refrain from making derogatory remarks to their children about the targeted parent, that they do not engage in behaviors which undermine the other parent's relationships with their children, and that they do not model for their children maltreatment of the targeted parent. Even when alienating parents acknowledge that they harbor animosity for their former partners, they nonetheless profess that they employ great restraint in concealing from their children their negative feelings. They further assert that they employ heroic and extraordinary efforts to support and encourage their children's visits with the other parent. Ultimately, the alienator concedes failure in overcoming their child's "independent and sovereign" resistance to having a relationship with their targeted parent.

The following remarks are some of the more fantastic excuses I have heard from alienating parents regarding their efforts to facilitate the visits over the "independent" objections of their children: "I try hard to get them to visit. But why should I stifle my teenager's ability to make decisions?" "I always encourage the visits by asking them if they want to go. I strongly suggest that they should go, but shouldn't I be encouraging them to think for themselves?" "I tell them that they should keep the visit, but shouldn't I respect their feelings if they don't want to go?" "You were a kid once. Don't you remember choosing to be with friends instead of family?" "They have a right to their feelings, and I should respect their wishes not to visit."

I concur that children—as with everyone—are entitled to their feelings, but they do not have a right to act inappropriately because of those feelings. They must be taught by their parents to sublimate hostile feelings so that they learn how to function in our culture. This means that they cannot use such feelings to justify behaving in a disrespectful and abusive manner. It is, additionally, a parental responsibility to guide children to

make responsible decisions; and in areas of significant magnitude, such as attending school, keeping medical appointments, visiting with their other parent, etc., it is within the scope of parental authority to decide. Some alienating parents discussed in this book disagree with my position: they fail to appreciate the importance of the relationship between their children and the other parent. These alienating parents thereby demonstrated a disingenuous "encouragement" of their children's selective declarations of independence by sanctioning their visit refusal; and the children's visit refusal satisfied the clandestine needs and wishes of their alienating parents. And so goes the complementarity of the symbiotic relationship between the alienating parent and child. The assertion by the alienating parent that she/he is encouraging her/his child's independence of spirit and cognitive development is merely a ruse which conceals the covert desire to sever the relationship between the other parent and their children. The professed helplessness of alienating parents to persuade their "independently thinking" children to maintain their relationship with their targeted parent is a deception: in actuality, alienating parents are quite effective in manipulating their children to do their bidding.

Each previously discussed child who was at least nine years of age spontaneously and repetitiously volunteered that they had not been even minimally influenced by their alienating parent regarding their attitudes, feelings, and behaviors towards their targeted parent. Each insisted, instead, that she/he had arrived at her/his own independent conclusions and decided on her/his own behaviors. And that, of course, is the issue: because it **is** the job of parents to shape their children's attitudes, feelings, and behaviors. It **is** the job of parents to socialize their children—beginning in the family. So even when alienating parents doth protest innocence in **caus-**

ing their children's vile attitudes, feelings, and behaviors for their targeted parents, alienating parents have a responsibility **to correct** their children's vile attitudes, feelings, and behaviors. They cannot be absolved from this responsibility.

A previously discussed preteen boy gratuitously, repetitively, and passionately affirmed (as if in preparation for a trial), "My mother is not trying to alienate me from my father." Two previously discussed preteen boy and girl siblings spontaneously volunteered in separate sessions, "My mother did not implant ideas in my head." They each similarly elaborated that they had independently reached their conclusions about their father without having heard a single negative remark from their mother's lips.

In the case of a previously discussed preteen boy, he spontaneously and irrelevantly volunteered in sessions that he was not being influenced by his mother. He explained to his father, "My mom is not controlling me. My mom is not trying to turn me against you." He further insisted that his mother did not influence him to object to his father's girlfriend, but the timing of his rejection was curiously coincidental with his mother's filing of a petition for sole custody–even before the ink had dried on the divorce agreement granting joint custody.

A preteen girl who was alienated from her mother repeatedly exonerated her father from having turned her against her mother when she spontaneously exclaimed, "My father wants me to have a relationship with my mother. He tells me to go with her if I want to. I choose not to go. It's not my father's idea. You keep blaming him. It's not him. It's me. I chose not to go with her."

In another case, two teenage boys frequently affirmed in the therapy sessions with their father their "independent" thinking in remarkably similar terminology. The older boy exclaimed the following declarations of

independence, "I don't know why you say mom is coaching us. You keep thinking our mom is making us do this. But she's not. It's like we're being told by our mother what to say. Like our mother is making us do this. It's just the opposite. Our mother tells us to go. She's not controlling our actions. Why do you think our mother is telling us to say bad things about you? But she's not bad mouthing you. That's the problem with you: you don't trust that it's our own thoughts." The younger boy elaborated on this theme in the following words, "It's our words! We are not alienated. We don't believe you when you say that you will stop saying we are alienated. We have told you over and over that our mother never did anything to alienate us. How many times must we say this before you are convinced?" At this point, the younger boy started to cry, and his brother was impelled to clarify the tears by stating, "His tears are not due to how we feel about our father. We are just upset because he does not believe us. It's going to make you angry to be told that you are alienated when you are not and when you assume that our mother is alienating us when she is not."

Me thinks these children do protest too much!

A number of alienating parents remained in my driveway to pick up their children after the session. Heaven forbid they should permit the alienated parent to have additional time with their children while they drove to and from the session. Do they need to be in rescue distance of their children should something awful happen to them in a therapist's office with their other parent? How does this nonverbal message impact their children's independence of thought?

You have to be carefully taught to hate and fear–a loving and dedicated parent! You have to be carefully and thoroughly taught. Just as King Lear had been blind to the love of his daughter, Cordelia, PAS children are "carefully taught" to be blind to their targeted parent's love for them and to their love for their targeted parent. King Lear's blindness caused his demise. To the contrary, the blindness of PAS children to the love for their alienated parent is reversible–but only with early intervention from the mental health and judicial communities when working collaboratively.

When it comes to the symptom of the "independent thinker phenomenon," the germane issue is not whether the alienating parent has been culpable in influencing the child's vile attitudes, feelings, and behaviors towards the targeted parent; the germane issue is that it is the responsibility of the alienating parent to utilize her/his parental authority to correct the child's "horrific" attitudes, feelings, and behaviors towards the targeted parent and to encourage that relationship.

Chapter 6

REFLEXIVE SUPPORT OF
THE ALIENATING PARENT

Why then tonight let us assay our plot.
–Shakespeare, *All's Well That Ends Well*

The symptom called "reflexive support of the alienating parent" is descriptive of the process by which PAS children uncritically and dogmatically align with their alienating parent, particularly when disagreements and hostilities arise between the parents. Because of the alienating parent's and child's entrenched historical coalition (in that it likely commenced when the family was still intact) it is often difficult to determine whether the alienator "hired" the child as a collaborator or whether the child "volunteered" for the job. It is usually a combination of both, but teenagers will likely volunteer while younger children are recruited. As the reader will discover in the treatment chapter, family systems therapists labeled this coalition the "perverse triangle" whereby the child is manipulated by one parent into forming a coalition to the disengagement of the other parent. This interactional pattern acquired such a label because it is a dysfunctional behavioral pattern: when a parent and child collude (either consciously or unconsciously) to deprecate and reject the other parent, the child often develops severe emotional disturbances. The requirement of the coalition is a destructive demand for the child to choose between parents: it creates a double bind in that the child must either sever a relationship with the targeted parent or else incur the wrath and probable rejection of the alienating parent for refusal to do so. Should the child accept the seduction, the unintended consequence is an unavoidable self-loathing; that is, by rejecting a parent, the child is simultaneously rejecting herself/himself, being a product of that parent. A later chapter will discuss how instilling a PAS in a child is a form of child abuse.

When a typical family enters therapy for help with a problem, they are generally unaware of their dysfunctional interactional patterns, predominantly characterized by triangulation. A skilled systems therapist will enable the family members to identify these patterns and will then support the process of de-triangulating the child by coaching the parents to problem solve directly with each other. This restructuring of relationships enables the family to attain a healthier and more effective level of functioning and frees the child from the middle position between her/ his parents. In PAS families, however, the alienating parent has no interest in de-triangulating the child. Alienators do not wish to co-parent with their former partner or problem solve with them; they do not perceive the importance of their former partner to their children; they desire that their child adopt their feelings of animosity and disdain for their former partner in order to pursue their ultimate goal of severing the relationships between their children and their former partner.

In the face of parental disputes, PAS children express unequivocal support for and allegiance to the feelings, opinions, and behaviors of their alienating parent and absolute disregard for those of their alienated parent. They assert that their alienating parent possesses a veracity above reproach in every dispute while the alienated parent is always guilty of mendacity. Indeed, the enmeshment with the alienator is so powerful, that these children will interpret their alienated parent's struggle to defend against the alienating parent's humiliating behaviors and malicious accusations to be an attack upon them. This partially explains the catch 22 for alienated parents in mounting a defense against the alienator's spurious charges: their children will perceive these endeavors to be against them as well. And yet, if the alienated parent does not dispute the erroneous allegations against them, their inaction lends credibility to the claims.

PAS children, for example, uncritically align with the alienating parent even after that parent's allegations of domestic violence are dismissed and even when having failed to witness a single such incident. Whether it be issues such as child support, financial disputes, infidelity accusations, fallacious child abuse allegations, or any matter arising in the divorce proceedings, the PAS child will align with the alienating parent.

Baker (2009) reflected on her experience with the symptom and described alienating strategies when she stated the following:

> Whatever the targeted parent does is seen in the worst possible light; and whatever the favored parent does is seen in the best possible light. The child blames the targeted parent for everything: "It's your fault that the judge is mad at mommy. If only you had not lied or paid off the evaluator, then mommy would not be in so much trouble." If something bad happens to the alienating parent, the children are going to blame the targeted parent.

Baker expounded upon the facility of the alienating parent to manipulate the child when she made the following remark, "Alienating parents manage to make their feelings so very real to the child that the child loses the reality of his/her own feelings."

Issues surrounding the court proceedings always receive an inordinate amount of emotional reaction in PAS families and are highly indicative of the symptom, "reflexive support of the alienating parent." In virtually every case presented here—and in the many more which I did not cite—alienating parents "educate" their children about the court proceedings. The targeted parent is always characterized as being devilish while they, themselves, are presented as being saintly and victims at the hands of their former partners. Alienators are fully cognizant of the effect of this behavior: it gains their children's reflexive support for their position in every parental/marital dispute. Such allegiances are symbolized in the child's repetitive use of the words, "we," "us," and "our" instead of "I," "me," and "my."

The following are some examples of previously discussed children who uncritically aligned with their alienating parent in the financial and legal disputes with their targeted parent. One preteen boy advocated for his attorney to support his father's petition for residential custody even though the boy was aware that the petition was based on fallacious abuse allegations. An alienating father of a multisibling group asserted to them the spurious claim that their mother was attempting to have a clause written into their divorce agreement absolving her from the obligation to contribute to their college funds. The children uncritically accepted this assertion and subsequently reported to their attorney that they had no use for their mother. They cited this as the principal rationale. A sibling group berated their targeted father for repeatedly taking "**us**" to court based on a "fabricated" claim of alienation. In actuality, it was their mother who repeatedly filed meritless petitions asserting that the father was in violation of his child support commitments. A latency-age boy harangued his targeted father for repetitively "harassing" his mother for "putting her in court." In actuality, it was his mother who repeatedly petitioned the court to grant her sole custody and overrule the joint custody stipulation of the divorce decree. A preteen boy expressed the following to his targeted father: "Well you know, dad, your suggestion for how to divide **our** marital assets does not sound credible." An adolescent child informed the targeted mother that all contact between them would be held hostage to her consent to granting the father residential custody, with, of course, an appropriate child support award. In another case, two siblings advocated with their attorney in support of their mother's desire to move out of state even though that meant that their father could be only marginally involved in their lives. During a tirade against him, the older child excoriated him by exclaiming, "You ruined my life because you would not agree to the move." In another case, an alienating parent had shared the divorce documents with a

teenage child. In response, the teen exclaimed, "I will have to read both sets of court papers before I decide who I will side with." A preteen boy aligned dogmatically with his mother in support of her desire to move with him across the country. Although the boy had numerous friends and was engaged in many extracurricular activities, he stated that he nonetheless wanted to move because, "I'm just unhappy here. I have no connections here." (The reader can assume that his father was counted among those with whom the boy had no connections.) Using the father's girlfriend and her two daughters as a specious justification of his unhappiness, he added, "I can't live here knowing you are taking care of someone else's children. I'm not going to be part of that family." His absolute allegiance to his mother became even more apparent when he mimicked her rationale for moving," I am going with her because she can't find work here." The boy unswervingly defended his mother's assertion that she is unable to secure employment in New York, even though she has a Ph.D. in literature and had been employed as a college professor.

A latency age boy advocated with his targeted father on behalf of his mother regarding her request to move to the west coast with him in order to be near her extended family. The boy exclaimed to his father, "Why don't you want to move? Because you don't like Filipinos! But I'm Filipino, like mommy. I want you to go to jail, you Jewish person." The father denied that he does not like Filipino people, but the boy could not be disabused of this. When I asked him why he doubts his father, he responded, "He's lying. I know he's a liar." He subsequently exclaimed, however, in a rare moment of candor, "I know he must be lying because my mother said so." When I asked him for reasons why he believes his father should go to jail, he responded, "I can't remember why." But he had previously uttered to his father, "You are a bad father because you got the divorce."

The following is a small sampling of comments which PAS children have expressed to their targeted parent in the therapy sessions regarding the court proceedings: "You're lying when you say that you are not the one who goes back to court." "You have been taking **us** to court for (X) years." "Why were we in court?" "Why did you have dad served the subpoena when we were home?" "If you want to know the reason for not visiting you, it's because we don't trust that you will not take **us** back to court again."

It is quite common that alienating parents read to their children directly from the court papers or allow their children to read the papers for themselves. Fifty children discussed in this book were provided some information by their alienating parent about the events of the court proceedings–including a child who was as young as three years old.

Although financial and legal actions garner the most reflexive support, any marital/parental dispute will expose the cross-generational coalition between the alienating parent and the children. Whether it be whose extended family is gifted with the graduation tickets or which parent gets first dibs on holidays and vacations or who gets the prime seats at the child's recital or who makes medical decisions, or, or, or, and so on–PAS children grant their alienating parent the authority and deference to have it their way.

A latency age boy accused his targeted father of being "negligent" for not giving him money for his school lunches. In fact, on the school day following his sleepover at his father's, the boy went into a panic if his father failed to provide these funds: the boy was in double-bind with either having to forgo lunch or else disclose to his mother that his father does not provide him with lunch money. He would have chosen to starve rather than con-

front his mother; but his father rescued him by providing the funds on the days he was with him. Nevertheless, the boy held his mother entirely blameless regarding this ordeal, expressing to this father, "School lunches are not a covered expense in your child support payments. They are additional."

A preteen who had refused all contact with the alienated mother for a year defended the father after he had withdrawn from co-parenting therapy by exclaiming, "I don't see why my father has to come to the sessions with my mother. He never does anything wrong that he would need to correct." On the other hand, the preteen reprimanded the mother after a parental dispute arose by exclaiming, "You're supposed to be co-parenting with my father."

A latency age boy's reflexive support of his mother was observed when he interacted differently with his father in his mother's presence and when not in her presence: upon approaching my office door with her, he hung his head as if to convey displeasure about the visit; he avoided all physical and eye contact with his father, and he would not greet him. When safely on the other side of the door, however, his behavior so dramatically shifted that I thought for a moment I was observing them walk through a time portal! The boy was affectionate with his father, hugging him, kissing him, and sitting on his lap.

Two previously discussed teen brothers provided the following explanation as to why they had changed their established summer schedule with their alienated father: "We talked to our mother, and we agreed that the change we are offering you is much better for us and for her. We decided that it was good for everybody except for you." The teens then declared that the father had to "take it or leave it" as they would not make any exception to their unilaterally revised schedule. When the father's work commitments prevented him from complying with the revised arrangements, the children accused him of "intransigence," and they used it as justification for their year estrangement from him.

A teenage girl uninvited her alienated father to her high school graduation because the father "insensitively" expected to attend with his wife, who was detested by the girl's mother.

The following comments are just a small sampling indicative of this symptom and which were expressed to or about the targeted parent: "You cheated on my father, and he never did anything to deserve that." "You put your needs ahead of your husband's." "Technically, dad, the divorce agreement required that you address this matter in a six month's time or else you lose out." "If it wasn't you who called CPS on our mom, then who would it have been? Who else knows what goes on in our family? Who else would have lied about our mother?" "You failed to do your wifely duties." "You never kept the house clean. You never did laundry. You never cooked what my father liked. The house was always a wreck." "You are taking my father to the cleaners. Now I know why he can't buy me the iPad." "Daddy moved out and does not want us anymore." "Dad earned the money; so what if he emptied the bank account." "Dad, you made mom cry. I expressed my feelings to you over the phone. Why are you doing this to us?" "Mom was right when she called you a piece of shit." "Did you or did you not have multiple affairs?" "My father asked my mother for a divorce but went through my older sister to tell her. That was wrong to do." "There must have been something you thought mom was doing that you did not like. Why else would you have asked her for a divorce?" "If I were you, mom, I would be looking to get an apartment with one less bedroom because my brother will be the next to move out on

you." "I will not tolerate one more time your hanging up on dad and me." "My dad hurt me sometimes when I tried to say good night to my mom." "We don't trust that you won't keep badmouthing our father." "I can't remember anymore why I am sure that you called CPS against mom. It happened so long ago, but I know you must have done it even though I know it is pure speculation."

For the reader who is a parent, imagine hearing just one of these comments from your child.

It is quite common that PAS children will validate the alienating parent's spurious domestic violence allegations and refute the very real incidents in which the targeted parent had been physically abused by the alienating parent. Previously discussed multisiblings were afflicted with amnesia regarding several domestic violence incidences they had witnessed in which their mother, the alienating parent, physically abused their father, the targeted parent. During one such incident, the mother chased the father around the backyard while kicking him and punching him. On another occasion, she scratched his neck and pounded his head against their stone fireplace. On yet another occasion, the mother flung shoes at his head. The children adamantly denied having witnessed any of these incidents; but these incidents were confirmed for me by independent observers. Nevertheless, the children asserted that they had witnessed their father physically abusing their mother.

Because alienated parents live in constant fear of being falsely accused of domestic violence, their attorneys advise them to make audio recordings when in the presence of their estranged partners when they still live in the family home or when they are arriving for the visits with their children. Very frequently these children remain aligned with their alienating parent, even when that parent is contradicted by the audio recordings.

One alienated father played for his children several extremely clear recordings in which his children and his former wife could be heard cursing him and degrading him with the worst possible character assassinations. The children were conspicuously heard in the background, but they were nevertheless resolute in their insistence that they and their mother had never verbally abused their targeted father. When asked for their rationale for disputing what was clearly heard in the recordings, including names, they responded, "They are not us. They must be actors."

The previously discussed children who had accused their father of leaving them without air conditioning during a heat wave could not be disabused of this belief either. Even upon listening to an audio recording between their parents which confirmed their father's attempts to send a repairman, they still insisted that he did not make any attempt to have repairs made. Other children made similar remarks upon listening to audiotapes of their participation with their alienating parent in deprecating their targeted parent. The following are some of the typical comments: "That's not them." "It can't be us." "They don't sound like us." "That never happened." "She edited the tape." "Now you see how deceitful he is that he has to record us." "This is why we can't trust him. He can't be trusted to have a conversation with us without a recorder." And yet many of these very same children, at the behest of their alienating parent, secretly recorded their targeted parent in therapy sessions and during visits.

A word of caution to all therapists who treat and evaluate these families: videotape every session! But of course, do it openly after having discussed with the parents during the initial contact the rationale for doing so.

Another example of "reflexive support of the alienating parent" is exemplified when the children mimic the epithets about their targeted parent which they had heard expressed by their alienating parent. The reader, I am sure, has encountered situations in which family members thoughtlessly spew "technical jargon" at one another, sometimes in jest, sometimes out of immaturity, and sometimes out of unappreciated sarcasm. Such jargon as "psycho," "mental case," "wacko," "moron," "loony bin," et al., fall into this category. As offensive and objectionable as these words are, they are generally not meant to inflict pain, and the recipient may take it with a grain of salt. But this is not the case when the words are spewed at the targeted parent by the alienating parent and their reflexively aligned puppet children. Many of these children uttered to me that they agreed with the diagnosis by their alienating parent–none of whom had medical training–that their targeted parent is "mentally ill," "narcissistic," "passive-aggressive," "an alcoholic and a druggie," "violent," "borderline," and so on.

A previously discussed young man revealed his reflexive support of his alienating father when he regurgitated his father's "justifications" for having physically abused the targeted mother. The young man exclaimed to her, "You argued with dad. You didn't know how to shut up. You're a wacko." He further chastised his mother because she had sued his father for child support on behalf of his younger sister: "Daddy has to go bankrupt because you took **us** back to court."

PAS children generally remain stubbornly loyal to the alienating parent even in the face of compelling and credible evidence to the contrary. In Shakespeare's play, *As You Like It,* the hypocritical and melancholy Jaques–one of several characters pretending to be other than themselves–masterfully represents the condition of being untrue to oneself. It is likewise with the PAS child who is an actor progressing through the stages of this syndrome by playing a part that is also untrue to herself/himself. The role is not authentic to the player; it is, instead, a highly scripted role in a tragic drama written by the alienating parent, who is simultaneously director and co-actor. Just like Jaques, the PAS child lives in a world which he/she does not freely inhabit and plays a role that is essentially ego-dystonic—and which nonetheless exacts a substantial price.

Chapter 7

CRUELTY TOWARDS THE ALIENATED PARENT WITH NO REMORSE OR GUILT

Ingratitude . . . more hideous, when thous show'st thee in a child.
                    –Shakespeare, *King Lear*

This was the unkindest cut of all.
                    –Shakespeare, *Julius Caesar*

PAS children typically exhibit toward their targeted parent a cruelty so wounding that the serpent's bite pales in comparison. The wounds cut so deeply that every emotional and physical fiber of their targeted parent becomes ensnared. I have commonly observed targeted parents tremble and to shrivel in response to their children's cutting words. Pouring salt in their parent's wounds, these children reveal no remorse or guilt for having caused such pain. Indeed, Gardner (2001) exemplifies the cruelty as being so extreme that the children are completely unaware of the effects of their "sadism" (p. 189) on their targeted parent.

When treating the targeted parent, I repeatedly find myself in the awkward position of having to counsel them to search for a measured response to their children's cruelty. Although I help targeted parents recognize that their children's maltreatment is a consequence of having been manipulated by their alienating parent, it is, nonetheless, difficult for them not to react in kind.

PAS children reveal to their targeted parent an ingratitude for presents, child support, vacations, trips, bar mitzvahs/bat mitzvahs, communions, confirmations, sweet sixteen parties, coaching their sports teams, missing work to attend their recitals, providing a comforting hug when rejected for a date or for not having made the cheerleading team, having sacrificed their own night out with friends to be available for chauffeuring to that special party, taking valuable time and energy to invest in their lives and activities, and so on. To the contrary, targeted parents are "rewarded" for their efforts and investments by being remorselessly denigrated and rejected by their children.

Two previously discussed siblings cheered each time their father sobbed about how much it hurts to have lost any kind of relationship with them, let alone a meaningful one. Mimicking their mother's words, they snapped at him in session, "You should have thought about the consequences before you abused us and mom," and "You got what

95

you deserved." Without acknowledging in the slightest that their behavior was indefensible, they kicked him in the groin, punched him in the head, threw water on him, spit at him, and slapped him in the face. They were trying to hurt him seriously as if he were a punching bag. And let us not dismiss that they routinely cursed him. Many times after physically abusing him, they had the audacity to call the police to have him arrested on the spurious claims that he had abused them! I was incredulous at the ever-escalating level of cruelty which they displayed towards him and at the pleasure they took in the pain which they had caused him. In updating the information for this book, the father shared with me that his children have continued to express their remorseless contempt and cruelty for him, and they have refused all visits for the past several years.

Another previously discussed sibling group expressed to their father, "You don't deserve to have a relationship with us because you are a poor excuse for a father." They were unmoved by his expressions of pain due to their visit refusal for a period of many months, and they laughed when he sobbed about their lost relationships.

In the case of a previously discussed girl whose contact with her father had been severed for several years, she responded to his tearful expressions of grief about their estrangement with the following words, "You always overreact. It really wasn't that bad." The girl completely dismissed his father's pain, and she further exclaimed to him, "You deserve to be alienated due to your history of abusing **us**." She physically assaulted him a number of times, and frequently then called the police to have him arrested.

Two previously discussed brothers, who attended the family therapy only because it had been court ordered, displayed a complete indifference to their father's emotional expressions of regret that they had become ensnared in the divorce proceedings, albeit at their mother's instigation. In session, their father sobbed the following, "I love you very much. I miss you very much. I would do anything for you. You have no idea how it hurts to lose the relationships with your children." The children nevertheless, revealed no affect in the face of these vulnerable comments. They shrugged their shoulders in response, indicating a total dismissal of their father's pain, and they justified their visit refusal by stating, "You brought it on yourself."

A previously discussed girl sat motionless and unmoved throughout multiple therapy sessions in which her mother sobbed about how much she misses her and how hurt she is that there had been no contact for more than a year. The girl responded to her mother's tears by rolling her eyes, looking away, and exclaiming to her, "Get on with life without me." She uttered that she, herself, had shed no tears and did not think about or miss her mother at any time during their estrangement. She then volunteered, "I am behaving perfectly okay. I am being taught good values by my father."

Forty-nine children discussed in this book were verbally abusive to their targeted parent, and of the 49, 18 were also physically abusive. None of them acknowledged guilt or remorse for their maltreatment nor did they agree that their behavior was inappropriate. Indeed, they generally justified their actions by asserting that their targeted parent deserved the maltreatment due to one spurious justification or another. It is astounding how these children remained stoic and without affect in response to their targeted parent's expressions of utter vulnerability about having been forsaken by them.

If a parent treated her/his child in the abusive manner by which PAS children treat their targeted parent, that parent would likely suffer the consequence of becoming indicated by CPS. However, when these children maltreat their targeted parent, there is no consequence to them or admonition from the alienating parent—the only parent with any leverage over them. Many times they are rewarded. The result is that they remorse-lessly persist in their abusive treatment in an ever-escalating manner.

What does the reader surmise about how these children are being taught to deal with authority?

Chapter 8

PRESENCE OF BORROWED SCENARIOS

Fie, fie, you counterfeit. You puppet, you!
—Shakespeare

Because it is so illustrative of a programming, the symptom called "borrowed scenarios" is highly indicative of the presence of the PAS. When interviewing PAS children, one is inescapably impressed with how scripted they sound and how effectively they employ language, concepts, and terminology commensurate with a cognitive stage well beyond what is typical for their actual age. If the interviewer is unknowledgeable about the PAS and its symptoms, the interviewer would likely conclude that these children are child prodigies! However, when the PAS-aware interviewer goes where most interviewers fail to go by requesting that these children define their words and explain the meaning of their phrases, they are unable to do so. Their precocious charade then collapses like a house of cards.

In addition to the sophisticated use of language, another indication of borrowed scenarios is the commonality of expressions between those of PAS children and those of their indoctrinating parent. Indeed, the litanies of deprecation uttered by these children are often indistinguishable from the litanies expressed by their alienating parent. A further indication of the presence of this symptom occurs when PAS children reveal an intimate knowledge of events that they could not have witnessed or of which they have had no personal experience, such as events that occurred before their birth. It is only because of the alienator's programming that these children became privy to such information, which is usually inflammatory, exaggerated, or completely fabricated about their targeted parent. Numerous mental health professionals, including Gardner (2001), have coined a metaphor for situations in which a child speaks but the parent's words are spoken: these children are the "puppet or marionette" (pp. 164, 184) of the ventriloquist alienating parent.

A previously discussed latency age boy used expressions that are indicative not only of "borrowed scenarios" but of all the symptoms identified by Gardner. In my initial session with the boy and his mother, he exclaimed, "I hate my father." Instead of discouraging this feeling by communicating to him that it is unhealthy to abhor a parent, she validated it when she expressed, "See." She then provided additional "justification" for her son's feeling when she alleged that his father had a protracted history of hitting

99

him. This history was a total fabrication. The boy then declared in puppet-like mode, "Yes, he would hit me." I subsequently met with the boy alone in an attempt to explore the extent of his father's alleged physical abuse. In characteristic mode for PAS children, he was unable to cite even one example in which his father had employed corporal punishment as a form of discipline or any examples of actual physical abuse. He characteristically responded, "I don't remember." He eventually exclaimed to me, "I know he must have hit me because my mother said he did." Although the mother was not permitted to participate in the session, her sanctioning of the boy's resistance set the tone for the sessions, which were horrific and painful for the boy, for the father, and for the therapist. The boy repeatedly exclaimed to his father, "I hate you." He announced, "I don't have to be here if I don't want to." The boy felt at liberty to express these thoughts because he was standing on his mother's shoulders. This interpretation of the boy's declaration was subsequently validated when the mother acknowledged to me that she had informed her son—on the advice of her therapist—that he could elect not to attend a visit if he felt "afraid of his father." Further evidence of the boy's programming by his mother was revealed when he spewed the following at his father, "Didn't anyone ever teach you to love? It's all your fault: you put **us** in court. It's your fault for the divorce. You're getting the divorce." These comments were made with such pain and passion that it would have been a correct interpretation that the boy expected to be divorced along with his mother. He continued his harangue of his father by exclaiming, "You're evil. You're mean. There is always a problem with you. You need to change if you want to see me. It's not right to be taken away from your mother." The boy was unable to cite any examples of how his father is

"mean and evil" or how he needed to change. He was further unable to explain the meaning of the concepts he had expressed. For example, when his father asked him what he meant by, "didn't anyone ever teach you to love," he shrugged his shoulders and looked perplexed. The boy's entire dialogue was too sophisticated for the cognitive development of a latency age child. During another session, the boy persevered in deprecating his father in highly precocious concepts. He exclaimed, "Who's more important: your students or me, your child? You're always putting your students first." In this message, he was reflecting his mother's repeated brainwashing that his father prefers the extra income from tutorial jobs instead of visiting with him. But she was nonetheless aware that the father needed the extra income to support their two separate households as she had refused to secure employment in order to help with finances. The boy rejected his father's attempts to disabuse him of his perceptions, and he showed no interest in his father's expressions of pain upon hearing these comments. In subsequent sessions, the boy confirmed that his mother had shared with him the details about the court proceedings and that she had expressed to him that his father was scheming to take him away from her. (There was a bit of projection in this comment as the mother had once absconded with the boy when he was an infant, and the father had to incur huge expenses to locate them and have a court order their return.) This father had always been a loving father and was very involved in his son's life and activities before separating from the mother. The only explanation for the boy's hurtful comments was that he was expressing the thoughts and doing the bidding of his alienating mother. This case exemplifies the symptoms which are indicative of a PAS, including denigration of the targeted father, frivolous rationalizations, absence of guilt and ambivalence, reflexive support of the alienating parent, and finally the presence of borrowed scenarios.

In the case of a previously discussed preteen girl whose parents were in a dispute regarding the father's request for more time with her, she mimicked her mother's rationale for fewer visits–her mother having affirmed in a previous co-parenting session that "children need the consistency of a base to work from." In the subsequent family session, the parents began to argue about this, and the girl interrupted to exclaim to her father, "I need a base to work from." When I asked the girl to explain what she meant, she first looked at her mother and then responded that she did not know. She next spontaneously exclaimed, "I don't mind splitting the time more equally, but I can't say this without making one of my parents very angry." The girl's courageous remark is clearly indicative of speciousness of the PAS child's enmity for the targeted parent.

A previously discussed teenage girl frequently declared to her father, "I shall never forgive you for everything you have done; you have not earned the right to be forgiven; you do not deserve to be forgiven." As with another unrelated, previously discussed girl, she sounded more like a scorned wife than a daughter. She could not cite any of the events for which she was unable to forgive. On several other occasions, she sounded like a broken record by repeatedly exclaiming to her father the following opinion regarding the family therapy, "The family therapy is a waste of time as you are not changing." Regarding her father's individual therapy, she declared, "You are not benefiting from your anger management therapy." Her mother had previously cited these criticisms to me in front of her children. Indeed, many of the children discussed in this book expressed similar precocious concepts, sounding again more like a jilted lover than like children. Regarding

another incident in this case, the mother had reneged on her agreement with the father to split the cost of the girl's iPad. In a haughty tone, the girl exclaimed to her father, "You would have incurred the entire expense if you truly loved me." During other sessions, she and her sibling reproached their father for, "having taken **us** back to court." This was in reference to an ongoing financial dispute being litigated between the parents. (Becoming imaginary defendants in legal proceedings in which the targeted parent is the plaintiff seems to be a common fantasy among PAS children!)

The following were comments made by previously discussed unrelated latency age children: "The family therapy is messing up our family." "My father should get married again and have more children so that he can forget about me." "My father treats me like a piece of paper to be thrown away." "Go away, daddy. You hurt us and took advantage of us." "Go away. I checked my schedule and you are not on it." "My day is already filled with commitments so I can't visit." "You should get on with your life and forget about us." Another previously discussed latency age child was watching the *Sleeping Beauty* movie with her father, and she exclaimed to him, "The prince is not coming back to give her a kiss. He will abandon her."

Several previously discussed unrelated puberty age children made the following remarks in session to their targeted parent or to me: "My dad left because he wanted his freedom." "Does he really think he is doing right by us?" "My dad committed adultery. He is not being a good role model for his children." "My civil rights are being violated by being forced to visit." "He filed me away in his file cabinet like I was an unpaid bill." "He's time-frazzled." "He is a poor role model as a father and for the male gender." "He is terrifying when he stands there and watches me play." "My father stalks me." "He subjects us to slave labor." "He has a problem with his anger management skills." "You're brainwashing me!" "My dad promised he would never leave when I was first born." "My dad became jealous when I tried to kiss my mom goodbye."

The following remarks by previously discussed unrelated preteen and teenage children were offered specifically to justify visit refusal: "I'm a young adult; this is my decision as a young adult." "He used to be a fun loving guy. It's his character. That's the problem." "I have the right to decide where I live once I turned a certain age. I could decide about visits." "I'm growing up, and I figured out that I could decide for myself." "I think it is reasonable for me to decide this now that I am a teenager." "I have the right to live where I want to live. We're not young kids who can't choose." "We have our rights, we have our rights." "It's my decision to visit or not." "I have my HIPAA rights so I can refuse to see her if that's what I want."

Another common refrain expressed by PAS children which exemplifies how they resemble one another, is the request that their alienated parent "change" before they will resume a relationship. Nevertheless, they are unable to be precise about what changes are being requested. The following remarks were expressed by the children discussed in this book: "You must become a changed person and take responsibility for what you have done." "It's past things that **we** don't like. I think you should know by now what you've done." "How many more times do I have to tell you what to change? I can't keep repeating myself." "You sound like a broken record when you keep asking me how you need to change. Why can't you remember what I told you?" "I don't remember anymore what you need to change, but I know it must be bad if I still feel this way. Go ask mom what you've done. She'll tell you." "You sound like a broken record by continu-

ously asking me how you have to change. Just change. I can't be more specific." "It's the same things you keep doing over and over." "If I have to tell you one more time, I'm really going to get mad. Just change everything you're doing when you see me getting mad." "You know what to do!" "You will need to change before we can have a meaningful relationship." "Your problem with anger makes it difficult for me to deal with you. This is why we have a problem with you."

Thirty-eight children discussed in this book expressed the requirement for their targeted parent to change in order for them to agree to visits and to a relationship.

When previously discussed alienated parents made suggestions to their children about how to improve their relationship–such as planning interesting activities, deciding where to eat, and offering to purchase their necessities and desires, they were battered with the following hurtful rejections: "You don't build a relationship while we eat." "You can't buy me with clothes." "It's really not possible to eat our way into making up." "If you buy me that dress, it will make you feel better but it will do nothing for me." "You don't build a relationship with Adidas sneakers." "I don't want to have a relationship with someone who lies." "You can't have a relationship based on dishonesty."

A number of previously discussed alienated parents were accused by the children of cheating on the alienating parent, even when the reverse had been the case. Alienated parents were confronted with the following remarks from their children who were discussed in this book, "My mom told me it was wrong and illegal to date someone." "Did you forget that you are not yet divorced?" "Mom says you cheated on her numerous times throughout your marriage. How many affairs did you have?" "Daddy says you have a boyfriend who's trying to break up the family."

Twenty-nine children discussed in this book "indicted" their targeted parent for cheating, and one of these children was as young as five years old.

PAS children–regardless of age–appear to have a precocious understanding of the nature of relationships. All of the above statements reflect a cognitive development far beyond what the child who expressed the comment could appreciate or understand. None of the above children were able to explain what was meant by their respective comment nor could they provide specific behaviors or incidents that would exemplify the comment.

In what situation exclusive of the PAS has the reader observed a child speaking thusly to his parent? Not so coincidentally, many of the remarks were strikingly similar to the issues and expressions announced to me by their respective alienating parents.

The symptom of "borrowed scenarios" is more readily detectable in younger children as they are less adroit at protecting the programming ventriloquist parent and because the symptom is so noticeable when a younger child mouths an enhanced facility with language. Nevertheless, when provided the therapeutic environment to interact with their alienated parent, many of the adolescents discussed in this book bared their insincerity and confirmed that the origin of their comments was from the ventriloquist alienating parent.

The plagiarized yet disingenuous expressions of PAS children resulting from the manipulation at the hands of the alienating ventriloquist parent was best expressed by, William Shakespeare when he declared, "Fie, Fie, you counterfeit. You puppet, you.

Chapter 9

SPREAD OF ANIMOSITY TO THE EXTENDED FAMILY OF THE ALIENATED PARENT

A little more than kin and less than kind
—Shakespeare, *Hamlet*

This symptom is akin to visiting the "sins" of the alienated parent upon her/his parents and relatives. That is, the vilification and rejection of the targeted parent usually will extend to her/his entire family of origin. These relatives, such as grandparents, who had a previously loving relationship with the child will now be inexplicably rejected. The PAS child utters no remorse regarding such rejection and expresses no feelings of loss for the termination of these relationships. When these relatives attempt contact with the child, their efforts go unanswered, and all requests for visits are refused.

A previously discussed sibling group who had moved out of state resisted visiting their paternal grandparents, paternal uncles and aunts, and their cousins. On the rare occasion when they did, they acted-out so horribly that they were asked to leave early and were not readily invited to subsequent family events. They had confirmed for their attorney that they were in agreement with their mother's request to move out of state, and they had provided as rationale, "We have no family here."

A previously discussed preteen girl refused to attend the 65th wedding anniversary of her grandparents—the parents of the alienated mother. The girl remained outside the uncle's home for hours in a snowstorm rather than participate in the celebration. One by one, each of the relatives—aunts, uncles, cousins, and the grandparents—left the party to coax the girl to join in the festivities, but to no avail. She defeated each one of them. These were relatives with whom the girl had had a loving relationship before the onset of the alienation.

A previously discussed teenager announced to the targeted father, "I don't have to deal with anyone who has anything to do with you." And just like that, the teen stopped visiting the paternal grandparents, with whom the teen had a loving relationship before the onset of the PAS.

Many targeted parents discussed in this book reported to me that their children made fun of their extended family by referring to them as being bald, old, toothless, gray, and so on. Grandparents were suddenly addressed by their first names. These were relatives with whom the children always had a loving relationship.

The behavioral problems of 22 previously discussed children were so severe during the visits with the extended family of their targeted parent that the parent had no option but to terminate the visits prematurely because the children had become so aggressive and disagreeable. These events were reported to me as having occurred on Christmas, Easter, Father's Day, Mother's Day, on birthdays, and on anniversaries. In one particular case, a girl ordered her alienated grandmother to leave her high school graduation ceremony! Indeed, 13 targeted parents discussed in this book shared with me that their former partners had interfered with and frequently prevented visits and contact between their children and their extended family during the marriage. This probably should have been an early indication to the targeted parents about the intentions of their former partners. And why the targeted parent permitted the alienating behaviors during the marriage is a treatment issue.

Chapter 10

ADDITIONAL ASSESSMENT CONSIDERATIONS

Four additional diagnostic considerations supplement the characteristic eight symptoms already discussed, and they provide additional insight into assessing for the presence of the PAS. As these considerations are neither necessary nor sufficient for diagnosis, they will be only briefly discussed.

The first additional consideration is called "transitional difficulty" occurring at the time of visits, and this refers to the degree of resistance which the child exhibits when transitioning from the care of the alienating parent to the care of the targeted parent. In situations in which the PAS is mild, the resistance is negligible, if at all. In cases of severe PAS, resistance to the visits is so formidable that frequently the visit has to be canceled. The degree of transitional difficulty in the moderate category falls somewhere in between that of the difficulty in the mild and severe categories. The probability of the visits occurring is greater than in the severe category but is not at all assured as in the mild category.

The following is an example of transitional difficulty at which time both the mother and her latency age son were in the severe stage, but was reversed for the boy as a result of meaningful and frequent contact between him and his father. The events occurred as follows: just prior to the first therapeutic visit

with the father, which was also their first contact after five months of suspended visits, the mother called to inform me that her son did not want to attend and that she thought it would be best to cancel the visit. I responded that I intended to comply with the court-ordered therapeutic visits, and I implored her to rely on her parenting expertise to bring the boy to my office. When they arrived, the boy was "performing" for her: he shrieked that he did not want to see his father, and he resisted entering my office. The mother announced to me in front of him, "I told you he did not want to come." The mother's declaration empowered him to escalate his tantrum. He began to flail about and verbalized his opposition to the visit by expressing that he was afraid of his father. He repeatedly stated, "I hate him, I hate him, I hate. I'm afraid of him. I never want to see them again." The mother continued to encourage the boy's resistance to the visit by expressing that he is entitled to his feelings and that every therapist she had spoken to prior to me had stated that he should not be forced to see his father against his will, especially if he's afraid of him. I refused to be co-opted by this mother, and I informed her of the time that the visit will end. She departed with great reluctance, but her son continued to act out his mother's wishes by becoming physically aggressive and verbally abusive to his father.

Behavior during the visit is the next assessment consideration. In the case of mild PAS, the child is typically pleasant and cooperative, and it can be anticipated that the visit will be uneventful. In the case of severe PAS—as in the case just discussed—the child's behavior often creates extreme pain and consternation for the targeted parent. The behaviors of these children can be appalling to the point of physically abusing their targeted parent and destroying their property. In such situations, the targeted parent frequently makes the painful decision to terminate the visit prematurely. This is a double-bind for them because they will be accused once more of not taking full advantage of their visitation time. Several targeted parents described to me situations in which the police terminated the visit prematurely because their children had called 911 and made spurious allegations of child abuse. The result was that the children succeeded in manipulating the arrest of their targeted parent thereby selecting the time for termination of the visit. As an unfortunate consequence of such history, some targeted parents themselves sometimes failed to schedule visits out of fear of spending a night in jail. Behaviors of other children in the severe category were the polar opposite: several children discussed in this book disengaged totally from their targeted parent and secreted themselves in their rooms for the entire visit, failing to interact with anyone in the house-

hold. The withdrawal was so resolute that these children failed to abide by even the minimum social amenity of uttering "hello" and "goodbye" to their targeted parent or to other family members in the home. And yet, I initially worked with many of these children, many of whom had interacted very warmly and affectionately with their targeted parent at the time that family therapy had been initiated. So who helped to push these cases into the severe category? The usual culprits where the professionals in the mental health, child protection, law enforcement, and judicial systems who had been co-opted by the alienating parent, thereby emboldening that parent.

The behavior of the children in the moderate PAS category falls somewhere in between the behaviors of children in the mild and severe categories, but these children generally do not become violent or so provocative that subsequent visits are canceled or that their targeted parent becomes subject to arrest.

Bonding with the alienating parent is the third consideration. With mild PAS, there is a strong, healthy relationship. With severe PAS, the bonding, or more accurately, the enmeshment, is significantly deleterious to the child. Moderate PAS, again, falls somewhere in between.

Bonding with the alienated parent prior to the alienation is the last consideration. This behavior is the same with all degrees of the PAS; the bonding was strong, healthy and minimally problematical, if at all.

Chapter 11

THE CONTINUUM OF THE
PARENTAL ALIENATION SYNDROME

All the World's a Stage.
—Shakespeare, *As You Like It*

The PAS is a progressive syndrome which will inexorably travel from the mild to the moderate to the severe stage. Because it is a progressive syndrome, every case of PAS will not necessarily fit neatly into one of these stages. Rather, a case may overlap stages as it pushes forward should there not be professional intervention. Early diagnosis is therefore imperative, and remedies must be swiftly applied. This caveat is particularly pertinent to the judicial system, whose authority may be the only means to interrupt the probable outcome. Short of the alienator spontaneously ceasing from the alienating behaviors–a circumstance that seldom occurs–the reversal of the PAS will require the collaboration of the professionals in the systems which impact child custody. I have previously referred to these systems, and once again, they are the mental health, law enforcement, child protection, and judicial systems. It has been my experience that reversal of the PAS and prevention of its progression can be achieved with surprising swiftness under two conditions: that an experienced PAS-aware family therapist provides

the treatment and that the aforementioned systems afford the therapist a level playing field between the alienating and alienated parents.

Although each of the three stages may vary appreciably from each of the other two, some degree of most, or all of the eight symptoms is typically present in all three stages. The designation of a case to a particular category depends upon the symptom level in the child even if the alienating parent is further along the PAS continuum; but the level in the child can be expected to increase should the programming of the alienating parent continue unabated.

MILD PAS

Children in the mild category exhibit relatively superficial manifestations of Gardner's eight symptoms. They demonstrate only minor resistance to visits; they relate only a few tales of woe about their targeted parent and there are minor occurrences of denigration. The contact, involvement, and interaction between the targeted parent and child serve as an antidote to the programming by the alienating parent and is a major force to inhibiting the progression of these children into the more severe categories. Disrespectful and aggressive behaviors towards their targeted parent are virtually nonexistent. When in the absence of the alienating parent, the child and their targeted parent share a mutually loving relationship. The triangulation of the child into the parental dyad in service of the alienator is generally only a minimal transactional pattern. There is usually contact with the alienated parent's extended family and friends, and these relationships, as with the targeted parent, are loving. Children in the mild category generally have a strong relationship with their targeted parent, usually inviting the parent to their social and extracurricular activities. There are virtually no incidents of cruelty and therefore no reason to feel guilty. There is little cause and motivation to assume a stance of ambivalence, reflexive support of the alienating parent, or a charade of independence. What they may exhibit is a reservation about expressing their positive feelings in the presence of their alienating parent so as to protect that parent from feeling threatened by a close relationship with their other parent.

MODERATE PAS

All eight of Gardner's principal symptoms are likely to be present to some degree in this category, and the intensity is closer to the severe category than to the mild. The campaign of denigration is prevalent, particularly at the moment of transfer for visits. These children report more rationalizations for the deprecation of their targeted parent than do children in the mild category, and the rationalizations are frequently preposter-

ous, frivolous, and damaging. Lack of ambivalence is pronounced, and the independent thinker phenomenon is quite perceptible. These children demonstrate greater partiality to their alienating parent, especially when the parents have disagreements. The scheduling of visits is highly problematical as these children demonstrate formidable resistance, which is unambiguously supported by their alienating parent. Children in the moderate category present with little or no guilt regarding the pain they cause their alienated parent. The use of borrowed scenarios is substantial. While children in the mild group express loving feelings for their targeted parent's extended family members, children in the moderate group have appreciably repressed their loving and positive feelings. These children will, however, interact more agreeably with their targeted parent when not in the presence of their alienating parent. When visits therefore do occur, they are more likely to be uneventful in that the children are reasonably manageable.

SEVERE PAS

Children who are in the severe category will likely present with all eight symptoms, which will be manifested to a significantly impairing degree. These children become hysterical at the prospect of visiting with their targeted parent. Because alienating parents are "empathetic" to the desires of their children, they support their child's visit refusal. Gardner (1998) describes the severe PAS child's resistance to visits as follows: "Children in this category may become panic-stricken over the prospect of visiting . . . their blood-curdling shrieks, agitated states, and rage outbursts may be so severe that visitation is impossible" (p. 122). Should visits occur, these children generally act provocatively, aggressively, destructively, and disrespectfully. When listening to children in the severe category, the interviewer can expect to hear outlandish and vile accusations about their targeted parent and phony expressions of hatred for them.

It is the typical course of this syndrome that the alienating parent and the child will obtain the same degree of PAS severity. There are, however, situations when this is not the case. Some children are able to resist the programming and therefore do not progress as far along the continuum as their alienating parent. Factors such as age, intelligence, ongoing and meaningful involvement with the alienated parent, judicial authority, the child's own recollection about the family's truths, family therapy, influence of peers, and education all account for these exceptions. Nevertheless, time is on the side of the alienator. Without intervention–generally therapeutic coupled with judicial support–it can be pretty much guaranteed that the PAS child will eventually reach the same stage as the alienating parent. The reader must remember that the alienating parent has handed the PAS child a script which was written and produced by that parent about the family drama and for which the parent has directed the child to play a leading role. Therefore, when determining time frames for remedy of the PAS, TIME IS OF THE ESSENCE.

Chapter 12

THE ALIENATING PARENT

Almost as much has been written about alienating parents as has been written about the PAS child, and the literature is, at best, confusing and contradictory with respect to their mental status, their motives for the alienation, their receptivity to treatment, their ability to put the needs and feelings of their children above their own, and whether or not it is possible to gain their collaboration in reversing the PAS.

This author will offer her contribution to the controversy in the chapter on treatment. In the meantime, however, before we rush to judgment about the individual client/patient who presents before us, she/he must be accorded respectful and humane treatment devoid of the presumption of preconceived ideas about her/him. As with any other client or patient who voluntarily seeks our help or is remanded by the courts, the identified alienating parent should expect to be treated with neutrality, sensitivity to her/his feelings, compassion about the pain of the divorce and break-up of the family, appreciation for the anticipated difficulties of being a single parent, and with the belief that he/she has the capacity to change out of love for her/his children. Before we sit in judgment of the alienator, we need to ask ourselves if our own motivations have always been pure, our behaviors always above reproach, and our feelings always altruistic and noble.

The following classifications of the alienating parent are broad generalizations which do not account for the idiosyncratic differences and qualities of the individual who presents before the therapist. I offer these categories only as a general overview, and then I request that the treating professional immediately discount the characterizations whenever in the process of making an assessment of the alienating parent. So, in keeping with this caveat, I preface the portrayals of the classifications with the following cautionary words: it has been described in the literature that: the alienating parent is also classified along the continuum of mild to severe.

Alienating parents in the mild category only minimally engage in a denigrating campaign and behaviors to interfere with the relationships between the other parent and their children. Their primary goal is to preserve their relationship with their children rather than to sever the children's relationships with their other parent. They recognize that alienation from the other parent is not in the best interests of their children, and they perceive the other parent to be somewhat important to the child-rearing process. Therefore, they usually apprise the other parent of their children's medical, educational, and social developments. They are generally cooperative with the court orders and assure that the visits occur. They are, nevertheless, intent upon retaining residential custody. They recognize that protracted court litigation will cause grief to all family members and is particularly detrimental to their children. Their efforts to co-opt professionals to support alienating maneuvers are minimal. In general, the programming of alienators who remain in the mild category is a temporary response to the agonies of divorce, to the uncertainty of the future, to the frequently concomitant diminution in their standard of living, or to their temporary feelings of rejection. They may merely be reacting to the immediate turmoil and crisis that impacts most people enduring the anguish of divorce and family break-up. Very often their alienating behaviors will diminish or cease entirely as soon as the legal proceedings are resolved and they adapt to this transitional development in their family's life cycle. Frequently they are quite amenable to therapeutic intervention for the purpose of facilitating a civil and respectful co-parenting relationship and are receptive to modifying alienating behaviors when they appreciate the detrimental effects on their children of even the slightest demeaning comment about the other parent.

PAS alienators who are in the moderate category are more focused on effectuating the severing of the relationships between the other parent and their children than they are focused on maintaining and strengthening their relationships with the children. The campaign of denigration is prominent although the alienator is likely able to distinguish preposterous allegations from those which are not. There is a strong desire to withhold visits from the other parent, and, although these alienators will attempt to circumvent court orders, they will eventually comply out of fear of judicial penalties. The programming in the moderate category is

formidable, and a range of exclusionary tactics are employed.

Alienators in the severe category are resolute about effectuating the complete severing of the relationships between the other parent and their children. In order to achieve this goal, these alienators will employ extreme tactics, even to the point of circumventing the law. They generally harbor great antagonism for their former partner. If they are unsuccessful in obstructing a visit, these alienators employ shameful measures to disrupt the visit and to convey to their children that their other parent is dangerous and cannot be trusted. In order to achieve the goal of effectuating the alienation, the severe alienating parent will distort, exaggerate, and/or misrepresent any and every situation in order to diminish her/his former partner. She/he may have directly observed the particular situation, or she/he may rely on the reporting of the child, regardless of the age or immaturity of the child. In the extreme, the severe PAS alienator has diminished capacity to engage in a civil and respectful co-parenting relationship with her/his former partner, and this is the single most important variable for a child of divorce having a good immediate and long-term outcome. Alienating parents in the severe category do not perceive their children to have feelings, ideas, and wishes unique unto them. As a consequence, they believe that their children share their rage for the other parent.

Now that the reader has a superficial knowledge about the alienating parent, please forget this superficial knowledge and instead be curious about this parent just as you would about any unknown, idiosyncratic client or patient who presents before you.

Dr. Havlicek concurs with my cautionary caveat; he stated in his interview that the alienating parent cannot be neatly stereotyped into this or that pathological category. He recommended that the motives of the individual sitting before the evaluator or therapist be discerned. He described three motives which, upon such determination, he then assigns alienators to a differential category: (1) those whose motive is the receipt of financial support for retaining physical custody; (2) those whose motive is vindictiveness due to anger about the divorce or due to the denial and projection of guilt; and (3) those whose motive is enmeshment/codependency with the child. He stated that alienators whose motives fall into the first or second category are amenable to the treatment process. Alienators in the third category, who are generally overlooked by evaluators and therapists according to him, are the most difficult to treat. Nevertheless, children require that the alienating parent not be overlooked for intervention any more than the alienated parent should be, according to Dr. Havlicek.

I agree with Dr. Havlicek about the profession's moral imperative to engage with both parents. I believe that there is an important caveat about diagnosing: it is more art than science. A diagnosis is wide open to impression and to interpretation—or misinterpretation, depending upon your point of view. I have found that it is best not to prejudge because this becomes a trap which will bind us to realizing self-fulfilling prophecies. (If one walks around with a hammer, everything looks like a nail!)

I have, therefore, resisted attributing pathological labels to the alienating parent. It is no more justifiable to stereotype them as a group for pathology based solely on a categorization any more than it is acceptable to stereotype according to race, sex, religion, nationality, and so on. To attribute a pathological label is a trap because it informs the therapist in terms of pathology, limitations, myopia, hopelessness, and blame thereby binding the therapist to low expectations for remedy and change. It focuses the therapy on weaknesses instead of strengths; negatives instead of positives; pessimism instead of optimism; derision instead of respect; and rescuing instead of encouragement of growth, autonomy, and self-reliance. It fails to recognize that children require the relationship with their alienating parent as much as they do with their alienated parent. If the professional healer of the PAS were to write off the alienating parent, it would be isomorphic with the alienator's co-opted professional having written off the alienated parent. This is not how **I** was trained as a structural family therapist.

The opportunity to become rehabilitated and to receive the benefit of the doubt is afforded to parents who have been neglectful or abusive to the point that their children had been removed from their homes. So too, the ethical standards of our profession require that those of us who treat the PAS family must accord alienating parents the like opportunity—not just because it is compassionate and responsible—but because it is in the best interests of the child. This is what their children desire and need. Just as the overwhelming majority of foster children, upon "graduating" from the system, seek out their biological parents, then we must arrive at the inescapable conclusion that PAS children covet their relationships with both of their parents. Let us recognize that children do not view their alienating parent as a walking *DSM-IV* code on axis II. The professional should not do so either.

Chapter 13

THE ALIENATED PARENT

Alienated parents generally find themselves in a double-bind situation: if they pursue a relationship with their resistant children, they are labeled aggressive or insensitive to their children's feelings. But if they do not pursue their visits, they are accused of abandoning their children. Alienated parents must frequently make a calculated decision about whether to appear for visits because of the risk of arrest due to being falsely accused by the alienating parent or their children of menacing or threatening behavior. And then there is the concern of how to relate to their children out of fear that a gesture of affection will be misinterpreted as inappropriate sexual contact, should there have been a history of fallacious sex abuse allegations. Alienated parents are accused of showing no interest in their children when they do not appear at their games; but when they have appeared, they are humiliated by being ignored or advised to leave or labeled as a stalker. Another dilemma for alienated parents is to resist responding in kind to their children's hostility and deprecation. It is often a no-win situation, and that creates frustration and anger and a helplessness in deciding the best course of action in these very convoluted situations.

Major (2006) sums up the targeted parent's double-bind situation as follows:

It is common with PAS that alienated parents are in a chronically defensive position. They are continuously defending themselves against one wild accusation after another. Instead of being proactive, they are most likely to become passive. In the face of overwhelming hostility from the other parent, target parents cope by trying not to rock the boat. Tension builds. Something snaps and people react. Families with PAS are volatile families. (p. 281)

As I stated earlier in the book, a family therapist recognizes that there is a complementarity between the alienating and alienated parents and this means that they had co-created each other throughout their relationship. In other words, the alienating parent was accorded greater power due to either the passivity of the alienated parent, the alienated parent's conflict aversion, the alienated parent's desire to shelter the children from serious parental blowups, and so on. And the alienating parent's need for control has disempowered the alienated parent. All couples must negotiate the power distribution in the relationship, and each couple will reach an idiosyncratic agreement on a balance of power that is appropriate for the two parties. Although the power arrangement of each couple is, for the most part, successful in maintaining an effective homeostasis in the relationship while the parents are together, the power imbalance becomes unacceptable to the alienated parent upon separation should the alienating parent engage in the campaign of alienation. The experienced family therapist is capable of facilitating the separated parents to renegotiate a power redistribution that is acceptable to each and which provides for a meaningful role for the nonresidential parent in the children's lives— but provided that there is a level playing field between the parents. It has been my experience that the power imbalance alone within the parental subsystem is usually not so severe that the alienated parent becomes a victim of the alienating parent. I maintain, instead, that the outcome of the alienating parent's maneuvers would not be nearly as horrific, victimizing, effective, and successful were it not for the support that the alienating parent obtains from the professional rescuers in the mental health, child protection, law enforcement, and judicial systems. It is when the alienator is emboldened by the rescuers in these larger systems that the profound victimization of the alienated parent transpires. In order to guarantee adherence to the best interests of the child, the professionals in these larger systems must cease from enacting this role. The multidisciplinary professionals who were interviewed for this book made recommendations for systemic changes which minimize the adversarial aspects of addressing child custody and visitation, and which affords a level playing field between the parents for treatment and adjudication of this family development known as divorce.

Chapter 14

JENNIFER'S SAGA

A modern-day version of Gaslight's femme fatale.

I was impressed with his degrees and work experiences and his volunteer work for civil rights. How much more could a gal be looking for?" So we began to date, and after a time, we began to live together. His two children from his prior marriage were staying with us more and more frequently. I soon became pregnant with our daughter, at which time my husband-to-be informed me that he intended to seek custody of his older children. I willingly agreed to support him in this venture, although I knew that he would have pursued it even if I had I objected. I quickly became the primary caretaker for them. I remember having Dr. Spock at my side at all times as I was simultaneously breast-feeding, potty training, keeping up with socialization and education at school, and reading Dr. Spock because I had three children all at once. I, as a person, disappeared. Several years later my son was born, and it became yet more stressful and challenging. My husband controlled everything: what I bought for the kids, what I cooked, what we watched on TV, even what I wore. He negotiated me down as to how much I could spend on food and necessities for the family. I took the kids to all medicals; sent them off to school; conferred with the

schools; took them to their activities; and supervised all homework. When I agreed to support him getting custody of his children, I expected him to be a co-equal parent. But he was not. The around-the-clock demands upon me were exhausting. He never expressed any appreciation for how I took care of his two older children. It never occurred to me to leave him—I so loved having a family and home.

I felt so vacant that I asked to see a therapist, and he denied me that. I maneuvered to see one on the sly, but he found out, and this intensified his anger. His anger built up, and one night he repeatedly punched me so hard that he gave me a black eye. He had never been physically abusive before, but that night he threatened to break my arm. I called the police, but they did nothing as he denied doing it, and then the police said it was my word against his. There was no evidence as my face only later swelled up and became black and blue. Red marks on my neck where he had tried to choke me did not initially appear either. I was living in so much fear, and things were so tense that even my two-year-old son noticed. On one occasion my son commented to me after seeing my husband walk by me, "Call the police!" He could barely speak, and these were the first words out of his mouth. He could sense the storm starting to brew in his father. There was never a moment of tenderness or affection from my husband. He told me I contributed nothing to the family. I was slowly losing myself and my mind.

I finally persuaded him to go to marriage counseling, but things deteriorated because he did not like what the counselor articulated. After one session, he made me walk while he drove himself home. I arrived home to discover that he had locked me out. He had the children help him move furniture in front of the door to block me from coming in. I again called the police, and again they were entirely unhelpful, suggesting that I leave because he was so incredibly angry. I did not want to cause a scene in front of the children, who were already quite upset, so I left. My daughter, who is now 26, was eight years old at that time, and, except for a brief two weeks when she stayed with me due to a fight with her father, I never lived with her again and had no contact. In fact, we had no relationship at all during this entire time. My husband allowed me to take our two and a half-year-old son as he had no one to watch him while he was at work. My daughter was lost to me. Over the years, he brainwashed her to be afraid of me, and he convinced her that I had abandoned her. He refused to let me speak with her whenever I called her, and he never gave her any cards or presents that I sent to her. He disparaged me to her by telling her that I was promiscuous and that I was a pervert alleging I have sex with animals. I filed multiple petitions to enforce my visitation with my daughter, but she never came. He had convinced her that I was the mother in *Mommy Dearest*. He told the judge that she refuses to visit, and the court accepted this explanation. I had to repeatedly take him to court to collect child support for our son, for failing to support my

visits with our daughter, and for threatening my future.

A law guardian was assigned, and she listened to my daughter wail against me at the behest of her father. There was a total lack of understanding by the law guardian of how my daughter was being poisoned against me; she concluded that there must have been something I had done to make my daughter feel so alienated and hostile towards me. None of the professionals would force her to visit me when she was afraid of me. But what astonished me most was the court's ruling on custody based on the forensic evaluator's recommendation. She concluded that my daughter was being beaten by her father with a "psychological cudgel" but that she should nevertheless remain in his custody. The rationale given was that it would be too hard for my daughter to live with me as the waters had been too poisoned. The evaluator was saying that it was too late for my daughter, but they were granting me the custody of my son in an attempt to placate me for the loss of my daughter. I was stunned! Imagine, the evaluator knew that my husband was emotionally abusing our daughter, and yet she awarded her to him. How does this make any sense?

To this day, my daughter believes that her mother walked away from her. Since the day when my husband had put me out of our home, the only interactions I had with her occurred when she came to my home to verbally abuse me and physically attack me. The first incident transpired in her early teens when she was screaming on my front lawn that I am a whore and a horrible person and other vicious things. The next time I saw her was when she was about 21; her father had spent a night in jail for failure to pay child support for her brother, and she came into my home and pounded on my chest so hard that I was black and blue from shoulder to shoulder. I became convinced at that time that I had lost my daughter forever because she had become her father and had internalized the very perceptions, anger, and hostility that he had for me. When she was 24, her father unexpectedly died. I had hoped that this event might improve our relationship, but she became even more distant.

My son did not escape unscathed either from the parental alienation syndrome. He still entertains the idea that I'm not there for him; that I don't show up; that I don't pay him money that he thinks he's entitled to; that I had promised him things and then didn't follow through. Yet, when I brought him to various therapists, they would ask him for examples of this. And he couldn't think of any because this was all being drummed into him by his father. He would tell the therapist, "I can't remember." He still has the belief today that I am the kind of person who promises things and then disappoints.

If there was one thing I would tell the professionals who read this book, I would say to them that I'll never understand how they all awarded a child to a man whom they knew to be abusive to her. What do you think will be the outcome when you turn a female child over to a father who had abused her mother? I don't see that there was justice to this. I still sit here and don't know. I wish someone would tell me why they did that because they caused so much damage. I lost a daughter, and she lost a mother. And she is now essentially an orphan as a result of her father's alienating deeds.

UPDATE: there have been positive developments in this case, which are discussed in the chapter on treatment interventions as Jennifer and her daughter have begun the exciting reunification journey.

Chapter 15

JIM'S SAGA

A Tale of Two States.

It was the worst of times: in my opinion, things became twisted right after the birth of my youngest daughter. It seemed that once we had the children, my wife no longer had use for me. I was a sperm donor and nothing more. I would arrive home from work at a reasonable hour to find my wife ushering the children into bed. She had already fed them dinner and given them their baths. When I protested that I wanted time with the girls, she stated that I am an uninvolved father. But on weekends, when she wanted to be off duty, she "allowed" me to have the girls. Things continued to deteriorate rapidly. One night, my wife called the police on trumped-up charges that I had threatened her. The police admonished me! That was the beginning of the end. My wife then obtained a restraining order based on spurious allegations about this event. There was absolutely no indication that I had done anything wrong. With the restraining order in place, she continually threatened to have me arrested, and she could have done this without any proof that I had violated the order. She had only to say she was afraid. We separated soon after that, and she always made the visits difficult or impossible. The girls and I would be having a good time, and their

mother would call. Instantaneously, the girls became upset, disrespectful, and disruptive. At other times, my wife called up and "counseled" the girls that, if I became abusive to them or if I threatened them or if they were afraid of me, she would come for them. As a result, my disciplining of them generally morphed into abuse, as they saw it. They called their mother, who then warned me she would call the police if I did not release them to her immediately. She encouraged them to act-out knowing that disciplining created a double-bind for me. I lost my authority as a father. I became identified with being an abusive person. The kids' disruptive behaviors eventually resulted in my wife filing a CPS report on an exaggerated incident resulting from my attempt to restrain my younger daughter from a physical tantrum. This incident was enough for CPS to charge me with abuse. Lacking the funds for an expensive trial, I pled guilty on the advice of counsel. That was the biggest blunder I think I made in my entire life. CPS then insisted that my visits be supervised by them, and they were no better than my wife. They told the girls that, if they were afraid of me or wanted to end the visit early, they should tell the caseworker. Of course, every time I needed to discipline them, they became afraid of me, and my visit ended. CPS humiliated me just as my wife had done. In the end, I lost meaningful time with my kids. The abuse order further afforded my wife the opportunity to persuade the children's lawyer and divorce court to allow her to move out of state. My wife then used the order–even after it had expired in a year–to prevent me from communicating with any of my daughters' new schools and medical providers, even though there was nothing in the order which prevented me from acquiring this information. I was excluded from all parent/teacher conferences, medical appointments, and sports activities. I had to fight for every piece of information I received about my children's educational, medical, and social circumstances. I was never invited to any of the birthday parties. My ex-wife used that order to convince everyone that I had a long history of abusing my children. She used it to indoctrinate my children against me, and they now thoroughly believe that I had abused them during their entire lives. She undermined my authority with the girls by taking them off any punishment I had given them, and this conveyed to them that I was an ogre. She repeatedly put the girls in the middle of the divorce issues by having them lobby me for additional financial support. At other times, she threatened in front of the girls that she would file criminal charges against me if I objected to any decisions she made about them. The clothes she sent on the visits were always inadequate, soiled, wrinkled, and never appropriate for the season. But of course, that was only when she kept the visits. One of conditions of her being allowed to move out of state was that she must bring the girls to regular visits so I could see them. I don't think she kept even a third of those visits. There was always an excuse. Her counsel to the girls was to discuss with me about the anger that they had

for me due to a history of abusing them.

The court systems in both states were a joke. I was shuffled back and forth between jurisdictions and admonished by each jurisdiction whenever I attempted to file petitions to remedy the violations of my parental rights. The state in which my daughters resided asserted that the sending state should not have granted permission for the children to move out of its jurisdiction, and the originating state asserted that they gave up jurisdiction once the girls had moved away. I believe that I was penalized for bringing these petitions because each jurisdiction resented the petitions. Even though the receiving state recognized PAS as a legitimate syndrome, the judge failed to impose any meaningful remedy. He basically slapped my ex-wife on the wrist. He chastised her for alienating the children from me and for not keeping the visits; he admonished her that he would transfer custody if she did not cease this behavior; but in the end, he imposed no penalty when she perpetuated the PAS. The judge obliged my daughters' wishes to remain with their mother and was reluctant to give me custody because of my daughters' expressions of fear of me. So how much could the judge have really understood about PAS? My girls had been brainwashed against me and were doing their mother's bidding when they were questioned about what they wanted. Why didn't the judge recognize that they were not expressing their true feelings for me? If visits had been enforced, it might have made a difference. In the end, I was heartbroken, bankrupt, and no more connected to my girls. There was no talking to my ex-wife about her alienating behaviors. She insisted that I had to develop anger management skills as my abusive behaviors were the cause of the alienation from my girls. And my girls have suffered severe consequences.

If I had one thing to tell the judges,

lawyers for children, police, and CPS workers, I would tell them to look below the surface; don't believe what you hear; and certainly don't believe what you hear if you speak to only one side. You can't even believe what you hear from the children, as they have been brainwashed. You really need to spend more time with them to figure out how they really feel and whether or not they are being unduly influenced by one side. I am convinced that had I been granted cus-

tody and the authority that goes with it, that the girls would have responded positively to me. Once out of the claws of the alienator, it is remarkable how quickly feelings get turned around!

What the system did to me was to rob me. I was robbed of the two most important things in my life. I feel like I was raped! I feel like I was violated! I don't believe there is any hope for the best of times.

Chapter 16

BOB'S SAGA

A Not so Funny Thing Happened on the Way to Visit My Kids

I grew up without a father and I always knew that once I became a father, I wanted to give my children everything I didn't have. I was involved in every aspect of my daughter's life: taking her to the doctor, changing her diapers, getting up with her at night, feeding her, and playing with her. My wife and I did not agree about many things, and I wasn't sure how long this marriage would last. She then pressured me for another child, and my son was soon born. The marriage continued to deteriorate, and I decided to move out when my children were preschoolers. I believe it became my wife's goal to hurt me. She began to exclude me more and more from the children's lives, and my son developed an estrangement. When I came to pick him up, he began to cry. Instead of reassuring him that it was okay to come with me, she made comments that exacerbated my son's anxiety by telling me in front of him that he is afraid of me. I pleaded with her to reassure him knowing that he would take his cue from her, but she refused. She sabotaged all my visits. She obtained sole custody, but the court at least mandated my visits. She agreed in court to comply with the visits, but whenever I came for my kids, my son began to sob hysterical-ly, and she did not allow them to come with me. She once called the police, and, even though I had come prepared with my family court order, the police told me it was worthless. They did nothing to ensure my visit. All they could see was a hysterically crying child in my arms and who was comforted as soon as his mother pulled him away. She should have been arrested for violating the court order. She then suggested arranging for transfer at a toy store, expressing that my son might go more readily in that setting if I bought him a toy. But it was a trap, and I fell for it. As soon as I picked up my son, she inflamed him with fear that I would upset him, and he again began to wail. My wife pulled out a video camera and filmed the entire event, which she subsequently produced in court as evidence that my children were afraid of me. Whether some store employee called the police or my wife had prearranged it, the police arrived to restore order. I again left without my children in tow.

So I went back to court and, after multiple adjournments and the passage of time, the judge ordered my ex-wife to comply with the visits. The visits started, and my children could not wait to come to see me. Their mother tried to control everything. She told me what to do with them, what to let them watch on TV, whom they could play with, what to feed them, what family could visit when they were with me. She subjected my kids to the Inquisition after the visits. Sometimes she called me within ten minutes with criticisms about what happened during the visits. Within ten minutes she was able to pump my kids for this information. And if she didn't like what I did with them, she punished them. Now that was a real incentive for them to want to keep visiting! And that's what happened: the kids stopped coming. I returned to court, and the judge agreed to order family therapy. We had to keep changing therapists each time the therapist told my wife that she could not dictate what went on in my home. My wife made multiple CPS reports against me, which were all unfounded. But my visits were suspended for months at a time during the investigations. She kept all medical and educational information from me.

It's been two years now that I haven't seen my daughter, and she states she has no interest in seeing me but has been unable to tell any therapist why she feels this way. Her mother tells her that it is her right not to come. My son states that he wants to see me, but he fears reprisals from his mother and sister if he insists on coming. Even when my son told one therapist that he wanted to see me, his mother later called her to tell her that he did not mean it. I don't even receive a phone call on Father's day or my birthday, and they don't take my calls to them, ever. That is extremely painful.

If I could tell the police anything, I would say, "If you have a court order for visitation, enforce it." In New York City, if the custodial parent does not comply, they will arrest her. There is such a burden for the father to prove his importance to his children. This is

not fair. Sometimes he has to prove that he is not a neglectful or abusive father because the mother can go to court and make the wildest accusations against him. If you don't have a lot of resources, what recourse do you have? Why should he suffer not seeing his children just because he doesn't have $100,000 to pay an attorney? I would tell the judge that fathers must have equal importance to their kids. It has to be fair. They should make parents stay in the peace program until they get it. In the end, it's the children who suffer; they are the losers in the system. You can't lose a parent and be okay. I've lost more than three years with my kids. And why? Because nobody wants to enforce anything. Because nobody wants to believe that PAS exists. But it's real! I have lived it! The cops won't enforce the court orders, and the judges and lawyers won't hold anyone accountable. Do something! Fine her! Throw her in jail! Because if the situation were reversed, if I did not pay child support, they would do it to me.

My daughter needs a father. She's a teenager, so she needs me. I worry that she's going to have difficulty adjusting to relationships, especially her relationships with men because her father was cut out of her life. You could be bitter, but this is about the kids. The only thing my kids know is that their mother hates me, and that I don't like what she does. I am not even sure that this damage can be undone. All they have ever seen are the lies and deceit and manipulation and control. That can't possibly be good for them; it can't possibly have a positive effect on their future relationships. I worry for them.

I'm just numb to it all at this point. The only way I can function is not by thinking about it. (Bob falls silent, and tears begin to stream down his face.)

Chapter 17

JOE'S SAGA

A Reenactment of Franz Kafka's The Trial.

My wife and I were not getting along. She asked me to move out, and I complied with her request because the fighting was so unhealthy for our children. But I came back regularly to stay involved with my children. During one of these visits, she told me she wanted a divorce, and I thought I just got shot in the chest. I started crying, and she screamed at me to get out of the house. After that, she refused to talk to me even when I called about the children. That's when she began her campaign against me. She told our children that I was sick and abusive. My whole life was devoted to my children and to my wife. I didn't know what I would do without them, and I was worried about how my children would be without me. I took this very hard. My wife flat out told me she was going to do everything possible to sever my relationships with the kids. This was a bad dream, but the real nightmare was yet to come when I was informed by the police that I was being investigated for having sexually abused my daughter. It was a horrible ordeal, and I lost all rights to visiting with my children for years. During that time, my wife made sure that I was excluded from knowing about and participating in my children's health, education, and social activi-

ties. She was following through with ridding me from their lives. Even before the allegation, my wife did everything in her power to prevent my visits by alleging phony domestic abuse charges, which were all dismissed. CPS sent me to multiple therapists. I think it was a total of seven. I was referred to all kinds of experts, who all exonerated me from the allegation. My daughter was examined, and there was no finding that she had been sexually abused. Nevertheless, I was, incredibly, found guilty of having sexually abused my daughter–based solely on my ex-wife's belief that it happened. So on the belief, supposition, and aspirations of a highly prejudiced and invested party, I was found guilty. I felt like I was Josef K. in Kafka's, *The Trial.* My predicament was truly surreal!

My daughter had to go to therapy too. Over and over, it was drummed into her head that her father had sexually abused her and that she had to "talk it through," in order to get past it. How was it helpful to my daughter to be indoctrinated with this incredible lie? Who does that? I am listed as a sex offender, which means that I am labeled. And I am prohibited from working in several occupations in which I could earn more income.

If I could send a message to the judges and law guardians and to CPS, I would tell them that you can't just automatically believe what the mother says; you have to scratch the surface and find out her motives. And you can't assume that she is the better parent just because she is the mother. Look at the entire situation. She had the advantage for gaining custody because she was home with them. I was penalized as the father because I was out working to support them. How does that make any sense? I listened in the courtroom to all the other cases, and it was automatic, time after time, I would hear, "Give the mother custody; she is home with the kids." It shouldn't be this way. We are equal parents. We both take care of the kids. The point is that I was deprived for years of a relationship with my children, and they were deprived of a relationship with me, based on the fantasy, the untruths, and the wildly concocted allegations of a vindictive person. The system must change the way it evaluates and decides custody of children because it does not now protect their best interests.

The professionals who did this must be held accountable for what happened to my children and to me so that they cannot do it to anyone else.

Chapter 18

DAN'S SAGA

A Plea for the Wisdom of King Solomon.

When my wife and I initially separated, things went rather smoothly regarding our cooperation in parenting. Visits with my children were unobstructed for about a year. But inexplicably, my ex-wife began to schedule interesting activities during my visitation time so that my kids did not want to come with me. At other times, there was an excuse as to why the children couldn't come. When I discussed with her about the children's failure to come for visits, she responded that they did not want to go. She always gave them a choice about whether to visit. She never made it clear to the kids that they had to go on the visits and that they would suffer a consequence for refusal. That's what has to happen. But then again, if she had supported the visits to begin with, the kids would want to come. It was always a fight with her. Holidays were always refused. I had to go to court to have visits mandated. That was not what I had wanted. I had chosen to live near my kids just so that I could see them more often. I had wanted joint custody, and I had hoped to split physical custody so that we each had the kids 50 percent of the time. My desire was for my kids to feel that life would not change much for them despite the divorce. Their mother initially accepted the proposal for 50/50 physical custody, but she reneged when she discovered that her child support would be greatly reduced with this arrangement. It was all about the money for her. In the end, the court granted me only the customary visitation schedule for the noncustodial parent. Where is the wisdom that nobody recognized that a 50/50 split in residential custody–so that the kids can have the needed time with each of the two people who had been the most in their lives before the divorce–is really the best for them? But of course, that wisdom did not rule the day. But even this modest visitation arrangement was sabotaged. Once the visits were court ordered, she called them five times a day when they were with me. She interrogated them as to what happened in my home, and if she didn't like certain things, she would call me to complain. She made them feel like they were spies in my home because I needed to be investigated.

At the moment that my ex-wife made it into an adversarial proceeding the campaign against me commenced. My children told me that they heard their mother disparage me to friends and family. My kids overheard a conversation in which it was expressed that it was a shame that I had not been seriously injured during an accident. My kids were told that I had multiple affairs during the marriage. It wasn't true, but how do you tell your children something like this even if true? My children also told me that they don't have to deal with anyone who was connected to me, so they stopped seeing any of their relatives on my side of the family. There wasn't a single time in which I had input into a decision about my kids. I was kept in the dark about all school functions, medical conditions, and social activities. I always had to make diligent efforts to find out these things. I was not listed as an emergency contact with schools. I had to provide proof of my identity to get their report cards. I found out about their medical conditions only when the bill arrived. When my daughter received an award at school, I had to play hide and seek with her in order to congratulate her. Whenever my ex-wife and I had disagreements regarding what to expect of the kids, she overruled me and told them that their father was unrealistic. If she was present at an event, my kids ignored me. She does not acknowledge that I breathe, and the kids see that. I always told my kids to respect their mother, but I don't get the same respect in return.

My ex filed numerous CPS reports against me, and they were all unfounded. But while CPS was investigating, my visits were suspended. My kids started growing more and more cold to me, and they became more and more distant. The visits gradually decreased until they finally stopped altogether. It is been several years since I have seen them, and they refuse to talk to me.

If I could tell the judge anything, I would express that, of all the experiences in my life, and I have suffered a lot of abuse, nothing hurts me more than losing my kids. The system is designed in such a way that the non-custodial parent, which usually means the father, has no recourse. It is not a level playing field. I am sure that there are plenty of fathers who don't deserve visitation, but look at each of us as an individual. It is just assumed that the mother will be the primary caretaker. It is just as hard on the father that they don't have time with their kids. The courts need to mandate joint custody, with a 50/50 split of physical custody whenever possible. They need to look at the efforts that fathers make to be involved with their kids. And they also need to evaluate the negative effects on kids when they don't have a father actively participating in their lives. When the courts favor the mother as they do, they give her the opportunity to further the PAS. They need to understand that the PAS exists; it's real; I know, I live it every day of my life. My kids live it every day of their lives, and likely will for the rest of their lives. No one can tell me we have a court system that looks out for kids. My kids have suffered a lot and they have lost a lot of advantages. You can't have good self-esteem if you feel that you were abandoned by your father. This situation can't have a good outcome: if my kids eventually see me as the concerned and committed father whom I am, they will have to believe that their mother has lied to them for most of their lives. So great, then I become the good parent, and their mother becomes the bad one. Either way, my kids get hurt. My kids end up suffering. And me too, but them more so.

Chapter 19

JOSE'S SAGA

Parting is Such Painful Sorrow.

I missed all the red flags. From the very beginning it was her way or the highway: where to live, what to buy, when to start a family. I gave in because I wanted to please her. This became the basis of our relationship. She overruled me on all parental decisions. I was becoming a stranger to my children even though I was a very involved father. I had to weigh getting a divorce: I don't love her, but I love my children. So I stayed. But my kids started pulling away anyway and they were being made to fear me.

Then we separated, and the preposterous lies became worse. The children accused me of not supporting them. My wife petitioned for several orders of protection based on fabricated allegations, and all were eventually dismissed. She filed multiple reports with CPS, the worst alleging that I had sexually abused all of my children. Another report alleged that I physically abused them. They were all unfounded, but I lost valuable visitation time with my kids—time I needed to counteract the malicious and fabricated brainwashing. I never would have imagined that she could be so effective in alienating my kids. They just stopped visiting, and they never returned my phone calls. I had to go to court several times to enforce my visits.

And when they finally came, they were rude to me and to all my relatives. They were not nice to anyone associated with me. They made it plain that they were not happy to be with me. It was very hard parenting kids who treated you like this. No matter what I paid for or how expensive it was, nothing was ever appreciated. I pleaded with my ex-wife to communicate with me but to no avail. I never received information about my kids' school, medicals or extracurricular activities. She wanted to exclude me completely. They disregarded my punishments with their mother's approval. I had no authority with them during my visits. She never sent appropriate clothing on the visits. I repeatedly received disrespectful e-mails allegedly from the children but which were written far above their cognitive level. These e-mails would state that I was a dangerous, terrible father. The children were difficult except when I took them away on trips. Away from her influence, they were my old kids again. But other than that, I have no relationships with my kids.

If I could have the ears of the judges I would tell them they have to give more time to fathers. I mean quality time. I think it begins with time. You have to make it clear to the mother that if she exhibits any behaviors which interfere with the father's visits or if she behaves in a way that supports PAS, she will be reprimanded severely and she will lose time with her kids. Reverse the time! She was able to get away with her alienating behaviors because it was not made clear to her that she would suffer consequences. Impose jail time on the mother if she does not make the kids attend the visits with their father. That's when the kids started visiting regularly. But you have to do it early on, before the PAS progresses so far that it passes the point of no return. The alienating parent must understand the consequence of PAS behaviors will result in the loss of custody. I would tell the lawyers for the children and therapists, in particular, that they must become aware of the existence and signs of the PAS. Therapists are supposed to be the first line of defense, and most therapists do not understand how the PAS operates, if they even understand that it exists. They accept the word of the mother and the kids who are parroting her, and they think the father is an abusive monster from whom the kids need to be rescued. Therapists need to know PAS exists; it is real, and it is destructive not only to the alienated parent but more importantly to the children. Therapists, especially, should understand that children are very impressionable and that it is so unnatural to hate a parent; therapists should be suspicious and curious about what is really going on when a child expresses hatred for a parent. CPS must not be biased against the father based on what the mother says. Otherwise, he is presumed guilty and struggles to prove himself innocent.

To the parents who are victimized by the PAS, I would say to never give up. It's hard, and it hurts. It kills you. The worst thing to do is to pull back because that only gives free rein to the alienator. If you don't co-parent, there is a high probability that the kids are going to hate you. Children cannot grow up healthy if they hate a parent.

Chapter 20

MITCH'S SAGA

All's Well That Ends Well.

My ex-wife was very controlling and liked to get her own way, but I didn't catch this at the beginning. The marriage fell apart after the birth of our second child. I felt like she had gotten what she wanted from me, and my sole function was to bring home the money. I felt like a sperm donor. I did everything for my kids; I was an involved father. We agreed to separate when our children were young. Initially, I was just as involved with my kids, but that changed as soon as she found someone in her family to watch the children while she worked. After that, when I attempted to visit, it was never convenient for her. Holidays were always hers to pick and choose, and I just got the leftovers. I always had to beg her to see them, and then I would owe her something for the privilege. I requested that there be a regular visitation schedule with the kids, but she refused to cooperate. At that point, I consulted an attorney, who filed a petition in family court to guarantee my visits. Despite the granting of the petition, visits rarely took place. My ex frequently had an excuse why the kids couldn't come. Other times, she was not home when I arrived to pick them up, or she kept me waiting for hours before releasing them. I couldn't plan my life because I never knew if the kids would be coming.

My ex-wife filed several petitions alleging physical abuse in my home, and she requested to terminate the visits by court order. Her multiple petitions were dismissed, and she was ordered to comply with the visits. She criticized everything in my home, and she interrogated the kids about what occurred in my home and what we did on the visits. My kids felt like they worked for the CIA. She called me frequently and screamed at me that I was an unfit father. I could hear my kids in the background listening to this. I felt like I was under a microscope. The kids began to mimic their mother's concerns, and my ex-wife coached them to tell me that they did not want to see me. Soon they again stopped visiting either because they refused to come or because their mother kept them hidden away in the house whenever I came to pick them up for my scheduled visits. I had attended the peace program, and they recommended not causing a scene in these circumstances as it only creates anxiety for the children, so I drove away. Despite the Family Court order, my kids again did not visit for more than a year. I returned to court and obtained a mandate for family therapy so that I could bond with my children, who were now alienated from me. My ex was also mandated to participate as recommended by the therapist. But she did everything in her power to sabotage the therapy: she resisted making her appointments, then she missed most of her appointments, and she frequently withheld the kids for my appointments. The PAS unaware therapist did not address the lack of visiting; instead we spent a year "exploring" my children's purported "enmity" for me. My children's lawyer had a PAS-aware therapist assigned, and that made all the difference. With the assignment of this therapist, things changed rapidly. The therapist addressed my ex-wife's behaviors, and she helped me to address myself. I felt resentment towards my children even though I knew that their anger for me was not their own. I looked at them, and I would see my ex because they were conveying my ex's nonsense, criticisms, and antagonism. It was awful getting to the point where you blame your children and resenting them because you can't deal with their hostility. Yet you know it's not them. It takes a lot of energy and therapy to diffuse the situation. Then you have to figure out what are the legitimate issues in your home and what stems from the criticisms from the other home. Only a knowledgeable therapist in PAS can facilitate the healing process.

Today, things are much improved. The kids keep their regular visits, and they are much less manipulative and surly. As a result of the therapy, their mother is no longer the switchboard between them and me so that I work things out with them in a way that doesn't put me at a disadvantage. I know there is still some brainwashing going on, but I handle it better as a result of the therapy. I know that my kids will be susceptible to gravitating towards relationships which mimic the relationship they each have with me.

So if we do not preserve and develop an even more open, honest, and loving relationship, I doubt that they will find it in their marriages.

I would tell the therapists who think they know about PAS that they probably don't. They need to become educated about this syndrome because they are the ones who can apprise the children's lawyer and the judges as to what is actually happening with them and the family. The therapist who is knowledgeable about PAS will recognize that it is exceedingly unlikely that children can genuinely feel such loathing for a loving parent and particularly when they are unable to provide any credible explanation for their feelings.

If I had the privilege of talking to judges, I would tell them that all this drama could likely be avoided on the first or second court date if they just conveyed to the custodial parent that they will impose fines and/or jail time if they interfere with the visits with the other parent and if they attempt to alienate the children. If therapy is ordered, they must cooperate or suffer severe consequences. Why should I need to spend thousands of dollars just to have a relationship with my kids? I pay child support; I have always paid it; my kids are cared for and are safe with me. Why should I have to go through all this drama just to have a relationship with my children? This is my right; it is not a gift to me to see my kids. The judges need to support the rights of noncustodial parents and recognize the importance of fathers to their children. I have a right to unhampered visitation with my children and to have relationships with them. But this is not only my right; it is the right of children not to be deprived a meaningful, consistent, satisfying, and enjoyable relationship with their father.

Chapter 21

WILLIAM'S SAGA

A Pound of Flesh.

She micromanaged everything from the day we got married, and I just got tired of hearing her mouth. So I capitulated and let her do everything her way. Once our children were born, she had no more use for me. She made me feel like a sperm donor. I became persona non-grata to her. But I was always involved with my kids; I played with them; took them to the park. I arose in the middle of the night to take care of them. Nevertheless, it was always a fight with her about the parenting, and she would win. She complained I never did enough with the kids and then criticized whatever I did do. Everything I did was wrong. It was nasty, and it was in front of the kids.

I feared that she would concoct a scheme to rid me from her life, and she succeeded at this surreptitiously: she alleged to the police that I had intentionally thrown something at her but which she knew to have been an accident. I was arrested on the spot and jailed for the night. When I was released a day later, I returned to my home only to find everyone and everything gone—my wife, my kids, and all the marital assets. She emptied all our accounts and disappeared. I had to hire a private detective to locate my children. It took a year and $100,000 to find

them, to have them ordered returned to New York, and to obtain an order for visitation. I lost a year out of my children's lives, and they lost a father during that time.

But even though I had a court order for visits, she never complied. I could wait for three hours, and she then refused to release the children to me. She was always calling the cops on me alleging that I was violating the order protection, so I always risked being arrested. She was so cagey that she would call me to help with the kids, and then she called the cops alleging that I had threatened her. Fool me once, shame on you. Fool me twice. . . . What was really surprising and disheartening was when the cops caught her in lies, they stated, "It is no big deal." She used the order of protection—which was only in regards to her—to prevent me from obtaining any information about my kids from their schools and medical providers. I was granted joint custody, but I still had to go through hoops to obtain this information. I was told that I needed a note from the mother in order to obtain this information. Despite the joint custody order, some medical providers just refused to talk to me, let alone consult me about my kids' treatment. Behind my back, she put them on heavy medications with many side effects, and I could not object once I discovered this. I could not pick up my kids at daycare without her permission. One time I attempted to do so, she called the cops, who prevented me from taking my children. She was at work, and I was able to care for them—as per my right of first refusal. But that was not to be. I was made to feel like I was a kidnapper of my own children. She called CPS on me multiple times, and every case was unfounded. My only right was to pay child support or go to jail.

If the judges and lawyers are fortunate enough to find this book, I would say to them that fathers are important to their kids, and kids need to be connected to their father. The way the system is now, fathers have no rights. The judges must do a better job at finding out what's really going on in a case, and they must understand that alienation is real. I lived it. My kids lived it. And they suffered because of it. You can't just take the mother's word for what has happened. Judges really need to be sure that the allegations are true before ordering an order of protection because it is used as a weapon to keep fathers from having a relationship with their children.

Chapter 22

LINDA'S SAGA

Growing up with Richard Cory and Dorian Gray.

My initial conception for this book was entirely different from what is presented here. I had not realized that my counter-transference–deriving from my own victimization by the PAS–was blinding me to presenting a constructive and encouraging guide to remedy this family interactional pattern. The inspiration for the change to the book's focus must be credited to Patricia Minuchin, Ph.D. After I had described to her in 2010 my initial conception, I was awakened by her poignant response, "Linda, did you forget all your training at the Minuchin Center?"

So this is my story. My training at the Minuchin Center for the Family taught me that I cannot expect my clients to risk being vulnerable–this being essential to realizing change–if I am unwilling to do likewise. Loyalty to the principles and efficacy of my family therapy training demanded that I risk the same exposure as did all the others who participated in revealing their painful sagas.

My sister and I were victimized by the PAS at the hands of our mother and her mother, who had lived with us until I was 14 years old, at which time my parents separated. My entire childhood was truly a double-bind because my grandmother, who was the relentless deprecator of my father, was also the parent from whom I received my principal nurturing. My father was a workaholic who was at his business seven days a week/14 hours a day, and my sister and I virtually never saw him. My mother was self-involved, which also translated into little meaningful involvement with her children. My father's disengagement from the family permitted my mother and grandmother to engage in the alienation process–to which my father was utterly oblivious. I only recently discovered the clue to his obliviousness: each of his parents had severed their relationships with their respective siblings as the resolution to disagreement. Emotional cutoffs were thusly normalized for my father by his parents. There were many triangles in my family: my mother and grandmother against my father; my mother and sister against me; my grandmother and mother against me; my grandmother and sister against me; and the rare moments when it was my father and me against everybody else. But due to his workaholism, these moments were rare, and I was generally the odd one out.

I can recall the deprecating comments as if they were uttered yesterday. During the time when we were all living together, my grandmother repeatedly proclaimed that my father could never afford to keep us in our home and that it was her income which covered the mortgage. When my sister and I were in our teens, my grandmother thought it prudent for us to become aware of our father's emotional history so she shared that he had tried to check out on us by attempting suicide at the time when we were barely into our latency years. On yet another occasion, she determined that it was indispensably vital for us to appreciate that our father had wanted to abort one of us. Subsequent to my parent's divorce, an incident occurred in which I had asked my mother to please lower the sound of the football game which she had been blasting in an attempt to entertain a boyfriend, and she retorted, "Why bother studying anyway? Your father will never have enough money to send you to college."

Well, the reality was that neither parent had planned for my college. So at 18 years of age, I moved to my father's home in New York City in order to attend the City College of the City of New York, which was then tuition-free. I remember the feeling of passionately hating my father as I began this new journey in my life with him but yet anticipating it with pleasure so as to escape my mother. My hatred for him, however, evaporated overnight and quickly developed into loving admiration for the father whom I only then discovered. He was concerned, committed, involved, and encouraging. He shared with me the enthusiasm for what I was learning in my studies, and he inspired me. He inculcated me with my present value system of the importance of family, of caring about others, about fairness, about equal opportunity, about shared social responsibility.

A year later, my sister joined us—also with the intent of acquiring a free college education. But this new journey did not mean to her what it had meant to me, and she soon made the painful decision (painful for my father, that is) to withdraw from college. My parents and grandmother conspired together (misguidedly but united nevertheless) to keep her in college by refusing to provide her with shelter if she chose otherwise. But unilaterally and surreptitiously, my mother accepted her back in her home and further never revealed her participation in the scheme. My mother's double-cross led to an eight-year estrangement between my father and sister, who still believes to this day that her father had rejected her. I last saw my father in 1991, six months before he was gone. He expressed to me then, in one of his rare maudlin moments, that the biggest regret of his life was having lost those eight years out of my sister's life and the years out of the lives of three grandchildren.

Several years ago, I had added the use of the genogram to my treatment interventions, and I then became curious about my own. Simultaneously, my paternal aunt required nursing home care, and being her closet relative, I closed down her apartment. In her belongings were address books, and I thereby discovered my genogram. I became aware of relatives whom I did not know existed due to the normalizing of my father's self-imposed estrangement from his first cousins. I was able to contact more than 55 second and third degree cousins who then informed me of my unknown family history.

The normalizing of emotional cut-offs began in my grandparents' generation, was passed onto my father, and has now contaminated my generation: My sister has denied us a relationship for almost a decade. The loss is profound. I think about her, her children, and her grandchildren more than I care to admit. The last time we spoke, I had conveyed to her that alienation is an intergenerational family behavioral pattern and that she is modeling it for her children. Nevertheless, she confidently responded, "They will not be affected." She remains married to the same man for more than forty years, and I hear that my two nephews and niece are happy and well-adjusted. I am pleased about that. I had hoped to discuss with her the material in this chapter, but her contact information is unlisted. I did speak with my niece, who agreed to inform her mother of my desire. I have not heard from my sister as of the completion of this book.

I, too, have been able to maintain a thirty-two year marriage–my second. And three parents contributed to the rearing our emotionally healthy, self-sufficient, successful, and well-adjusted son. But I can tell the reader this: when a child goes through life with an alienation hovering over her/his head, it is like a cloud of sadness and a cloud of deprivation because the involvement of a parent had been wanting. And just like a cloud, the sadness and emptiness periodically comes and goes.

Chapter 23

TREATMENT INTERVENTIONS

What's gone and what's past help should be past grief.
    —Shakespeare, The Winter's Tale

The wisdom of Shakespeare to move forward and leave grief behind is the task that unites all therapies. But the various therapies accomplish this task by very different methods. Gardner (2001) suggested a way when he proclaimed, "A picture is worth a 1000 words. . . . An experience is worth a million pictures" (p. 348). I could not concur more with his axiom. Having been trained by the world-renowned and highly respected child psychiatrist, Salvador Minuchin, founder of structural family therapy, I believe in the power of family members to heal each other through their experiences with each other. It seems so marvelously simple to appreciate that we are most likely to change for someone whom we love and who loves us. I have found in my 43 years of practice that no quantity or quality of words between an individual and the therapist—who is nonetheless a stranger—can possibly have as powerful and as meaningful an impact as when the therapist provides, instead, an environment in which emotions and experiences are released among family members. No therapist, however competent and well intentioned, can possibly recreate a relationship with the patient that rivals intimate family relationships—particularly the meaningful parent/child relationship.

It seems so evident, then, that the crucial player to assume the deprogramming role is the "formally" loved and loving alienated parent. Indeed I assert that the deprogrammer who has the greatest potential for success is the alienated parent—who is not only the holder of the family's truths but who has had the loving relationship with the child. The role then for the therapist is to serve as a catalyst who encourages and guides the creation of healthy, corrective transactions between the alienated parent and the child as well as among all the family members.

Despite the logic of the argument to treat the entire family system so as to facilitate the healthy reorganization of its relationships and to capitalize on the innate love that parents and children have for each other, the literature on treatment suggests a counterintuitive approach. From my review of multiple treatment recommendations, the focus for intervention is generally the child alone, and a professional assumes the task of the deprogramming process, typically utilizing a cognitive and/or behavioral treatment modality. I found very little emphasis in the treatment literature for identifying the family system as the primary focus of intervention, either in its entirety and/or with its various subgroups. Nor is the alienated parent utilized as the prime mover of the deprogramming process. When the professional becomes the deprogrammer, the relationship between the therapist and the child is intensified resulting in the further weakening of the emotional connection between the alienated parent and the child. I am therefore suggesting in this chapter a novel approach to treatment of the PAS family, and this approach is called family systems therapy. Through the use of case examples, I will be specifying later in this chapter recommendations for treatment using one particular school of family systems therapy called structural family therapy although I am by no means suggesting that this systems approach is superior to any other systems approach. It is simply the approach with which I am most comfortable. I will demonstrate through my treatment summaries how this treatment modality capitalizes on the family members' unique ability to heal each other. I will be suggesting that the family system as a whole as well as its various subgroups be the target of intervention in order to reverse the alienation. These subgroups include: the targeted/alienated parent and the child(ren); the alienating parent and the children; the parents together with the intention of capitalizing on their love for their children to motivate them to develop a civil and respectful co-parenting relationship; the entire family system once the co-parenting therapy has reached the point at which World War III will not break out in front of the children; the therapist and the alienating parent in order to obtain that parent's cooperation and collaboration and to explore and attempt to resolve the underlying causes for the alienation; the therapist and the alienated parent. The work with the alienated parent will support the develop-

ment of coping mechanisms so that anger—a natural response to the alienation—is not transferred to the children from their former partner; will identify the best strategies for the deprogramming and for rebuilding the relationships with the children; and will help determine how to interact with the other parent for the benefit of their children. In some cases it may also be useful to enlist the assistance of extended family members and friends.

There are other rationales for targeting the entire family system for intervention. As the reader discovered in the previous chapters, the characteristic dysfunctional transaction of PAS families is the cross-generational coalition between the alienating parent and the child(ren) to the exclusion and disempowerment of the other parent. As such, this interactional pattern, being created and maintained by the family system, cannot be ameliorated by targeting the child alone. That would be as fruitless as attempting to improve a football team's passing game by singling out the quarterback for intervention to the exclusion of the receiver; or attempting to mediate a dispute with the participation of only one party; or coming to the peace table with only the vanquished party in expectation for concluding a peace treaty, and so on. To treat the child alone would be as futile as giving a patient antibiotics for an infection and then returning her/him to the environment with the germ that had caused the infection. Well, you get the idea. Another self-defeating, unintended consequence to singling out the child for treatment is that the child's self-esteem is attacked by the inference that he/she must be the problem as only she/he is sitting in the therapy chair. When the parents are not simultaneously in therapy, the child interprets this to mean that the parents are emotionally healthy and their behaviors are appropriate—despite all the vitriol and disrespect that had transpired between them and was modeled for their children. How about that for more confusion! Now let me play the devil's advocate: I stipulate that the child therapy becomes "successful," and the brainwashing is reversed. Is it then the child's responsibility to change her/his parents? This would not bode well for facilitating healthy family hierarchy.

The philosophical underpinnings of family systems therapy is the certainty that symptoms reside within the family system and are observed in its organization—in its patterns of interactions; in the coalitions which are formed; in how the subsystems function; in how power and status are distributed and regulated among the family members; and in how distance and closeness are regulated. It is the family's dysfunctional organization which maintains the symptoms of its member who is the identified patient. Systems therapy rejects the notion that symptoms reside intrapsychically or within an individual but are instead maintained situationally by one's intimate relationships. It inescapably follows that, because the family regulates and impacts the behaviors, attitudes, thoughts, and feelings of its members, then the target for intervention must be the family system. In my professional opinion, effectiveness of the treatment of the PAS family has been limited by the utilization of some form of individual treatment. In order to confirm my contention, I will discuss how an individual versus a systemic treatment approach is differently operationalized. I shall begin by summarizing some of the traditional individual treatment modalities while recognizing that the commitment of these therapists to publicizing the PAS have enabled me to make my contributions to the treatment of the PAS family.

In order to afford Dr. Gardner the well-deserved recognition for his pioneering work in diagnosing and treating the PAS, I shall begin with a discussion of his treatment recommendations. In his book, *Therapeutic Interventions for Children with Parental Alienation Syndrome,* Gardner (2001) first enunciated the crucial characteristics of the therapist who must be "hard-nosed" and "have a thick-skin" (p. 35) rather than assuming the traditional stance using "sympathy, empathy, and an understanding approach to treatment" (p. 36). Adopting a supportive stance, according to Gardner (2001), is not only ineffective but is actually detrimental to the treatment of PAS children because doing so only serves to "empower them and indulge their psychopathology, thereby making them worse, all under the guise of proper treatment" (p. 36).

Here, here! I am in complete agreement with Gardner about the necessity for the therapist to be challenging. The reader will soon discover that the use of challenge is an indispensable intervention of family systems therapy, subsequent, of course, to an appropriate joining process. Dr. Minuchin (1981) described this process as "joining and challenging" (p. 49). But Gardner and the family therapist employ challenge very differently, as the reader is about to discover. So, let us return to the discussion of Gardner's intervention strategies for the PAS child and how he employs the concept of challenge.

Once a duly confrontational therapist is identified, Gardner (2001) suggests interventions to be utilized by the therapist for each of the eight symptoms. These interventions reflect, generally speaking, an individual, cognitive modality to effectuate a deprogramming. These cognitive restructuring techniques, according to Gardner (2001) have the goals of: (1) creating doubt in the child about her/his perceptions of the alienating and alienated parents; (2) heightening the child's shame, embarrassment, and guilt about how she/he maltreats her/his targeted parent; and (3) punctuating for the child how she/he is being inappropriately and selfishly used by the alienating parent (pp. 111–118).

Gardner (2001) further suggested that encouraging the child to confront the alienator might be attempted but does risk reprisals because the alienating parent will likely become defensive (pp. 118–119).

The following is a summary of the principal cognitive interventions recommended by Gardner (2001) for each of the specific eight symptoms of the PAS. He suggested deprogramming for the campaign of denigration by appealing to the child's intelligence. He described this intervention as:

> Another maneuver that may be useful when debriefing PAS children is to appeal to the child's intelligence. The particular focus here is to encourage PAS children to use their cognitive processes to differentiate between fact and fantasy, between reality and unreality. (p. 117)

Other cognitive approaches to debrief for this symptom is to appeal to the child's innate understanding of her/his need for the alienated parent or what Gardner (2001) referred to as "the organ transplant principle" (p. 127). He also suggested debriefing for this symptom with the graphic use of metaphors, such as portraying the child as the "puppet or parrot" (pp. 112–113) of the alienating parent. This intervention serves to appeal to the child's subliminal awareness that she/he is being used by the alienating parent. When deprogramming for frivolous rationalizations, Gardner recommended that the therapist utilize the cognitive technique of expressing incredulity about the absurd statements the child expresses regarding the alienated parent (p. 145). To debrief for lack of ambivalence, Gardner (2001) recommended cognitive measures which help the child understand that it is human and not monstrous to make mistakes and for the therapist to express doubt about certainty; articulate the limitations of seeing the world

in terms of black and white; and discuss the difficulties one will encounter by being closed to disagreement and controversy (pp. 156–157). Regarding the independent thinker phenomenon, Gardner suggested using the metaphor of the "puppet or robot" (p. 164) of the alienating parent to challenge the child's blind adherence of the alienating parent's point of view. He further encouraged the therapist to use the Socratic method (my interpretation) by asking the child a series of questions which are designed to encourage independent thought rather than to robotically accept the brainwashing of the alienating parent (pp. 168–171). In addressing reflexive support of the alienating parent, Gardner uses cognitive deprogramming comments which indicate that the child does not have a mind of her/his own (pp. 181–184). When deprogramming for absence of guilt, Gardner uses himself as the moral educator of the PAS child. He described this role as follows:

> The PAS child must be helped to reestablish the sense of immorality that comes from betraying a family member. This principle has to be replanted in the child's conscience. . . . The PAS child must be helped to develop not only more guilt regarding the denigration of the victimized parent, but less fear over defying the programmer. (pp. 233–234)

Gardner views the therapist as the instrument of this reeducation and redemption, and he outlined a series of questions as to how the therapist can be an effective educator. With the symptom of borrowed scenarios, he suggested that the therapist assume the role of a Columbo-style "ignorant-interrogator" (p. 268) and engage in a polemic with the child by expressing curiosity about the child's understanding of her/his comments and use of terminology. This cognitive approach is designed to create embarrassment for the child when she/he is unable to convey an understanding of her/his comments. To deprogram for the spread of animosity to the extended family, he suggested invoking guilt in the child by discussing memories of her/his alienated parent's extended family and having the child imagine how the extended family must feel now that contact has been discontinued (pp. 285–286).

Gardner's approach to treatment would have to be predicated upon a well-established joining process between the child and the deprogramming therapist, and this process is likely to be quite lengthy. In the meantime, the brainwashing by the alienating parent is likely continuing unabated.

Despite Gardner's recognition of the power of the "experience," he did not capitalize on it to the maximum. And although he recognized and encouraged the alienated parent to play a role in the deprogramming process, he still assessed that role to be an adjunct to the therapist's role as the principal deprogrammer. Gardner stated his judgment about this as follows:

> Healthy living experiences, however, are the most effective antidotes to the delusions regarding the targeted parent's allegedly noxious and/or dangerous qualities. Much more time should be spent providing the children with experiences that negate the validity of the false accusations. The victimized parent can be engaged by the therapist as a **therapeutic assistant** [emphasis mine] in the deprogramming process. (p. 57)

What a shame! Gardner was almost there. Although Gardner assessed as "useful" (p. 182) the infrequent family interview, which could include both parents, its utility was for the therapist's edification to "smoke out the truth" (p. 182) rather than utilizing it as an opportunity to facilitate healthier family in-

teractional patterns. Again, Gardner was almost there but failed to capitalize on an intervention which family therapists have long determined to be extremely useful and effective. But where I find Gardner to have fallen signifcianclty short was in his approach to the alienating parent, whom he assessed, as a group, to be typically untreatable (pp. 295, 314–315). The reader will soon discover from my treatment summaries that disregarding and minimizing the alienating parent limits and often undermines the effectiveness of the therapy.

In their book, *Children Held Hostage,* authors Clawar and Rivlin (1991) suggested a treatment that is undertaken by a professional who also utilizes a cognitive orientation to achieve a deprogramming. They describe their approach as follows: "The deprogramming can be undertaken most effectively after a thorough understanding exists of the actual indoctrination techniques and the rationale behind them" (pp. 131–132). According to Clawar and Rivlin (1991) there are 14 factors to be assessed and understood in order to achieve an effective deprogramming, and I summarize them here: knowledge of the themes and content of the programming; knowledge of the motives of the alienator; knowledge of the techniques of the alienator; knowledge of duration and intensity of the programming; evaluation of the extent of the damaging effects on the child; evaluation of the resources available for the deprogramming process; establishment of joining with the child by the deprogrammer; knowledge of possible risks to the deprogramming; recognizing and addressing the "point of no return;" awareness for the potential for "shutdown;" introduction of supportive materials; environmental modification; reeducation counseling; evaluation of the degree and type of changes resulting from the deprogramming process (pp. 131–132). I cite these to indicate the cognitive orientation of their recommended treatment. Should the reader deem this approach to be useful, an in-depth description of the 14 factors can be found in their book.

Upon gaining this comprehensive understanding of the 14 factors, Clawar and Rivlin indicate that the professional deprogrammer will then be in a position to utilize this understanding to reason the child through a reversal process (pp. 147–148). This process is analogous to the Socratic Method (again, my interpretation) in which the deprogrammer asks the child a series of questions regarding the family's history aimed at leading the child to reach her/his own conclusion that her/his recollections of the targeted parent are distorted. By doing this, the therapist also seeks areas in which to create cognitive dissonance about what the child has been brainwashed to believe and what the facts actually support regarding the events which had occurred between the targeted parent and other family members.

In this model, the therapist has the arduous task of becoming fully aware of all the bits and pieces of the family's history so as to avoid the pitfall of being accused by the child of ignorance, stupidity, or even insanity. Indeed, Clawar and Rivlin acknowledge this momentous task when they stated, "This means that, of course, the deprogrammer must have at hand as complete a history of the facts as possible" (p. 147).

There are, thusly, several noteworthy limitations of this treatment approach, according to this author/therapist. Firstly, there is the implausibility for an outsider becoming that familiar with the family's history as to be proficient in defending against all the curve balls that will inevitably be thrown by the child. It is further improbable that any acquired knowledge by an outsider about the family will be as extensive as what is known by the alienated parent. And this punctuates

an extremely significant drawback to this therapy: the underutilization of the alienated parent. Although Clawar and Rivlin acknowledge the importance for the child to have "abundant positive contact with the target parent" (p. 130), they nevertheless do not ascribe to the target parent a principal role in the deprogramming. Such contact is more of an adjunct to the important therapy which occurs between the child and the professional deprogrammer. And finally, Clawar and Rivlin offer few suggestions for working with alienating parents because, according to these authors, they are "poor candidates for reeducation and counseling. . . . They were largely other-blamers" (p. 153).

Another suggested form of treatment which has been discussed in the literature is a modified form of exit counseling, which was developed to deprogram cult members. It has the goal of changing the child's belief system in the context of a trusting relationship with the therapist. This therapy is also a form of cognitive therapy, and it attempts to help the child make more informed decisions upon receipt of new information from the therapist. The therapist attempts to educate the alienated child about the manipulation and victimization of brainwashing techniques and of mind control, explores with the child about how she/he has been adversely affected by the alienating parent, facilitates an understanding of the need for both parents in order to live a healthy life and adjust appropriately, and examines with the child how she/he has made undue sacrifices for the alienating parent. The therapist is also charged with helping to improve the child's self-esteem and support the child's pursuit of her/his own goals, models respect and a noncoercive relationship, confronts the child on her/his coercive and manipulative behaviors, meets with the child and alienating parent together so that the child can observe the parent's hypocrisy when the parent behaves differently in the presence of the therapist, helps the child to gain confidence in her/his own thinking and feelings, and so on. This therapy also designates a therapist as the principal deprogrammer.

Ludwig Lowenstein, Ph.D. (2006) recommended a therapeutic approach which will enable the alienated child to develop the ability to think independently, to develop a conscience about her/his treatment of her/his alienated parent, to perceive her/his alienating parent realistically, to alter her/his negative feelings for and perceptions of her/his alienated parent (pp. 296–299). Lowenstein summarizes his treatment approach by stating, "Changing behavior relies on changing the attitude or cognition of the child" (p. 298).

These cognitive, individually oriented treatment approaches have the ultimate goal of readying the child for a relationship with her/his alienated parent. As the reader will learn from my treatment summaries, I do not believe that it is possible for anyone—even a professional therapist–to have nearly the same potential as do the parties themselves, in contact with each other, to become ready for a relationship with the other. Every time I hear the unsubstantiated platitude for a therapist, "to prepare the child for contact with the alienated parent," I want to erupt. Children do not possess the cognitive facility for abstraction so they cannot participate in a theoretical discussion about what an appropriate relationship entails; nor can they comprehend a desire for something in the abstraction. Children think very concretely; it is not until early adolescence that there is only the beginning stage for the facility for abstract thinking, which does not significantly mature until the end of adolescence. Thus you will hear an eight or nine-year-old exclaiming, "Step on a crack, break my mother's back." There is method to the madness of having no one younger than the age of

eighteen sit on a jury. A child, therefore, cannot have a discussion about desiring a relationship with someone who is in absentia; nor can a child participate in determining what to expect from the relationship with that "someone." That "someone" needs to be concrete, in person, in the flesh and blood. The therapist cannot, therefore, prepare the child through intellectualism for the rebuilding of a relationship with someone else. To be able to do this is a fantasy perpetuated by an adversarial child custody system in order to appease the parties and deceive one another into believing that the alienation is being addressed. Individual therapy will not be able to resolve this–at least not in a meaningful and timely fashion. To do so is also a fantasy perpetuated by the mental health community–partially out of ignorance, partially out of an opposing belief system about the power of the therapist and about how people change, and partially to assure our continued employment. I have lost count of the number of preposterous requests I have received asking me to treat a child whom I have never met in order "to ready them to reunite" with a parent, whom I have also never met and know nothing about. I am being asked to treat a relationship without having observed and examined it! Would a doctor diagnose for a disease without observing/examining the patient? Family systems therapists must educate the judge and the child's attorney about our uniquely effective approach to treatment.

Further compounding the ineffectiveness of an individual treatment modality is the necessity to rely on self-reporting, which is highly unreliable in general and is exponentially unreliable when it comes to an alienation. This is not only because of the cognitive immaturity of the child; it is because it is the rare child, indeed, who possesses the ego-strength to resist parroting the wishes of the alienating residential parent. My mental

health colleagues must become more attuned to this dynamic. It has been my experience that all too many in the mental health
profession are PAS unaware. They further
the alienation by demonstrating empathy for
and validation of the child's negative feelings
for the alienated parent and become determined to rescue the child from that allegedly abusive parent. Generally, the therapist is
co-opted by the alienating parent, who had
initiated the therapy and brings the child to
the therapist. The alienating parent's goal for
the therapy is not to facilitate an amelioration of the alienation but rather to obtain
professional support to further it. I assert that
no therapy would do less harm.

I was impressed with many of the treatment recommendations of Richard Warshak,
Ph.D. In his book, *Divorce Poison,* he recognizes the necessity to work with the alienating parent and does not assume that they, as
a group, are unreachable, unworkable, and
incorrigible. Warshak (2010) affirms, "Therapy with alienating parents helps identify the
fears, hurt, and shame that often lie beneath
the anger that drives divorce poison. It provides a safe forum for the safe release of hostilities" (p. 244). Warshak affirmed that therapy with the alienating parent is multifaceted
in that it provides outlets for sublimation of
anger, explores other avenues for needs fulfillment, educates about the detrimental effects to the child as a result of the alienation,
helps the parent to recognize the child's age-
appropriate/stage-specific needs, and provides a forum for communicating that transfer of custody is a possible outcome should
all other remedies fail to enlist the alienating
parent's cooperation in reversing the alienation (pp. 244–245). Warshak also offers
many valuable suggestions to the alienated
parent as how to become proactive as well as
how to respond more effectively when put
on the defensive. Some of his very valuable
suggestions include, but are not limited to:

1. not visiting the sins of the alienating
   parent on the child by responding to
   the maltreatment with retaliatory comments, anger, and punitive behavior;
2. maintaining contact regardless of how
   efforts are rebuffed (pp. 37–38, 164);
3. not provoking the other parent and
   refraining from competitive behavior
   for the child's affections;
4. crediting the other parent for her/his
   importance to the child for the positive
   aspects of her/his parenting (p. 90);
5. correcting misinformation without
   blaming the sender of the information
   (pp. 102, 149–150);
6. providing the child with empirical evidence, such as videos and pictures, to
   remind the child of involvement (p.
   104); and
7. not tolerating being maltreated. (p.
   146)

I find these suggestions–and numerous
others–extremely constructive and creative.
But Warshak's therapy also relies principally
upon the therapist to be the instrument for
reversing the alienation, should the step be
taken to seek professional intervention. Also
utilizing an individual, cognitive treatment
modality, Warshak reserves the deprogramming role for the therapist. Warshak describes his therapeutic intervention as follows:

The therapist tries to help children extricate
themselves from their parents' battles. Alienated children need to achieve a more balanced
view of each parent rather than a polarized
view of one parent as saint and the other as
sinner. The competent therapist is a voice of
reason and balance. He listens carefully to the
children and shows them that he understands.
But he also gently confronts their corrupted
view of reality. He encourages the children to
judge for themselves the accuracy of each parent's allegations. Therapists are often in a bet-

ter position to do this than target parents are. (p. 246)

Although I freely stipulate that targeted parents would likely benefit from coaching by a professional when engaging with their children in the deprogramming process, I will nevertheless demonstrate by my treatment summaries that the targeted parent must nonetheless assume the role of the principal deprogrammer, even if the process occurs within the safety of a therapist's office. This approach will send a powerful message to the child in that the authority of the therapist validates and supports the alienated parent's position in the family hierarchy and as the holder of the family truths. The approach has the additional advantage of conveying to the child that the targeted parent merits status, given the "therapeutic" position accorded to the parent within the therapy session.

I could not disagree more with Warshak's contention that the therapist is in a better position to counter the alienation. And I further emphatically disagree with Lowenstein's assertion that behavioral change results from insight. The discussion to follow about family systems theory will validate the refutation of these two contentions. Indeed, family systems theory upholds that change occurs through experiences and interactions with our intimate relationships which will then alter insight, attitudes and feelings. Indeed, if Gardner is correct about the impact of the experience—and I affirm that he is—then a treatment modality which capitalizes on the emotional experiences and corrective interactions between the alienated parent and the child must be more effective. To underutilize the alienated parent in the role of the deprogrammer is mystifying, especially given that every PAS-aware therapist affirms the critical importance for the alienated parent to be involved in every aspect of the child's life.

Another significant disagreement between individual versus systems theory is the definition each assigns to environmental modification. To individually oriented therapists, it means either the transfer of custody to the alienated parent or a significant reduction in time with the alienating parent in the situation in which the therapy fails to reverse the alienation. But to a family systems therapist, environmental modification means the replacement of the family's dysfunctional interactional patterns with corrective patterns that no longer maintain the alienation. Family systems therapy thus requires that the family unit—as opposed to the child alone—becomes the target of intervention. And to demonstrate the effectiveness of family systems therapy in treating the PAS family, I will be summarizing 16 treatments using a structural family therapy approach.

But before presenting these summaries, this orientation will be more readily comprehended if I place systems therapy in its historical context. Returning to Dr. Gardner's axiom regarding the magnitude of having "an experience," the original founders of systems therapy recognized, as early as the 1950s, the importance of "an experience" to the diagnosis and treatment of mental illness. Observing how their patients and their family members experienced each other through their interactions with each other, these early systems therapists reached the conclusion that the family's transactions played a role in the formation of the identified patient's symptoms. This hypothesis regarding the family's role was arrived at upon observation of their psychiatrically hospitalized patients as well as of institutionalized children, who, when they improved, another family member became symptomatic; or who, after having returned from a family visit, had regressed. It became inescapably evident to these psychiatrists that the family's interactions were somehow connected to the symptomatology of its patient member. Based on further observations of the family's transactions, these psychiatrists expanded their theory to indicate that the family system required a symptomatic member in order to maintain its homeostasis. In other words, these psychiatrists, most of whom began their careers as psychoanalytically trained and who were by and large working independently from each other, increasingly theorized that the locus of pathology was not internal to the individual patient but rather internal to the family experience or, in other words, how the family members interacted with each other. Before there were schools of family systems therapy, each with defined principles for understanding the context of the patient's symptoms and unique intervention techniques, these psychiatrists concluded that the patient's family played a significant role in creating and maintaining the IP's symptoms.

Merely talking to the IP alone, of course, would not reveal the family's organizational patterns that required her/him to be symptomatic because such interactional processes occur unconsciously, covertly, and perfunctorily. Diagnosis and treatment therefore demanded that the IP must be more deliberately observed in interaction with her/his family. Amelioration of the symptom would necessitate the presence of the entire family in the therapy so that each member understood how the family system required a symptomatic member. Without this collective understanding, the members would likely unite against the IP in her/his attempts to relinquish the symptom. These early systems founders thus began to work with the entire family in the here and now, observing each member's experience with each other. And thus began the exciting adventure which led to the founding of what today we refer to as the many schools of family systems therapy. I will summarize a few of the principal

schools of family therapy, but they are no means exhaustive of all the rich work that has been achieved in the area of family systems therapy.

Psychiatrist Carl Whitaker, who initially trained in psychoanalysis and who is perhaps the most renowned among the founders of experiential family systems therapy, began in 1943 to include in the therapy the family of his schizophrenic patients. He expressed in his book, *Dancing With the Family,* that to provide "an experience" is a preferable form of therapy to any individual form of talk therapy. Whitaker (1988) stated:

> The whole idea of symbolic-experiential therapy emerges from the fact that while we think about and talk about things on one level, we live on a level that's a very different territory. Symbolic therapy, then, is involved in the effort to move directly into the level of living, not settling for the realm of thinking, talking or reasoning. It's a therapy where you're not dealing with the data the family presents as data. It's not an education. The old saying, "nothing worth knowing can be taught" comes to mind. (p. 78)

To juxtapose the familiar forms of treatment, such as insight-oriented, cognitive, and other talk therapies, against Whitaker's experiential approach, one just needs to consider our clichés regarding the credibility of actions over words: actions speak louder than words; put your money where you mouth is; words are cheap; put up or shut up; well done is better than well said; people may doubt what you say, but they will believe what you do; nothing diminishes anxiety faster than action; and so on. Should the reader not yet be convinced, Whitaker buttressed his case for the rejection of talk therapies in favor of experiential therapy when he asserted, "I've yet to meet the person who's been able to grow emotionally via intellectual education. True emotional growth occurs only as the result of experience" (p. 85). Whitaker continued:

> My view of families is that the members are massively interconnected. I have very little confidence in the notion that ideas are information that can lead to growth. In order for real change to occur, the family needs to engage each other emotionally. They need real experiences, not cerebral insights. (p. 49)

Augustus Napier, Ph.D., (1978) a protégé of Whitaker and an experiential family therapist, describes the advantages of the experiential approach over traditional therapies as follows, "This approach assumes that insight is not enough. The client must have an emotionally meaningful *experience* in therapy, one that touches the deepest levels of his person" (p. 283).

Experiential systems therapy, as employed by Whitaker and Napier, produced a therapy which provided an environment for family members to release with each other their repressed emotions–the repression of which these therapists believed were at the root of symptomatic behavior and emotional distress. By supporting an experience in which family members reveal their material in the presence of each other, these therapists believed that the outcome would be enhanced family functioning and diminution of symptomatology. In other words, the experiential therapist focuses on creating an environment in which each member can express and experience with every other member their respective desires and hopes as well as their disappointments, fears, anxieties, sadness, anger, and so forth. In his 2004 book, *Family Therapy: Concepts and Methods,* Michael Nichols, Ph.D., summarizes the experiential approach to family therapy:

> Here the emphasis is on expanding experience. The assumption is that opening up individuals to their experience is a prerequisite to breaking new ground for the family group. The underlying premise of experiential therapy is that the way to promote individual growth and family cohesion is to liberate affects and impulses. (p. 207)

Minuchin (1981) commented on Whitaker's approach to therapy as follows:

> Whitaker sees the family as a system in which each member is equally significant. Each member must be individually changed to change the whole. Consequently, he challenges each family member, undermining each person's comfortable allegiance to the family's way of apprehending life. Each individual is made to experience the absurdity of accepting the family's idiosyncratic world view as valid. . . . Whitaker's assumption seems to be that out of his challenge to form, creative processes in individual members as well as in the family as a whole can arise. Out of this experiential soup, a better arrangement among family members result. (pp. 64–65)

Walter Kempler, M.D., (1971) another relatively early experiential family therapist who was initially trained in the psychoanalytic method, articulates the necessity for "the experience" in the therapy as follows:

> To witness another member of the family exposing, for instance, some fear or anxiety in preference to a defensive pose of bravado, usually elicits a new response from the observer. The others suddenly see through the defensiveness and respond with compassion and understanding as they feel less threatened. (p. 137)

To illustrate how the experiential therapist would differentially approach the presenting problem than would an individual talk therapist, I allude to a case of Whitaker's (1988). An adolescent girl was brought to therapy by her parents due to her suicidal ideation. An individual therapist would explore with the girl the extent of her suicidal ideation, including how long she has had the thoughts, how often she has the ideation, whether or not she has a plan, and so forth. If the reader is a therapist, you get the idea. Whitaker's treatment orientation can be summed up with one question he asked of the girl, "Whom do you think may want to see you dead?" One would assume that in this situation Whitaker had been well joined with the family; but then again, maybe not! His objective in asking this question is to reframe the symptom from an individual, intrapsychic and pathological perspective to one of a nonpathological, interactional interpretation indicating that the family system is somehow involved with maintaining and/or requiring the girl's symptom.

Although I am generally not as bold as Whitaker to approach a family with such a question, I can say that I certainly have experienced in my practice the phenomenon which he was punctuating. In the case of a 16-year-old girl who had been cutting herself daily for years and who had several hospitalizations for suicidal ideation, I explored with her in the presence of her parents the context for her behaviors by probing for how the family relationships were maintaining her symptoms. The family context was inescapably revealed by her following comment, "I know my father did not want me to be born." The girl further expressed that her father was repeatedly verbally abusive to her, as well as to her mother, and these family transactions provided daily credence and encouragement of her fantasy and for her behaviors. No amount of individual "therapist talk" with this girl would have been successful in dissuading her of the fantasy or to relinquish her suicidal ideation. The therapy without a doubt had to be approached systemically so that her father ceased his verbally abusive treatment of her, and that he

disabused her of her fantasy that he desires that she go out of existence. And of course, the mother's passivity as well as her situational depression, which she was modeling for her daughter, also needed to be addressed.

The essential difference between experiential family therapy and the individual talk therapies–which also encourages and supports the unleashing of emotions–is that in experiential therapy the family members are a critical component of the therapy because the family system is somehow involved in the survival of the symptom; in other words, experiential therapists do not consider expression of material to be therapy when in the absence of the other family members. This is a significant departure from traditional individual therapies in that the emotions which are released in the session are shared among the family members with the goal of increasing the emotional intensities and intimacy among the family members. The transference consequently occurs primarily between family members and not between the therapist and the individual patient.

Each of the various schools of systems therapy utilizes the here and now, objectively-observed experience–as opposed to the subjective recounting of the there and then memory–in ways different from each other and from the school of experiential therapy. But, the significance of "the experience" to family systems therapists and what unites all of these therapies, is that the IP's significant, intimate relationships are included in the therapy and are a critical component to and of the therapeutic process. The other significant characteristic that unites all family systems therapists is that they locate the symptom within the family system and not within the individual who is labeled the identified patient.

Murray Bowen, M.D., a psychoanalytically trained psychiatrist, became another early founder in the 1950s of family systems therapy when, like the other psychoanalytically trained psychiatrists, he experienced how the family system and the symptom mutually maintained each other. Bowen (1971) expressed the following regarding the shortcomings of the philosophical underpinnings of an individual treatment modality:

> Individual theory was built on a medical model with its concepts of etiology, the diagnosis of pathology in the patient, and treatment of the sickness in the individual. Also inherent in the model are the subtle implications that the patient is the helpless victim of the disease or malevolent forces outside his control. (p. 160)

This is what I have come to believe as I progressed through my mental health and family therapy training: that a person does not build self-esteem while carrying the label of a patient. Because Bowen treated primarily a schizophrenic population, he was in the unique position to observe how they behaved when on a psychiatric ward but then behaved very differently when in the presence of the family. Unlike many of his colleagues, Bowen (1978) did not relinquish his belief that psychoanalytic theory is relevant to the understanding of pathology. But he simultaneously recognized the significant role played by interpersonal family transactions on symptom formation and maintenance. When treating the patient, he addressed the influence of intrapsychic conflict while concurrently including the family in the therapy in recognition that member interactions impacted symptom development. Indeed, Bowen believed so strongly about the family's contribution to symptom formation that, when he hospitalized a schizophrenic patient, he also hospitalized the entire nuclear family! Bowen had initially believed that mental instability resulted from an overly enmeshed mother/child relationship which

had failed to progress beyond the stage of symbiosis. He later revised his assessment of pathology to include the concept of pathological triangles in recognition of the father's contribution to the development of an emotionally disturbed child. He described the triangulation process as that which permits tension between the parents to be diffused by the child, who is either hired by one of the parents as an ally in a coalition against the other parent or else the child volunteers for the assignment after having been previously co-opted (pp. 198–200, 373–375, 478–480).

Anyone who lives with a child and a partner recognizes how frequently triangulation quite innocently occurs in ordinary family life, such as when one parent turns to the child during a dispute with the other parent and asks the child, "Isn't what I'm saying true?" I am reminded of such nonchalant behaviors as reflected in the two, all too humorous but all too real-life TV commercials, which play-off of triangulation. In the first, a teenage girl, standing with her father in the kitchen, comments to him about how old and disgusting their refrigerator is. The father looks at his ingratiating daughter with admiring eyes and responds, "You think?" The girl, leaving the kitchen and passing her mother on the living room sofa, collects a $20 bill from her as a reward for the lobbying efforts with her father.

In the second commercial, a dejected-looking mother is standing with her latency-age son in the living room, and the boy asks her, "What's wrong?" The mother responds, "I want new floors but your father won't let me get them." The boy runs to the staircase and yells up, "Hey dad, mom wants new floors!" In the next scene, the mother is standing alone in her living room gazing down and smiling at her new floors. Unexpectedly she hears a voice yell from upstairs, "Hey mom, dad wants a new motorcycle." The mother looks up, her affect indicating her thoughts: "What have I wrought?"

Do not be alarmed, reader! Your occasional request of your child for validation of your position in a disagreement with your partner will not produce a psychotic child. The development of severe pathology in a child requires that the triangulating coalition be a repetitive, routine, rigid, and a predictable pattern which has the destructive effect of disempowering and demeaning the other parent. An occasional slip of behavior does not create pathology, although healthy family functioning requires that such behavior be kept to a minimum.

Many systems therapists, including this author, deem the most significant contribution which Bowen (1978) contributed to family systems theory to be his assessment that pathology results principally from the formation of a triangle, which he assessed to originate in an emotional reactivity provoked by family members in each other. He labeled this the "undifferentiated family ego mass" (pp. 159–162, 203–206), and Bowen defined it as the members being emotionally fused with each other. This resulted in the suppression of individual autonomy and the subjugation of cognitive processes to emotions. Each member's emotional fusion or emotional autonomy was dependent upon the behavioral interactions with the other family members. The goal of Bowen's therapy was to promote the "differentiation of self" (pp. 529–547). Nichols (2004) summarizes how Bowen defined this concept along with its centrality to his treatment philosophy:

> **Differentiation of self**, the cornerstone of Bowen's theory, is both an intrapsychic and an interpersonal concept. . . . Differentiation is the capacity to think and reflect, to not respond automatically to emotional pressures, internal or external. It is the ability to be flexible and act wisely, even in the face of anxiety.

. . . In contrast, undifferentiated people tend to react emotionally—with submissiveness or defiance—toward other people. They have little autonomous identity; instead they have a tendency toward emotional fusion with others. . . . Asked what they think, they say what they feel; asked what they believe, they echo what they've heard. (p. 121)

(Does the suppression of individual autonomy and the thwarting of cognitive development sound reminiscent of the PAS child and does the concept of a cross-generational coalition/pathological triangle ring true of the characteristic interactional pattern of the PAS family?)

Bowen's description of the processes of triangulation became the foundation for the theories developed by other systems therapists, such as Haley, who incorporated it into his assessment of pathological systems; and by Salvador Minuchin, who assessed triangles to be the source of dysfunctional family organizational patterns.

The Palo Alto group, initially consisting of psychoanalytically trained therapists who subsequently transitioned into systems therapists, was founded by Gregory Bateson, an anthropologist. His pioneering work in 1956 with his colleagues, Donald Jackson, Jay Haley, and John Weakland, was with the schizophrenic population. As a result of exhaustive observations, these therapists connected the development of schizophrenia to dysfunctional family communication patterns, which they labeled the "double-bind." These therapists observed a no-win situation of repetitive conflicting messages and directives conveyed to the patient by the family with one message occurring on an overt level and then contradicted on a covert level either by the same family member or by another member of significance to the patient. This is crazy-making behavior, and the Palo Alto therapists concluded, therefore, that the seat of insanity does not reside within the individual but rather within the family milieu and how the members communicate with each other. In studying the behavioral and communication patterns of the schizophrenic's family, the Palo Alto therapists observed how the family system could not remain without a symptomatic member. That is, these therapists observed that, when the schizophrenic member improved, either another family member became symptomatic or the family system went into upheaval. These therapists thus became acutely aware of how the symptomatic behaviors of the IP served the purpose of maintaining the homeostasis of the family system. An example of this system maintenance is reflected in the following example: The parents engage in a heated argument, and their child then distracts them from their fighting and disunity by developing problematical and symptomatic behaviors. (Obviously, if the child is an "angel," the parents could not be distracted.)

Jay Haley, MA, who had been trained in the psychoanalytic method, is another of the several original founders of family systems therapy. He joined the Palo Alto group in 1953. Like the other psychoanalytically trained therapists, he had independently arrived at the identical conclusion: that the IP's symptoms were a product of a dysfunctional family system which needed the symptom in order to continue and that the patient became symptomatic to protect the family. He therefore cast doubt on the effectiveness of individual approaches to therapy whereby the IP alone is sitting in the therapist's office. Haley (1990) concluded:

> It is always an oversimplification to describe psychiatric symptoms as if they could be isolated from the general problems of society. The ills of the individual are not really separable from the ills of the social context he creates

and inhabits, and one cannot with good conscience pull out the individual from his cultural milieu and label him as sick or well. (p. 2)

Haley further expressed his skepticism about the effectiveness of individual treatment modalities as follows:

> One casual assumption common to many psychotherapists is the idea that change is brought about by increasing the patient's understanding of himself and his difficulties. Different therapists who share this general point of view will emphasize different types of understanding, but basic in psychiatric tradition is the idea that a person changes as he gains more awareness of what he is doing and why. (p. 179)

Haley suggested an alternative approach to treatment, which became the foundation of the school of strategic family systems therapy:

> It will be argued here that a patient's symptoms are perpetuated by the way he himself behaves and by the influence of other people intimately involved with him. It follows that psychotherapeutic tactics should be designed to persuade the individual to change his behavior and/or persuade his intimates to change their behavior in relation to him. (p. 6)

Haley arrived at his assessment as early as 1959 upon observation of the dysfunctional interactional patterns among hospitalized patients with their families. He then determined that the therapist could be committed to the accuracy of symptom diagnosis only after assessing the nature of the family's transactional patterns, and it logically followed, of course, that the family must become the target for intervention.

What was the dysfunctional pattern which Haley (1968, 1977) had identified? He observed the occurrence of a cross-generational coalition, which he called "the perverse triangle" (p. 37). He described it as an act whereby one parent co-opts a child into colluding with her/him to the isolation and disempowerment of the other parent. Haley believed that this coalition led to highly symptomatic and dysfunctional behaviors, to emotional disturbances, and quite frequently to schizophrenia because of the double-bind that was created for the child; that is, the request by a parent for this collusion foreclosed the child to any good options: either she/he must rebuff the other parent or else pay the penalty of losing the love and approval of the co-opting parent for failure to collude. An additional characteristic of this coalition/triangulation is that it operates on a covert level, keeping in the dark the ostracized parent as well as any professional attempting to intervene in the family. Were the seducing parent or the child to be confronted about the existence of their coalition, it would be adamantly denied. (Does the reader join me in seeing resemblances to the PAS family?)

The reader who is a parent must have observed this sequence of events at one time or another in their own nuclear family. I can certainly not profess perfection in having avoided all arguments with my spouse in front of our son, who then attempted to assume the role of referee or that his father or I had thoughtlessly requested his allegiance in a marital dispute. The occasional slip of behavior does not a psychotic child make. It is only when this pattern becomes habitual and rigid and when the child is not reassured–preferably by behaviors and not solely by words–that an occasional dispute does not mean annihilation of the marriage and that his choosing of sides is unwelcome.

Haley also became convinced that the identified patient's symptoms serve to maintain the homeostasis of the family system, which in turn maintains the symptom

through the organizational and behavioral transactions of its subsystems. Symptom reduction is achieved by intervening in the subsystems in order to affect change in the organization around the symptom. Minuchin (1981) describes Haley's systems approach to therapy as follows:

> The strategic school sees the family as a complex system, differentiated into hierarchically arranged subsystems. A dysfunction in one subsystem can be expressed analogically in another; in particular, the organization of family members around the symptom is taken to be an analogical statement of dysfunctional structures. By rearranging the organization around the symptom, the therapist can release isomorphic changes in the entire system. (pp. 65–66)

Strategic systems therapy is therefore concerned with making overt the family's covert interactional patterns. For example, the first spouse might accuse the second spouse of not communicating with her/him. By observing how they communicate with each other, the strategic therapist is in a position to reframe their interaction: the therapist affirms that the first spouse silences the second spouse by interrupting and overtalking the second spouse. Problem resolution, therefore, is achieved by reorganizing the dysfunctional subsystem transactions around the symptom rather than focusing on the symptom itself. Minuchin cites the following case example as illustrative of how this approach would be operationalized:

> To challenge the restrictive ways in which crystallized family systems prescribe a view of reality to the family members, Haley and Madanes suggest that the patients pretend that the world is different. A depressed husband is to pretend he feels depressed. His wife is to judge whether he is pretending. The control that the husband has kept over the wife, by not improving while remaining in a powerless position, is

changed to a game in which the spouses play different power arrangements. (p. 66)

In one of my cases of family home-based crisis intervention, I was working with a single father of four children, all of whom had been diagnosed with varying mental health issues. CPS was involved due to school refusal, and the children were labeled as generally unmanageable. The family lived in the home of the father's parents, which the father loathed because it compromised his sense of autonomy and because his mother frequently reminded him of his dependency on her. She criticized his parenting, and he had introjected her perceptions of himself. He resented her intrusions and control, indicating that she was a more competent parent than he.

I first attempted to work with the father's strengths by creating the environment in which his parental effectiveness with his children emerged in the sessions. This did have marginal results of his gaining greater control over his children and being able to motivate them to do their chores. I awakened his prior managerial skills which he effectively utilized on a job so that he could apply this expertise to his parenting. He nevertheless minimized his progress, and my efforts failed to create second order changes in the family as he credited me and not himself for the successes. His misperception of his competency was also unaltered. I felt myself becoming vulnerable to being sucked into the family's helplessness and hopelessness. I decided on a strategic intervention: I expressed to the father that I was impressed with his protectiveness of and loyalty to his mother. He looked at me with disheartening incredulity, and he inquired as to how I had reached this conclusion. (A conscious concern for his mother's feelings was no where on his long to-do list.) I conveyed that I had reached this interpretation because of his

repudiation of his expertise and competencies with his children in order that he can appear weaker and less effective in comparison to his mother. By doing so, she could then feel exonerated from her feelings of failure with her own children. I expressed that he was in a double-bind situation: being competent with his children meant disloyalty to his mother, but remaining loyal to his mother required him to be an incompetent parent. This remark was balanced perfectly between being ego-syntonic and ego-dystonic. The father expressed to me that I had hit the nail on the head in that his mother had previously acknowledged to him that she had failed with her children and was hoping for a do-over with her grandchildren. As I expected, my comment provided all the motivation the father needed to reorganize around the symptom. When I arrived a week later for the next home visit, all the children had since been attending school, and they were cooperative with their chores. More importantly, the father expressed that he felt confident that he would be able to deal with his children. When I asked him how he had managed to accomplish all this, his response was, "Easy, I just did." He maintained this progress for a significant enough time for his case to be closed. Being insightful, he had nevertheless seen through my intervention, and, when we summed up the family's progress during the termination process, he conveyed to me that he had recognized my "transparent" comment for what it was. But he nevertheless was jolted to the point of arousing his motivation to change.

Although rejecting the effectiveness of insight-oriented therapy, Haley (1963) nonetheless placed great therapeutic value in redefining the family's formulation of their presenting problem from an intrapsychic issue to a systemic one. He developed a technique called "reframing" (p. 139), which became an essential element of strategic therapy. As examples: a teen who is labeled a liar is reframed as someone who is preparing to become a fiction novelist or a poet. A nagging wife is reframed to mean she is attempting to connect with her disengaged husband. Combativeness between a couple is reframed as "foreplay." A boy who steals money from his mother acquires a special status when the therapist reframes his behavior by thanking him for bringing his parents in for therapy. The problem for which the boy intuitively knows his parents need help: their conflict in which his mother is furious with his father because he "steals" money from her food budget to support his gambling habit! (The boy's symptom is symbolic of the parental issue.) A girl who is presented as defiant is reframed as "loyal" to her parents because she distracts them from their conflicts so as to avoid a divorce. A girl's school phobia is reframed as "mom's helper" when she stays home to comfort her mother who is lonely and sad because her husband ignores her.

The technique of reframing was so effective that it was subsequently "borrowed" by several other schools of family systems therapy, including by Minuchin, who adapted it as an essential intervention in structural family therapy.

Haley (1973) is also credited for perfecting the art of paradoxical intervention, and in this treatment modality he capitalized on the oppositional nature of our species. The readers who have observed the temper tantrums and defiance of a two-year-old or can remember their own terrible twos is aware that contrariness emerges as soon as we discover a degree of autonomy and power. The paradoxical therapeutic maneuver is similar to "aligning with the resistance" in psychoanalytic treatment in that the therapist gives a directive to the family for them to exaggerate the symptomatic behavior in the hope that the members will unite to rebel against the therapist. It was as a result of observing closed family systems, which have highly rigid interactional patterns and organizations that inspired Haley to develop this intervention. When employing a paradoxical intervention, the family members are not given directives to cease their dysfunctional behaviors. Instead, they are directed to do more of it. The therapeutic "catch" or actual manipulation occurs because the family must either sacrifice autonomy by submitting to the authority of the therapist's directive to continue the behavioral dysfunction; or else they retain autonomy but only by relinquishing the symptom! The brilliance of this intervention is that, either way, the therapist wins. The goal of this therapy is to mitigate the symptom through behavioral changes rather than to rely on insight for symptom reduction.

An example of this therapeutic intervention occurred in one of my cases of a family who was overwhelmed by situationally maintained depression due to the contagion of negativity that was passed around like a baton among the members. This family, consisting of two parents and four children, were continually criticizing each other and finding nothing positive about anything that any of the members did. They overlooked their many strengths as a family unit, as subsystems, and as individual members. Even upon my exploring with them how they support each other and extend themselves for each other, they managed to discover negativity in every action and interaction. They were "presumably" seeking direction on how to eliminate their focus on their negativity. I was the fifth therapist from whom they sought help, and each of my predecessors had adopted the approach of guiding, cajoling, reasoning, directing, and pleading with them into a more positive outlook. Each predecessor failed. Halfway through the first session, I concluded that focusing on their positives would be more of the same. As Einstein had observed, the definition of insanity is to keep doing the same thing time and again and expecting a different outcome. So at the end of the first session, I informed them I was prepared to give a directive as they had requested. They expected to hear a recommendation that incorporated a positive focus, just as they had heard four times previously. Instead, I explained that I believed that their problem was that they were not negative enough! They all looked at me incredulously, and, in all seriousness, I nonetheless directed them to go home and attempt to double the efforts at discovering negativity in each other and in themselves. When the family returned for the second session, I was not at all surprised to learn that they had united to defy me and failed at doubling their negativity. In their efforts to defend against me by "submitting" and thereby doubling their negativity, they reversed their habitual transactions to such an extreme that–in spite of themselves–they focused on the positives in each other. I feigned disappointment, and I expressed caution that they might not be able to maintain this behavioral reversal. In spite of the therapist's expressed reservation, they continued to fight against being too negative, and they were very shortly engaging in various subgroup transactions, doing a variety of activities and interests.

A word of caution is in order about paradoxical intervention. It is generally accepted among systems therapists that such an intervention be reserved as the last resort when all else fails. It is employed with highly rigid families who are a virtual closed system. And it surely would not be used in certain situations, such as when the IP's symptom is that of suicidal ideation or because the family is mourning over a significant loss or is a result of a crisis situation.

Virginia Satir, MA, author of many books on family therapy and who also practiced at one time as an experiential therapist, began treating the entire family as early as the 1950s. She initially worked in private practice but subsequently joined the group of family systems therapists in Palo Alto, California. She, too, reached the conclusion after having observed her patient's interactions with the family that the cause of psychological distress resided in the family system—namely in their dysfunctional patterns of communication. She brought a warmth and a positive outlook to her family sessions, and this enabled the family members to connect with each other through their strengths, optimism, and support for each other. Mike Nichols (2004) aptly sums up her orientation when he declared:

> Satir saw troubled family members as trapped in narrow family roles, like victim, placator, defiant one, or rescuer that constrained relationships and sapped self-esteem. Her concern with identifying such life constricting roles and freeing family members from their grip was consistent with her major focus, which was always on the individual. (p. 31)

Does Satir's conception of family roles seem strikingly familiar to the roles in the family with an alienation?

Don Jackson, M.D., (1971) was another early convert to family systems therapy. He, too, relinquished his psychoanalytic orientation in adopting a systems approach to pathology as the preferred treatment modality. He assessed that symptom formation was a function of a person's situation and interactions with her/his significant others. He expressed his novel approach to treatment as follows, "In brief, we are much more concerned with influence, interaction and interrelations between people, immediately observable in the present, than with individual internal, imaginary, and infantile matters" (p. 17). Jackson adopted this orientation after experiencing the family and the patient in interaction with each other, thereby observing how symptom formation was a function of the dynamics of the family's dysfunctional interactional patterns. Minuchin (1993) described Jackson's conversion to a systems approach in the following words, "He argued persuasively that the individual was an artificial construct 'produced' by the simple process of ignoring his or her connections to the members of significant social networks" (p. 28). Jackson (1971) is credited with being the first to identify the family system's pull towards homeostasis, which he defined to include the concept of resistance to change as well as its support of stability and predictability. Jackson's significant contribution to the family therapy movement was his critical insight that the symptom of the IP preserved the homeostasis of the system (pp. 16, 28–29). I shall return to this concept when I discuss the child's function in the family system with an alienation.

The Milan School of systemic family therapy has been comprised of many therapists including Luigi Boscolo, Gianfranco Cecchin, Lynn Hoffman, Peggy Papp, and Mara Selvini Palazzoli, who began to practice as strategic family therapists beginning in 1967. Although influenced by the Palo Alto group, they operationalized strategic family therapy very differently by using a team approach. The Milan team had to make a practical adaptation to the delivery of treatment in that the location of their facility was inconvenient for their patient families to attend on a continuing basis. The team therefore adapted the strategic treatment modality by offering intensive daylong therapy, at the end of which time the family was sent home with a directive intended to produce a reorganization around the symptom. The family would return for follow-up in approximately a month or later. As with all the systems therapists, the Milan team approached the symptom with the conviction that it was a function of the family's interactional patterns, and they made this assessment overt to the family members, who nonetheless had arrived with the belief that the symptom resided within a particular family member. These systems therapists, Boscolo, Cecchin, Hoffman, Penn (1987) described their response to the family's definition of the presenting problem as follows, "The Milan team will accept it as a label like any other and convert it into interactional process, or descriptions of behavior. They are particularly alert for indications that the family understands that a person's illness is a way of behaving with others" (p. 186). The Milan team (1987) agreed with the Palo Alto group that symptoms result from the double-bind, upon which they based their intervention, which they labeled "the counterparadox" (pp. 6–7). The team's creative and unique approach was to make overt the family's repetitive, crazy-making, game-playing mixed messages. They expected that the exposure, subsequent reframing, and therapeutic directive would have a palliative effect. The reframing which the Milan team developed was to portray the symptom as having a protective and positive connotation. For example, little Johnny's misbehavior was a form of entertainment for his lonely and depressed mother, who was emotionally abandoned by her husband. Rationales were given as to why the behaviors should continue, again with the expectation that the family would unite against the therapists to relinquish the symptom.

Maurizio Andolfi, M.D., Claudio Angelo M.D., and Marcella De Nichilo, Ph.D., are second generational family therapists who developed interventions which are specifically attuned to very rigid and disturbed family systems. They uniquely combined the therapeutic approaches from the various schools of systemic family therapy, including strategic, paradoxical, experiential, and structural. Andolfi et al. (1983) accepted families for therapy whom Whitaker referred to as the "whales" of families–families who are so inflexible and troubled that they purge out one "Jonah therapist" after another in their efforts at resisting change. Such families are those who have, for example, a schizophrenic, suicidal, or anorectic member. These family therapists are particularly concerned about the deleterious effects of the triangle, which they also maintain produces highly dysfunctional family functioning and severe pathology in the children. In their book, *The Myth of Atlas: Families and the Therapeutic Story,* Andolfi, Angelo, and De Nichilo (1989) state, "As with any other relational triangle, coalitions are possible, more or less masked, that produce dysfunctional relationships" (p. 214). The authors expressed their particular concerns about these coalitions when they stated, "We are interested in exploring a particular theme: the resolution of conflict in triadic relationships and the influence that this conflict may have on the process of personal individuation" (p. 24). Like the systems therapists before them, these therapists asserted that the co-opting of the child in a cross-generational coalition portends serious detrimental effects to the child by circumscribing autonomy and inhibiting the individuation process. Andolfi et al. (1983) described the damage from triangulation as follows:

> This causes the progressive alienation of the individual most involved, with concomitant damage to *his* self and to his personal space. When this process tends to become irreversible, rigid, and undifferentiated, a pathological situation results. . . . In these cases each one becomes a creator and victim of the same "functional trap." The absence of clear interpersonal boundaries which results from this type of relationship is translated into the impossibility of either freely entering an intimate relationship or breaking away. Constantly

maintaining a safe distance and, contrariwise, entering into a fused relationship are the behaviors most common to these systems, where personal space is confounded with interactive space, the individual with the function he serves, *being for oneself* with *being as a function of the other.* The only possibility for coexistence may then become the intrusion into the personal space of others, accompanied by the loss of one's own personal space. (pp. 7–8)

To wit, the child loses all sense of self–emotionally, cognitively, mentally, spiritually, and even physically, as personal space and identity are violated. (Does this not sound all too evocative of the PAS child in coalition with the alienating parent?)

Lynn Hoffman (1981) also addresses the detrimental effects on the subordinate party (generally the child) in a triangle when she asserts what all children have a right to expect from their family: namely that it is the responsibility of the family to facilitate the child's developmental imperative for age-appropriate autonomy and the eventual separation from the family of origin. In families with dysfunctional triangles, however, the child is too emotionally handicapped for this to be achieved. Hoffman summarizes the cues which indicate the presence of psychotic or psychoneurotic symptoms as being:

1. a high degree of family connectedness
2. covert coalitions which cross generation lines
3. closeness and distance between family members determined by rules for congruence of coalitions
4. third parties interfering with or deflecting conflict or closeness between pairs
5. relationships with a high intensity factor. (pp. 136–137)

Nathan Ackerman was a child psychiatrist; was mentor to my mentor, Salvador Minuchin; was another very early founder of the family therapy movement; and had independently arrived at the conclusion that it was essential to include the entire family in the treatment. He practiced in the 1930s initially employing a psychoanalytic model but determining as early as the 1940s that the family system must be the target for intervention. He affirmed that it was futile to treat the individual in isolation from the family because doing so discounted the family's organizational and interactional influences on the IP. He did not forsake his psychoanalytic roots as he was equally concerned with the intrapsychic processes of the internal world as he was with the processes of the interrelational external world. He was equally concerned with the effects of the internal conflicts among the id, ego, and super-ego as he was with the effects of unresolved conflicts among family members. He was equally concerned with the individual's repressed feelings, thoughts, and aspirations as he was with the family's secret world, with its denial and evasive maneuvers as well as hopes and goals for its members. In combining his commitment to these two seemingly irreconcilable forms of therapy, Ackerman recognized that families frequently function by denying and avoiding disagreements and problems just as the psyche employs the defense mechanisms of denial and repression to avoid acknowledging conflict and unwelcome material. According to Ackerman, symptom resolution could be achieved by uncovering the family's submerged conflicts so that remedies can be decided upon and implemented. Ackerman exposed as overt what the family had made covert, such as how it organized into coalitions. By observing the family's interactions, which revealed how particular members joined with other members as various times and under varying circumstances in opposition to yet other members, Ackerman became alert to the reoccurrence of dysfunctional coalitions in

families with a sick member. And he determined that cross-generational alliances were generally dysfunctional, particularly to the detriment of the younger generation.

A hallmark of Ackerman's therapeutic style was how he used himself to join with the family in order to effectuate change. Although his psychoanalytic training would suggest that he would have remained detached and unrevealing like John Locke's blank Tabula Rasa screen, Ackerman became convinced that he needed to take risks–through judicious use of self-disclosure–if he expected the family to do likewise. He therefore revealed to the family his thoughts and emotional responses to events unfolding in the session, and this afforded a safe environment for the family members to expose themselves. Ackerman (1961) described the therapist's use of self as follows, "It is very important at the outset to establish a meaningful emotional contact with all members of the family, to create a climate in which one really touches them and they feel they touch back" (p. 242).

The following case exemplifies how Ackerman and Franklin (1965) combined a psychoanalytic assessment of symptomatology with a determination that the symptomatology was embedded in the family system and not within the individual. The patient was an alleged psychotic girl who believed that she lived on another planet called "Queendom," a place inhabited only by women. The family specifics were that of a disengaged father and an enmeshed mother/grandmother dyad with the grandmother ruling the roost similar to a queen mother. Drawing on his psychoanalytic training, which taught him about underlying themes, combined with his understanding of the family's powerful interpersonal influence, Ackerman brilliantly reframed the girl's preposterous fantasy to symbolize the family's preposterous dysfunctional organization.

The organization of the family's subsystems did not recognize any standing for men—as it was in "Queendom." The boundary around the marital/parental subsystem was diffuse, failing to denote them as a couple and as parents, and there was an inappropriately enmeshed subsystem between the mother and the grandmother. The mother/grandmother dyad minimized the father, who tolerated being devalued. The mother was not, in reality, psychologically married to the father as she had, preposterously, not "divorced" her overcontrolling and overinvolved mother. Using systems theory to assessing the girl's emotional state, it can be interpreted that her symptoms served to maintain the homeostasis of the family system as well as her parents' marriage: her illness was the one situation which kept the parents united and in touch with each other and was likely also the one situation in which her mother was distant from the grandmother.

Many second and third generation family therapists concur that how Ackerman used himself as a tool to enable the family to break down emotional barriers and resistances was his most significant contribution to family systems therapy. This creative therapeutic technique was "borrowed" from Ackerman by Minuchin and which Minuchin very effectively incorporated into his therapeutic style, despite being misunderstood by some critics to be cold, distant, and mechanical in his interventions with the family.

I have personally known Salvador Minuchin since 2002, and I was individually supervised by him for a year. I can attest that those who perceive him as cold and detached could not be more mistaken! He is, to the contrary, deeply caring and compassionate, committed to being helpful to his students and to his patient families, empathetic to the difficulties of his patient families, deeply troubled by man's inhumanity to man,

and concerned with the plight of the underprivileged among us. He is all of these qualities; and yes, those who know his work and know him professionally, have also experienced his brilliance, his facility at using humor to induce change, his profound understanding of human relationships and of the human psyche, his willingness to reveal about himself in order to persuade the family to take the risks required of them by the treatment process. Those who are fortunate enough to know him personally can also attest to his deep connection to his own family and to those students and colleagues whose lives he has touched and who have touched him. This is the Sal Minuchin I have come to love.

The systems treatment modality which he developed is identified as structural family therapy, and it is this systems approach with which I fit most comfortably. By no means am I asserting that structural family therapy is superior to any other systems approach. This modality simply is the best fit for me given my temperament, my abilities, and my learning curve. Any family systems therapist who is committed to their particular school of family systems therapy would be equally successful in treating the PAS family.

Because structural family therapy is the treatment modality with which I am most familiar, most comfortable, and have most utilized, I will be elaborating more about it than I had about the other systems modalities. I will begin by summarizing its main features, and I will provide case examples from my practice to illustrate how this treatment approach is operationalized. The PAS family will be represented in many of the illustrated cases. Finally, I will discuss why I advocate for using a family systems approach to treatment of the PAS family.

Minuchin (1974) contributed appreciably to family systems therapy by delineating the framework or structure into which the family organizes itself and which thereby provides an understanding or "map" (pp. 89–109) of the interactions of its members. According to Minuchin (1974, 1981), this structure is defined by the family's boundaries (pp. 53–56, 146–160)–the external boundary creating a parameter around the family as a whole, thereby separating it from the outside world, and internal boundaries occurring around its various subsystems. Healthy family functioning occurs as a response to the appropriate marking of boundaries: boundaries the nature of which are clear rather than blurred so the members are not confused about their position in the family hierarchy; permeable enough to allow for the appropriate exiting and entering of different family members and of outsiders under specific circumstances and at certain times in the family's life cycle; balanced between firmness and diffuseness so that interactions between the generations and between peers meet the needs of the individual members while simultaneously setting appropriate limits on and expectations for its members; balanced between being permeable and contained so that the family can appropriately regulate distance/disengagement and closeness/enmeshment; flexible enough to adapt to evolving circumstances, which are due either to normal family and individual developments or due to unexpected crises and trauma. Boundary marking establishes the inclusion/exclusion of various individuals within the nuclear family and from the outside world; that is, establishing appropriate internal membership of the various subgroups, such as the marital/parental; parent and child; and sibling. But each individual may have membership in several subgroups at different times when additional groupings are considered, such as gender, age, common interests, shared activities, relationships outside the nuclear family, and so on. Boundary marking determines what coali-

tions exist at various times and under what differing circumstances. For example, will the second parent support or undermine the first parent in the discipline of their children? If the second parent disagrees with the first parent's method of discipline, how will this be discussed, in front of the children or in the privacy of the marital bedroom? How does the marital couple protect themselves from unwarranted intrusions by the children and by other family members? Is each parent attentive not to hire a child as an ally in a marital dispute? How much influence from the families of origin is exerted on and tolerated by the nuclear family's functioning? Do the grandparents usurp or support the parents' authority with the children? What is the appropriate balance among "I" time, "we" time and "family" time for the particular idiosyncratic family? At different times in the family's developmental life cycle, each subgroup will alter the levels of enmeshment (closeness) and disengagement (distancing) depending upon the needs of the individual members at a specific phase and due to the family's developmental stage at the time. For example, when children are newborn and very young, the mother is likely to be extremely close with them–but hopefully not to the exclusion of the father, for whom she must make time if the family is to continue functioning in a healthy manner. The arrival of the first child requires a restructuring of family relationships as the couple transitions to a family–just as they learned to accommodate to and compromise with each other when they had transitioned from two autonomous "I's" to a "We." And now that my husband and I have become senior citizens, for example, we will need to plan with our son for the possible development in which the caretaking role will need to be reversed. Appropriate boundary formation allows for the execution of the family's tasks, which assures its survival and that of its individual members. These tasks would include, but are not limited to, the enactment of individual member's role performance; provision for mutual support and nurturing between the parents and the parents for the children; encouragement of timely separation/individuation of the minor members; the socialization and acculturation of the children; adaptation to changing circumstances and to unexpected crises; all the tasks required for the survival and maintenance of the family.

Each new transitional stage will initially create a temporary disturbance in the family's homeostasis as it adapts to the requirements of the next stage in the family's life cycle and hence to a higher level of family homeostasis. For example, as the child progresses through her/his individual developmental stages, the parents must encourage age-appropriate separation in preparation for the first day of kindergarten, which could otherwise create separation anxiety–for the parent, that is, as child separation anxiety exists only in response to the parent's conscious or unconscious request for the child's company. That is to say, the child's school refusal is a homeostasis maintaining behavior because it fills the emotional vacuum between the parents and thereby stabilizes the marriage. Adapting to the stage of adolescence requires that the parents surrender some of their authority to the teen by taking into consideration the teen's opinions and feelings before making final decisions. And once again a reorganization must occur in order to accommodate this next developmental stage. And so on, with each successive developmental stage, the homeostasis is initially disturbed and then regroups at a higher level of organization.

When a crisis, such as the loss of income, the death of a significant person, or divorce occurs during a stable phase, it is disruptive enough. But when it hits the family in the midst of one of its transitional stages, it is a double-whammy, and it has the potential to prolong the attainment of a new homeostasis.

A family's organization is dysfunctional when it fails to adapt to changing internal and external circumstances; is unable to promote and sustain the developmental needs of its members, particularly those of the children; becomes stuck in a developmental stage which has outlived its usefulness; when individual family members acquire inappropriate membership in a subgroup; when subgroups and/or individual members of subgroups form coalitions that are inappropriately enmeshed and support the disengagement, disparagement, and disempowerment of another member.

Given that Minuchin assessed individual family members are continually interactive with each other and affecting each other, it should come of no surprise to the reader that he, like the other systems therapists, came to reject confidence in psychoanalytic theory, which postulated that insight produces change. He maintained, to the contrary, that it is the experience of interactions among family members in the here and now–as opposed to the recall of memories about the there and then–that is principally how people change. Structural family therapy affirms that it is behavioral change which influences thoughts, perceptions, and feelings and not the reverse. In his rejection of the psychoanalytic method and of its conventionally accepted belief about the effectiveness of insight to ameliorate pathology, Minuchin (1993) pokes fun of its unsubstantiated philosophical underpinnings when he declared:

> We had been trained to look for a set of invisible internal dynamics regulating the visible behavior of individuals. We were certain that if we were curious, careful, skillful, and patient, sooner or later the patient would provide us with an Ariadne's thread to lead us through

the labyrinths of the mind. . . . We were deep-sea divers searching for motivation inside people, helping our patients to "own" their behavior and to see how they were the builders of their lives. (pp. 28–29)

The illogic of extracting the individual from her/his environment to perform treatment is expressed by Minuchin (1974) in the following comments:

> The resulting treatment techniques focused exclusively on the individual, apart from his surroundings. An artificial "boundary" was drawn between the individual and his social context. . . . As the patient was treated in isolation, the data encountered were inevitably restricted to the way he alone felt and thought about what was happening to him; such individualized material in turn reinforce the approach to the individual apart from his context and provide little possibility for corrective feedback. (pp. 2–3)

Minuchin is commenting here on two failures of individual treatment: that patient self-reporting is unreliable and that venting in isolation from one's relationships offers no possibility for change.

In disavowing the effectiveness of psychoanalytic therapy with its emphasis on interpretation of repressed material about the there and then and of other individually oriented therapies, Minuchin instead maintains that change results from current transactions between the individual and their intimate relationships, arguing that there is a reciprocity in intimate relationships. We are certainly familiar with this concept reflected in the familiar axiom, "every action has a reaction," and vice versa, of course. Minuchin (1974) asserts that there is no such thing as independent, isolated behaviors when one lives intimately with others. Because of the powerful effect which we have on our intimate relationships and which they have on

us, it follows that each family member has the potential to change the others, just as the others have the equivalent potential in return. People living in intimate relationships have leverage to motivate each other. A stranger, even in the person of an expert, does not have this leverage. Structural family therapy is committed to the tenet that we are likely willing to change for someone whom we love and for who loves us (pp. 2–9). Minuchin (1981) contrasts his belief about how change occurs with the individual conception about this:

> An individual therapist tells the patient, "Change yourself, work with yourself, so you will grow." The family therapist makes a statement of a different order. Family members can change only if there is a change in the context within which they live. The family therapist's message is, therefore, "Help the other person to change, which will change yourself as you relate to him and will change both of you." (p. 71)

This conception of how change occurs–that family members co-create each other–is Minuchin's most valuable contribution to family systems therapy, among his many notable contributions. Minuchin (1974) superbly illustrates this concept with the following metaphor:

> A therapist oriented to individual therapy still tends to see the individual as the site of pathology and together only the data can be obtained from or about the individual. . . . A therapist working within this framework can be compared to a technician using a magnifying glass. The details of the field are clear, but the field is severely circumscribed. A therapist working within the framework of structural family therapy, however, can be compared to a technician with the zoom lens. He can zoom in for a close-up whenever he wishes to study the intrapsychic field, but he can also observe with a broader focus. (p. 3)

I used this analogy with an alienated father of children discussed in this book and with whom I had been working together with his children to repair their strained relationship. The children's mother had refused to participate in co-parent counseling. The father called to request a session with his sister, who had remained in communication with his former wife even though he and his former wife were unable to pass a civil word with each other. They communicated only via e-mail and only regarding his pick-up time for his visits with their children—when she would permit the visits. She rarely allowed him extra time with the children, unless it met her needs, even though she accorded this "privilege" to the paternal aunt, who had no children and who had always loved her brother's children as if they were her own. The father felt understandably betrayed by his sister because of her ongoing relationship with his former wife, and he hoped to enlist my help in getting her to forsake that relationship. I expressed to him in the session with his sister that I fully understood his feelings—when looking through the lens of a magnifying glass. But, looking through a zoom lens, I envisaged the larger picture—that perhaps his sister had the leverage with his former wife and that perhaps this leverage could be turned to his advantage. His sister welcomed the opportunity of accepting this mission, and she was eventually able to persuade her former sister-in-law to participate in co-parenting counseling.

Minuchin (1974) elaborates upon his concept regarding the processes of change, which he characterized by three axioms. He states the first axiom to be:

> The individual influences his context and is influenced by it in constantly recurring sequences of interaction. The individual who lives within a family is a member of the social system to which he must adapt. His actions are governed by the characteristics of the system, and these characteristics include the effects of his own past actions. The individual responds to stresses in other parts of the system, to which he adapts; and he may contribute significantly to stressing of the members of the system. (p. 9)

The second axiom, according to Minuchin asserts that changes in family structure contribute to changes in the behavior and intrapsychic processes of the members of that system. The third axiom affirms that the therapist's entrance into the family system also impacts how the system will respond to and interact with each other in order to produce change (p. 9). Because family members have co-created each other, there is no assignment of individual blame or pathology, thereby averting the detrimental attacks on one's self-esteem that results from such negative connotations. Family members are not only responsible for each other but are also accountable to each other for how each behaves. This interactional cycle of behaviors is therefore inconsistent with the idea of linear causation and is more accurately viewed as a chicken or egg condition. Minuchin (1981) describes this fault-free condition as follows: "The concept of causality loses its rough edges of blame in a conceptualization that posits the indivisibility of context and behavior. Both the assignment of responsibility and the consequent allocation of blame recede into the background of a more complex design (p. 197)."

A systems definition of the problem should create grist for thought for the therapist who treats the alienated child using an individual treatment modality. When a child is thrown into the therapy chair while the parents remain aloof from the treatment, the child receives the message that she/he is the problem rather than the parents. This appears to me to be much like the rape victim being blamed for the rape attack. Because alienated children suffer from poor self-esteem due to the exploitation by their alienating parent, because their maltreatment of their alienated parent likely makes them doubt their decency and goodness, and because they have no good options out of the triangulation, how will their self-esteem be improved when they are labeled as disturbed and helpless?

To the contrary, a structural family therapist does not label someone as "passive-aggressive," for example, in response to a spouse's complaint about her/his partner who continually "forgets" to keep promises that were made. Instead, the therapist would seek an interactional definition of the presenting problem by exploring, in the presence of the spouse, how the complaining spouse had participated in allowing her/his spouse to act irresponsibly. Such an exploration might reveal that transgressions are repeatedly overlooked by the complaining spouse because, for example, "It is not worth the fight" or because the complaining spouse is conflict adverse or because the complaining spouse may be neglectful of her/his spouse, and so forth. The complaining spouse would be guided by the structural therapist to recognize her/his role in co-creating her/his partner.

Another very typical example of the co-creation among family members occurs daily in the office of every therapist who deals with children: the "impossible child" arrives with her parents, and one of the parents announces, "She's spoiled. She's oppositional defiant. She does what she wants." Let us imagine, hypothetically, that the family entered the office of an individual therapist, who will assume responsibility for changing the girl's behavior while she and the girl are secluded away in the therapy room, during which time the parents are sequestered in the waiting room. (Are not these the object

relations whom, as an adult, the patient will be referencing in a therapist's office as a there and then memory to be subjectively recalled and interpreted? It seems so much more revealing and effective to have a here and now experience with the object relations so that the interactions can be objectively observed and assessed by the therapist.) But let us return to this individual therapist and her patient, the "impossible" child. The therapist will accompany the girl to her office and initiate a regimen of play therapy in order to join with her. (Somehow I always thought that it was the parents' job to engage in "play therapy" with their child.) The therapist will suggest that the girl select a game, and let us hypothetically pretend that she selects Monopoly. They begin to play, and soon the therapist helps the child decide if she should buy Park Place; and later the girl will be helped to decide if she should buy a hotel, and so on. The therapist will look for an opportunity during the game that will enable her to discuss the girl's misbehavior. Then alas, the opportunity arises when the girl lands in jail! Finally, the therapist can begin a discussion of consequences for misbehavior. But the therapist must continue to devote additional time to the joining process because a therapist—who is a stranger—does not have leverage with the patient. Weekly play therapy could therefore continue for several months before the joining process is substantial enough, and during this time there is likely to be no mitigation of the presenting problem. But, alas, joining has climaxed with the girl, and the individual therapist will focus intensely on her misbehavior and attempt to help her develop internal controls. Perhaps the therapist will be lucky, and the child becomes cooperative—with her. But how does this ameliorate the parent/child relationship? I know of no research or evidence-based practice that verifies that the therapist's ability to control the child is transferable to the parents. In fact, it is improbable that the child's behavior will improve with her parents unless they gained the knowledge to do with her what the therapist performed. But obtaining such knowledge is unlikely because, remember, the girl's object relations have been sequestered in the waiting room, and due to confidentiality requirements of the HIPAA law, the therapist is unable to discuss the girl's progress with her object relations without her permission. (What does this do to healthy family hierarchy and to the parents' authority resulting from the requirement to obtain the girl's permission for the therapist to talk with her parents? I will NEVER understand this one!)

Now let us perform a "take two" on this case. The family instead enters the office of a structural family therapist, who will define and address the symptom very differently. In response to the parents' definition of the presenting problem that the girl is spoiled and oppositional, this therapist asks the parents the following questions, "Who spoiled her?" "How did two intelligent, otherwise very competent adults in other roles in their lives, relinquish their power to a child?" The structural family therapist is thus making the symptom interactional rather than intrapsychic and will therefore view the family system as the unit for intervention. The structural therapist encourages the parents to discuss together how to answer her questions. While observing their interaction or "enactment" (pp. 78–97) as Minuchin (1981) labeled the family's transactions, the therapist will ascertain what is occurring in the executive/parental subsystem that has been preventing the parents from accomplishing a relatively simple parental task. The structural therapist will be assessing the enactment to determine whether the parents are contradicting and undermining each other's authority regarding discipline. Does mom, for example, become a mother lioness to protect

her young because she perceives dad to be too punitive? Does dad become the 800-pound gorilla because he perceives mom to be too permissive? If dad is the sheriff, is mom the co-sheriff or is she the attorney for the defense? Are they detouring unresolved marital conflicts through their parental roles? Is guilt contaminating the discipline process because, for example, the child was sickly when born? Or perhaps, are the parents reacting in the extreme reverse to their respective overly-punitive childhoods? In the latest development in structural family therapy, Minuchin (2007) has deemed it relevant to the therapy to determine which lens from the family of origin history is being used by each parent to view the current world (pp. 9–12).

After observing the parents' enactment, the structural family therapist will make a tentative hypothesis about how the family's interactional patterns are maintaining the child's symptoms. When these covert processes are made overt by the therapist, the family gains the awareness about their unconscious interactional patterns, and they are held accountable by the therapist to implement the necessary structural reorganizational changes so that the symptom can be relinquished. The therapist conveys to the family in the first session what she/he has discovered about how their interactional patterns are maintaining the girl's symptoms, and she then encourages the parents to begin a discussion in the session about how to implement the necessary behavioral changes that will alleviate the symptom. The family is sent home after the first session with the message that the therapy must continue at home by implementing the changes which they had decided upon in the session.

I am hopeful that the above case discussion sufficiently illustrated how a systemic and an individual therapist would differently approach the same presenting problem with the former therapist placing the site of pathology within the family's interactional patterns while the latter places the site of pathology within the individual's psyche. This distinction in assessment clearly has opposing treatment implications.

Minuchin (1981) labeled the reciprocity of behaviors among the family members as "complementarity" (pp. 191–206). It signifies, for example, that one spouse is overfunctioning because the other spouse is underfunctioning and so the reverse; that a mother is inappropriately micromanaging a teenager, but the teenager is inviting the surveillance by acting irresponsibly which provides "employment" for the mother as a mother because her husband has underemployed her as a wife; that one parent is disengaged enabling the other to be enmeshed and so the reverse. This is interpreted to mean that when one partner expresses material about the other partner, she/he is also revealing material about herself/himself; when parents describe an issue with a child, they are also revealing an issue about themselves as a couple. (So, be careful, reader, to whom you reveal about your spouse and your children!)

The following is an example from one of my cases that is illustrative of complementarity as defined by Minuchin.

A man contacted me for help with his severe depression. After talking to him about it, I suggested that he come in with his wife as she would surely be involved in his treatment for a medical condition of equal severity. The man agreed to do so, but when he arrived, he was alone. The following dialogue transpired between us:

Gottlieb: I expected that you would arrive with your wife as we had agreed. What happened?

Man: Well, you see, it is really all about me.

Gottlieb: Okay, you tell me all about you, and I will tell you all about your wife.

Man: (Looking at me like I had three heads.) I am just so depressed that I often cannot get out of bed in the morning, and I'm not functioning at home or with our baby or at work.

Gottlieb: Yes, I understand. And I assume that your wife is a high energy person who tends to overfunction, must always keep busy, initiates doing things that do not necessarily need to be done, and, I suspect, does things before you would even have the chance.

Man: (Surprised at my understanding of his wife, whom I had never met. He nods in the affirmative in response to my comments.) It's just that I do everything wrong. I'm always messing up; and sometimes I feel like my wife has two children not one.

Gottlieb: Yes, I see. I guess your wife is quite comfortable slipping into the role of an omniscient mother who is always right, can't tolerate disagreement, and has a hard time hearing your point of view.

Man: (Completely incredulous at my knowledge of his wife, and again nodding in agreement.) But you see, it's my anxiety, as well, which keeps me from doing my share of the parenting and household responsibilities. I become panicky at the thought of having to do something.

Gottlieb: I suspect that your wife is not very good at asking for help; that she likes things done her way, and that she might even prefer to do things herself so that things turn out exactly as she desires, even though she complains about your inertia. I'll bet also that she fails to give you credit and show appreciation when you do pitch in to help.

Man: (Looking astonished.) Yes, that's exactly it. But my wife says that she is really doing much more than she should.

Gottlieb: I agree completely. I think that you and your wife have a terrible vicious cycle going. And I am also sure she's incredibly angry at you for all the work that you arrange for her. How does she kick you in response?

Man: I see what you mean! My wife will be at the next session.

This tongue-in-cheek redefinition (or reframing) of the man's professed intrapsychic depression to a description of a problem which is being maintained by the marital relationship is not an easy task to achieve. But it is nonetheless the necessary initial step in the structural family therapy. Minuchin (1981) describes the therapist's tasks in reframing the family's definition of the presenting problem from that of residing within an individual to that of a systemic definition of their complementarity:

To facilitate this different way of knowing, the therapist must challenge the family members' accustomed epistemology in three respects. First, the therapist challenges the problem–the family's certainty that there is one identified patient. Second, the therapist challenges the linear notion that one family member is controlling the system, rather than each member serving as a context of the other. Third, the therapist challenges the family's punctuation of events, introducing an expanded time frame which teaches family members to see their behavior as part of a larger whole. (p. 194)

In other words, when a family enters the therapist's office, they generally come prepared with a story that one member is the sick one or has the problem or is the one labeled as the identified patient. They do not recognize their transactional patterns, which operate on an unconscious level. They do not arrive announcing, "We are here because we have a dysfunctional cross-generational alliance in the family between my wife and our son." They convey instead a "myth" about themselves which describes an individual conception of the problem, and this conception reflects the family's obliviousness to how their transactional patterns maintain the problem for which they are seeking help. The myth supports the maintenance of the IP's symptoms, which in turn supports the homeostasis of the family. This is why Minuchin articulates, "The family is wrong" (p. 67). The structural therapist recognizes that the family's dance requires multiple participants, for example, a leader and a follower; the giver and the taker; a sender and a receiver; a firecracker, a sluggard, and a distracter; an antagonist, a pacifist, and a referee. The family's choreographed dance reflects the contributions from every member.

Because the family arrives with a story that is circumscribed and narrow, misses the larger explanation, and is preventing problem resolution, structural family therapy commences with a battle: a battle between the family's myth about itself and the therapist's reframe of the family's problem. This reframe will shift from an individual, intrapsychic, pathological description of the problem to that of a systemic difficulty in which each family member plays a role. The therapist creates confusion and challenge for the family. According to Minuchin, "The goal is always the conversion of the family to a different worldview—one that does not need the symptom—and to a more flexible, pluralistic view of reality—one that allows for diversity within a more complex symbolic universe" (p. 215). Enabling the shift from an individual perspective to a systemic conception—the "reframing" (pp. 73–77) technique is not effortless but is nevertheless essential to accomplish in the first session, which establishes the nature of the therapy.

By the time the family seeks help, they have likely struggled with failed repetitive attempts to rectify the situation, but the attempts are generally more of the same. For example, if mother has been the primary disciplinarian, she will increase her disciplinary efforts with the impossible child. It does not dawn upon the family that perhaps the disengaged father should become responsible for the discipline. Minuchin describes the family's failed, frustrating attempts at change as follows, "The solutions the family has tried are stereotyped repetitions of ineffective transactions, which can only generate heightened affect without producing change" (p. 67). The structural family therapist does not tackle symptom manipulation head on but rather focuses on the underlying family transactions that maintain it. If the dysfunctional transactions are altered, then the symptom will be relinquished as it no longer has a purpose; it is no longer required by the system for its homeostasis; and the substituted, higher family organization does not maintain it. The therapist uses the initial session to observe the interactions among the family members and thereby assess how each individual member, including the IP, maintains each others' behaviors. The therapist will make overt the family's dysfunctional yet predictable patterns of transaction and encourage the members to establish more satisfying transactional patterns which meet the demands of the family's current developmental stage. Minuchin defines the therapist's role: "The therapist takes the data that the family offers and reorganizes it. The conflictual and stereotyped reality of the family is given a new framing. As the family members experience themselves and one another differently, new possibilities appear" (p. 71).

In order for the reader to appreciate what a structural family therapist accomplishes in the initial therapy, including how to operationalize the art of reframing, I will illustrate using case examples from my practice.

In a family consisting of two parents, a four-year-old girl and a six-year-old boy, the school had referred the boy due to severe depression. The pediatrician had suggested an antidepressant regimen, but the parents wisely declined the remedy and sought therapy instead. The family entered my office and sat down, the parents seating themselves on opposite ends of the semicircle—as far apart as possible from each other—with the children occupying the seats separating them. (How the family seats itself may be indicative of their organization. The way this particular family seated itself might indicate a distancing between the parents, but this assumption must be confirmed by their enactments.) The father was so disengaged that one might easily have assessed him to be either severely depressed himself or mentally retarded. Knowing, however, that he was a professor at an Ivy League college, I quickly ruled out the latter. I was so taken by this "vacant" father, who appeared to be forsaken by his wife, that I intuitively asked him, "When was the last time your wife made you smile?" Overcome with astonishment, the father was unable to respond promptly. The identified patient however summarily bellowed, "Never!" (This comment provides validation for the expression, "out of the mouths of babes!") The parents glared at their son in amazement, and the mother then exclaimed, "I knew that we were the problem. This was coming for a long time. My husband and I should have been in this office a long time ago." The father confirmed what his wife had stated. I then thanked the boy for bringing his parents in for therapy! (I think this must have been my quickest reframe ever.)

It could not be more evident how the identified patient's symptom was symbolic of his father's situational depression, or better yet, symbolic of the depressed marital relationship. Each parent later acknowledged their respective situational depression, being maintained by a disengaged and unfulfilling marital relationship. Had this family been unfortunate to have contacted almost any other Long Island therapist—the overwhelming number of whom practice using an individual treatment modality—this boy surely would have been relegated to an antidepressant regimen, which would have not only allowed for the continued masking of the systemic issues but would have needlessly subjected the boy to potent drugs.

In another family, a single working mother applied for therapy for her preteen daughter, whom she described as "a thief" and "a liar." The mother further expressed concern that the girl was seriously underfunctioning in school, especially in light of her superior intelligence. Having had several unsuccessful individual courses of treatment, the mother was beside herself, was at her wits end with the girl, and had considered sending her to live with her father. During the exploration of the problem in the initial session, I discovered that the girl stole only her mother's money. In all other settings, she was symptom-free—her friends' parents frequently complemented her for her cooperation and politeness; and she did not steal from or lie to any other adults including her father, her stepmother, her teachers, or her friends' parents. After ascertaining this information, I first complemented the mother for teaching her daughter good values and ap-

propriate behavior. The mother appreciated this. I then commented that it appeared to me that the girl's behavior seems to be related to their relationship as it does not happen with anyone else, and the mother had to agree. She accepted my redefinition of the presenting symptom as an interactional behavior—there was not much of an option but to do so. (This is another advantage of family therapy over individual therapy: it is difficult to deny what has unfolded before the therapist's eyes.) With this reframe being accepted by all, the presenting problem shifted from a characterological and intrapsychic description of individual pathology to that of behaviors which are a function of the mother/daughter relationship. But the how and why these behaviors were serving the system were still a mystery to me as well as to the mother and the girl. I asked the mother to talk with her daughter to determine if they could solve the mystery. With the initiation of their enactment, the mother, quite predictably, returned to blaming her daughter for the stealing and lying. Nevertheless, I encouraged them to continue talking, and the system maintenance of the girl's symptoms was soon revealed. As is typical of single parents, this mother was enmeshed with her daughter, who was the mother's only social contact. The mother was from another country, and she had no family or friends locally; she was either working or was on duty as a mother. Lacking peer relationships, she looked to her daughter to be her emotional confidante; she frequently expressed her loneliness and homesickness to her daughter as well as disclosing her disappointments in the girl's father and in the causes for the breakdown of the marriage. At other times, the mother looked to the girl for the consideration and affection she was missing as a woman and time and again asked her daughter to get her a drink, get her a blanket, and to rub her feet. It was further revealed that the mother frequently prevented her daughter from her peer activities, presumably out of overprotectiveness but also out of loneliness whenever her daughter was away. I interrupted their quibbling about the presenting problem as soon as I had ascertained enough information from their enactment to provide a reframe of the girl's symptoms. I stated to the mother that it appeared to me that a better definition than "stealing" for the girl's behavior was that she was withdrawing her salary for employment as her mother's caretaker and therapist. This reframe generated giggles in the girl. The mother, who was somewhat less impressed, gave me half a smile but subsequently acknowledged that perhaps I was correct. The girl's symptoms were serving the system as she was able to distract her mother from her depression and loneliness. The mother and I contracted to meet for a few individual sessions, at which time I empathized with her about her loneliness, frustrations, and worries, having myself at one time been a single working mother. Our brief relationship opened her to the possibility of seeking satisfaction in peer activities. I explored her options about this and for discovering a life outside of her daughter. She stated that, after her very traumatic marriage, she was not interested in pursuing a male relationship, but she nevertheless acknowledged that she was considering returning to her church, where she did enjoy the interpersonal contacts. I acknowledged her fears for her daughter and addressed her overprotectiveness, which was rooted in worry that her daughter would also develop dysfunctional relationships with peers and later with men. A few additional sessions included work with both parents because the father was a support for the girl, but the mother had not previously perceived him as such. Although the parents were unable to develop a co-parenting relationship, it nevertheless brought father and daughter into a

more meaningful relationship and counteracted the mother's sole role modeling. (It also counteracted the mother's deprecation of the father.)

This structural intervention was respectful of the mother and understanding of the emotions of the individual family members. Quite to the contrary of what some critics have expressed about structural family therapy, it is not purely a matter of directing people to behave differently. A proficient structural family therapist would never simply express to this mother, "Stop smothering your daughter. You must help her to grow up and separate. Get a life. Case closed." As a structural family therapist, my goals are to interrupt the unhelpful and self-defeating interactional patterns among the family members; but I am also sensitive to each individual member as a human being who has feelings, opinions, ideas, hidden potentials, and valuable contributions to offer.

UPDATE: In precisely the same week that I was searching for the family to obtain an update to include in this book, the girl (I will call her Jane), now in her twenties, was searching for me. Talk about ESP! Jane and I met twice, once when she was alone and once when she arrived with her father. Jane had been seeking me out to refresh her memory about what had transpired in the therapy, particularly in the sessions with both of her parents. I inquired as to what the therapy had meant to her. She related that she had been sent to multiple individual therapists before seeing me, and each of those therapists made her feel as if she were defective, having plucked her out of her family situation and conveying to her that all was right with her world, except for her. She articulated that I had been the only therapist who established the problem as a function of the family's dysfunctional relationships, and my reframe had given her optimism that she was not a bad seed. So how did the optimism influence preteen Jane, who had been seriously underperforming in school at the time of the family therapy? Jane is now pursuing her master's degree in education! She recently began living with her father with whom she has become very close, and she continues to have a relationship with her mother.

Another family, (whom I describe as "the family who was stuck with peanut butter,") consisted of two parents and their two children, an eight-year-old boy and a six-year-old girl. They presented with a curious eating disorder in the eight-year-old boy: from the moment this child began to eat solid foods, he refused anything except peanut butter. Nine therapists preceded me in treating him, and all had failed to resolve the presenting problem of getting him to eat a variety of foods. In reviewing the treatment history, I ascertained that all prior therapies had made no attempt to discover the underlying family organization which was maintaining the symptom but rather focused on symptom management through a variety of individual treatment modalities including play therapy, behavior modification, and talk therapy. In preparation for the first session, I reread *Psychosomatic Families,* a book about eating disorders by Minuchin (1978). It discusses the organization and structure of eating disorder families, the central characteristics being overprotectiveness, avoidance of conflict resolution, enmeshment, and rigidity (pp. 51–63).

I began the intake session by commenting to the family that I had some doubts that I would be more effective than my nine predecessors, and I asked the parents what they thought might be different this time around. They each let out a sigh, were unable to provide an answer, and revealed exasperation and defeatism in their facial expressions. I was planting the seed that they will be the ones responsible for healing their son. I explored with them the efforts they had made

to get to their son to eat, and it became clear from this discussion that they felt terribly controlled by him. They had attempted bribing, cajoling, reasoning, persuading, crying, and at times expressions of anger–but he defeated them at every instance. The family was unable to plan any vacations or outings without checking ahead and arranging for the availability of peanut butter. Meals were always an ordeal because the parents battled with the boy to get him to eat what was served to the rest of the family, but he always triumphed. I was not so much concerned with the content of the parent's discussion, but I rather hoped that this exploration would have revealed the process of their communications, thereby denoting unresolved parental rifts. But this rigid family was defeating me in the presentation of themselves as the Brady Bunch. They insisted that there were no other issues in the family and that they function quite normally and satisfactorily, except for their son's predilection for peanut butter. The parents declared that they treat each other and the children with mutual respect and consideration for everyone's thoughts and feelings. They stated that they take into consideration the children's feelings and wishes in their decision-making. The parents affirmed that they compromise with each other regarding areas of disagreement and that neither tends to dominate the decision-making process. The children affirmed that there is nothing they wished to change about their parents. (How often is this the case?) Nothing I asked revealed the submerged marital conflict, which I knew, nonetheless, had to exist. I was getting nowhere and not very fast!

Attempting a different strategy, I expressed to the parents that their son's problem was indeed a mystery to me and that I had concluded that I would be unable to determine the cause or solution. The parents looked at me in dismay as they had announced that I was their last hope. I continued with my expression of impotency to cure their son, but I conveyed my certainty that they held the keys to a successful cure because they are the experts on their son. The parents declared that they did not believe they had the keys since they attempted and failed at everything my predecessors had suggested they do and which they had devised on their own. I remained firm in my conviction that they indeed had the key to unlocking their son's mystery, and I urged the parents to have a discussion with each other about the characteristics of peanut butter. Interpreting their incredulous nonverbal responses to my directive, I believe they would have immediately alighted from my office had I not been their last hope. But because of their desperation, they complied with my request. The mother began by stating, "It smells like peanuts, it's brownish, it's sticky, and, and it's smooth." At that moment, she looked at me as if a light bulb had gone off in her head, and she declared, "It's smooth! You know, our son never eats crunchy style peanut butter. He insists on smooth peanut butter every time." I asked her for the significance of this as I was sure it had relevance to the presenting problem. The mother explained that, just like the smooth peanut butter, she is a person who "likes to smooth things over." I immediately surmised that she was referring to her relationship with her husband, and my goal was to make this overt. I asked her with whom she "likes to smooth things over," and I received the response that I had anticipated: "With my husband." I now uncovered the chink in their impenetrable armor, and I intended to make explicit that the interpersonal relationship between the parents was maintaining their son's symptom. I directed the mother to speak with her husband about this, and she confronted him about his rigidity and his defensiveness when she expresses

to him a differing opinion. She could barely contain her anger that she needs his permission—as if she were one of the children—to make any routine decision of daily living. She further confronted him about his disproportionate anger if the children commit the slightest transgression, such as inadvertently placing one step on the front lawn as they walk on the driveway to the car. The mother was furious with her husband for years of pent-up frustration, which erupted like Mount Vesuvius, regarding his control over her and over the family. She advised him that for too long she had submerged her feelings and wishes in order to keep things "smooth" with him, and now she realizes that the children are suffering the consequences.

It should be clear to the reader that the symptom of the identified patient was indicative of the repressed/covert conflict between the parents. The symptom served to maintain the homeostasis of the system in that, while the parents focused on the boy, he succeeded in distracting them from their submerged marital conflict, which otherwise risked the dissolution of the marriage. The boy's symptom, which so intolerably controlled the family, was symbolic of how controlled the family members felt by the father.

I can hear the resounding incredulity of the reader, who doubts that there is any "reality" to the reframe of the IP's symptom. The reality is, there is no reality! At least there is none to me or to you, the reader. But there was a reality to the family. When I offer a reframe, I am not concerned with truth or integrity or reality. I am concerned only with imparting a new "story" that has meaning to the family; that enables them to see another perspective on the presenting problem—a perspective which requires a systemic change in the family if there is to be a problem resolution. But the real beauty of the reframe in this case example was that it came from the mother! At that moment, the mother, a family member, became my co-therapist, which always makes for a more successful therapy. This was no longer a therapy about and for a boy with an eating disorder. It became a therapy about and for a family with an organizational disorder. Can the reader hypothesize where this therapy needed to go? Take a few moments to think about this question. Figured it out? The family's dysfunctional organizational pattern required that the membership of their subsystems change so that the mother joins the marital/parental subsystem as an equal partner with her husband and departs the sibling subsystem; so that the children begin to relate directly to each other without their mother mediating their interactions; so that the children deal directly with their father without their mother's interfering overprotection.

The following family is an example of the very destructive results to all members, especially to the children, when cross-generational coalitions become hardened and are used for scapegoating. I treated this family in the mid 1990s when I was a PAS-unaware therapist. The family consisted of two emotionally estranged and antagonistic parents and their five children, who ranged in ages from five to seventeen years. The family had been supervised for many years by CPS and was currently receiving preventive services due to the multiyear school truancy of the seventeen-year-old son and due to his aggression towards his younger siblings. This boy, the next two oldest children, and their mother had formed a coalition against the father, whereby they demeaned and disqualified him. The mother accused the father of domestic violence but which he adamantly denied. I was not able to determine the veracity of the allegation for, although the older children confirmed their mother's story, CPS had no verification of such history nor were there any orders of protection in this family. In an early family session, the father alleged—and which the mother admitted—that she not only provides the 17-year-old boy with an open-ended stream of funds to hang out with his truant friends during school hours, but she further chauffeurs him to his hangout places because she feared for him driving with a suspended license. The parents began to argue with each other in a verbally abusive manner about why the mother enables their son. The father quickly gained the upper hand in the argument as the mother soon retreated and fell silent. The boy in question then jumped to his feet, violated his father's space, and threatened to kill him with a baseball bat after the session. The mother made no effort to restrain her son or admonish him for his maltreatment of his father. In response to the father's unanswered question to his wife as to why his wife rewards their delinquent son with money that enables his truancy, I provided the reframe that she is paying the boy a salary for fighting her battles with him. I then told the father that, if he wished his wife to cease enabling the boy, then he and his wife must figure out a way to solve their problems without his bullying her into silence. I told the mother that she is placing her son at great risk by making him her ammunition in her fight with her husband. I additionally took a firm stand with this family and told them that therapy is a privilege, an admonition borrowed from Minuchin (1993), who had conveyed this sentiment to one of his families in which there was domestic violence (pp. 65–87). I affirmed to the family that I would resign as therapist if the verbal abuse and physical threats did not immediately cease. I held the parents accountable for the hostility which they were modeling for their children and that I expected them to keep their children secreted away from their arguments.

As with this last family, I have observed some degree of the perverse triangle in every situation in which the family presents with marital/parental discord. The following is all too typical and repetitive of this interactional sequence: The parents bring teenage Johnny in for therapy due to his belligerence and argumentativeness–with one parent generally receiving the brunt of the hostilities. As the family engages in their enactment, mother and father soon become embroiled in a verbally abusive screaming match with each other about some issue or another. One parent peters out, and let us hypothesize in this case that it is the mother who becomes weary and falls silent. At this point "belligerent son," who is also her puppet ally, takes up her argument with his father, mouthing her issues almost verbatim. I interrupt at this point and punctuate the transactions I just observed. I then refocus the parents on each other and direct them to continue talking with each other in order to resolve their disagreement. When the parents again reach the point where they can no longer tolerate the tension, they break off their discussion. Teenage Johnny does not repeat his prior rescue of his mother, accommodating to the therapist who had objected. To fill the pregnant silence, the father then turns to his son and berates him for his belligerence. It is all too obvious what is happening here: mother is allowing son to fight her battles with her husband as she is a conflict avoider, but her son is an expert debater; father is transferring his unresolved anger for his wife to her ally, who also happens to be his son. To this systems therapist it is unmistakable that the family's interactional patterns are maintaining the boy's symptoms. Therefore, symptom amelioration will be achieved only if the parents resolve their conflicts directly with each other, thereby freeing their son from stabilizing the marriage.

Each of the above cases demonstrates that symptomatic behaviors do not occur in isolation of the family system and that triangulation is the dysfunctional interactional pattern at the root of the child's symptoms. When the perverse triangle is not interrupted early on, the destructive consequences to children are immeasurable. It disturbs healthy family hierarchy because the child becomes more powerful than the demeaned parent in the process of being elevated by the seducing parent to the adult level. Allies are equals after all. The child will then frequently engage with the outcast parent in a verbal battle that mimics the conflict occurring between the parents. When this behavioral transaction is repeated so that the child rigidly aligns with the same parent to the deprecation of the other parent, the child will invariably be at risk for severe emotional and behavioral difficulties. When conflicts between the parents escalate and are habitually detoured through the child to the rejection of one parent, then there is great potential to produce such severely disturbed behaviors and emotional symptomatology that the child may not be able to become a functioning, self-sufficient member of society. In the extreme situation, the result of the perverse triangle produces psychosis or any number of untreatable Axis II diagnoses, such as sociopathology.

As with the other systems therapists, Minuchin is quite concerned about the detrimental effects on children resulting from the formation of the perverse triangle. He developed a metaphor for this triangulating process: the child becomes the puppet of the ventriloquist parent because the child moves her/his lips, but the allied parent's words are expressed.

Does this all not sound eerily characteristic of the PAS family? The reader may recall that I cited numerous examples of these destructive cross-generational coalitions or triangles in each of my previously discussed PAS families: children mouthing the words of their ventriloquist alienating parent by labeling their alienated parent with groundless deprecations; children aligning universally with their alienating parent in all parental disputes or whenever a court action was proceeding to the point that they "fantasized" being a defendant along with their alienating parent; that there exists poor boundary formation with the children being inappropriately involved in the marital/parental issues; that the boundaries between the alienating parent and the child are diffuse leading to enmeshment while the boundaries between the child and the alienated parent are overly rigid leading to disengagement. Is it not true that the alienated child's autonomy is compromised? Is there not the presence of the double-bind in which the child must make an impossible choice?

The structural family therapist intervenes in the family to enable its members to relinquish triangulation. Symptom elimination is achieved by the reorganization of the family's transactional processes whereby the child is freed from a position between the parents and as a staunch ally of one parent. This is accomplished by coaching the parents to solve their conflicts directly with each other without detouring through the child. For example, in the common situation in which the mother feels emotionally abandoned by the father and consequently looks to her child to meet her emotional needs, the structural therapist will work with the marital couple to explore how they each are pushing the other away and how father can seduce mother towards him and away from their child. The structural therapist interprets this accordion dance–being in and out from each other–to be mutually maintained in that the mother is likely berating the father for his distancing rather than attempting to seduce him towards her.

In treating the PAS family, the closeness/enmeshment between the alienating parent and child must be challenged along with the distance/disengagement between the alienated parent and the child. A healthy family reorganization must be realized.

Efforts must be made to encourage the parents to develop a civil and respectful coparenting relationship with each other. I realize that this is not easy, but the therapist must convince the parents that being responsible and mature means demonstrating that their love for their children is stronger than their enmity for each other. The therapist must help the alienating parent to understand that the alienating programming of children is detrimental to them and is a form of child abuse. It is hoped that this knowledge will be the motivation to relinquish the alienating behaviors. It is also essential for the therapist to discover positive qualities in the alienating parent (as most people generally do have positive sides of themselves) as well as conveying a concern for whom she/he is as a human being with feelings, needs, and opinions. Efforts must be made to ascertain the underlying motivations for the alienating behaviors. Is it out of hurt because of rejection by the former partner? Is it the fear of losing their children's love because now the other parent has become the "holiday and charitable parent?" Is it the fear of being "unemployed" after having been the primary caretaker throughout the marriage and that the parenting job was the raison d'être? Is it that their customary lifestyle is being threatened with dramatically reduced financial support? Is it that they are overprotective of the child because of a sincere belief that the other parent is either too permissive or too punitive? Is it due to the insecurity of not knowing what the future brings? Is it a feeling of loss of control stemming from the unpredictability of the divorce proceedings and custody battle? Could it be revenge?

Knowing the motivations and underlying fears of the alienating parent provides one focus of the co-parenting sessions and of the adjunct individual sessions with the alienating parent. If the therapist is able to join with the alienating parent and gain her/his collaboration, then the possibility for change is exponentially enhanced. The alienated parent is encouraged in the sessions to provide reassurance to the alienating parent, as best as possible, given the new circumstances that will be the inevitable result of a divorce. The therapist must remain nonjudgmental so that alienating parents are willing to cooperate with the necessary family restructuring. In recognition of the alienating parent's needs, the therapist will explore with the parent how she/he can substitute healthy peer relationships and develop a life outside of the child in order to facilitate the child's autonomy. In essence, the therapist will help the alienating parent to rewrite her/his self-perception as a child rescuer by alternatively seeking healthy and emotionally satisfying peer relationships.

The therapist must help alienated parents to relinquish their self-perception as a victim by supporting their efforts to become more proactive and self-assertive in reshaping the transactions that have been occurring in the family relationships. I have lost count of how many alienated parents expressed to me that they had been wearing blinders during the marriage and thereby denied the alienation that was unfolding right before their eyes long before the marriage ended. Other alienated parents acknowledged that they had acquiesced to their spouses when they interfered with the relationship between them and their children because, "It was too much of an effort to keep fighting." As previously discussed, the alienated parent will be afforded the role of the prime mover of the deprogramming with the therapist serving as a catalyst to the process. The alienated parent

must be encouraged and supported in assuming involvement in the child's educational development, medical care, and extracurricular activities. Alienated parents must be helped to relinquish their anger for their former partner if she/he ceases the alienating behaviors and engages in the healing process. This is also not an easy task, particularly if the alienated parent's visits with their children were suspended due to false allegations of sex abuse or was incarcerated on fabricated domestic violence allegations. If the alienated parent had transferred anger for their former partner to their child ally, apologies must be given. The alienated parent must recognize that their child was manipulated to be a puppet of the alienating ventriloquist parent and did not have any good options in this situation.

The therapist must capitalize on restructuring the interactions between the child with each of her/his parents by intervening to reorganize the two parent/child subgroups with the goal of flipping them so that the child becomes closer to the alienated parent and more distant from the alienating parent. The therapist will accomplish this by refocusing the child and alienating parent on age-appropriate/stage-specific interactions while simultaneously supporting the alienated parent and child to rewrite together the family myths and misperceptions about herself/himself and about the family's history and to increase involvement with the child's current life.

In my individual supervision by Dr. Minuchin (2002), he often challenged me with his usual poetic license to help me think outside the box (both mine and the family's) to create a larger story that promotes growth. The following is one of his favorite metaphors posed to help the family rewrite their myths: "How do you select from the Joycean grammar of family interactions the bits that will be significant for the construction of the therapeutic alternative? How do you encourage authorship by family members? How do you promote acceptance of the new myth as a better edition of the previous one" (individual supervision of Gottlieb, 2002)? The following treatment summaries of my PAS families will hopefully help to answer this difficult proposition. Come travel with me on a journey to help them amend their respective stories; to choose another road to be taken; to help family members discover sides of themselves that embrace, encourage, and expand the other; and to help them appreciate a child's need and desire for both parents.

In order to protect anonymity, I will be providing minimal case examples of the symptoms of the PAS and few direct quotes or specific demographics. The reader should be reassured, however, that the children in these case summaries were all previously cited as examples of the characteristic eight symptoms.

During the initiation period when I was learning about PAS, I began to work with a family consisting of a young girl and her divorced parents who were referred by CPS and family court for therapeutic visits between the father and the girl. The girl was expressing fear of her father with whom she had no contact in several years because of a sex abuse finding, which I will not elaborate upon. I will merely remind the reader of the frequency of frivolous sex abuse incidents which are alleged in alienation cases. I scheduled the first session with the residential parent, who was the girl's mother in this case. This is my standard method for initiating treatment of PAS families. I learned an invaluable lesson from this case–the necessity to use the initial contact to attempt to gain the collaboration of the custodial parent. But because I had determined that this mother had caused such unwarranted grief to the father and to the girl as a result of her alien-

ating behaviors, I did not express to her that she was important to her daughter and to the therapy. I did not seek her collaboration in the treatment. I further assumed that my mandate came from CPS, which would be sufficient authority to facilitate the goal of reuniting the girl with her father. It was not. I informed the mother in the first session of how I intended to proceed with the case, and I did not seek her input, as an expert on her daughter, as to how to comply with the mandate for reunification. She consequently was not supportive of the treatment plan, and she predicted that her daughter will have an anxiety attack in anticipation of the therapeutic visits. Count on the alienator's prediction becoming a self-fulfilling prophesy! I quickly discovered this, and I thus reversed my intervention strategy with her. But I am getting a little ahead of myself. In the first session between the girl and her father, she expressed her fear and mistrust of him while simultaneously exposing her loving feelings for him because she smiled upon accepting a necklace from him. Her uneasiness mirrored her mother's prophesy that, "My daughter is having panic attacks about the visit." The father attempted to deprogram her from the perception that he is an evil person who had intentionally hurt her and had abandoned her. The session ended more positively than it began with the girl expressing that she was eager for the next visit. It was evident that she was in a psychological trap, caught between her parents: fearing that her mother would feel betrayed if she were to rebond with her father. I realized I needed to approach the mother differently, and I scheduled another session with her in order to gain her collaboration. She alone had the leverage to free the girl from this double-bind. This time I approached her as an expert on her daughter, requesting her input about whom her daughter is. I invited her to make suggestions as to how to facilitate the relationship between her daughter and her father and how to help the family to heal. I articulated that my objective was to facilitate the rebuilding of the relationship between her daughter and her father and not to support the transfer of custody, as she had feared. The mother further appreciated my recognition of her importance to her daughter as reflected in my offer to facilitate her and the father to develop a civil and respectful co-parenting relationship. It is significant that she was agreeable to this. One issue on her agenda for the co-parenting sessions was her insistence that the father apologize to their daughter. The father had been unable to disabuse the mother from her belief that he had sexually abused their daughter. At the same time, she agreed that it is time to move on and to convey to her daughter that she supports the rebuilding of her relationship with her father. We contracted to make one focus of the parental sessions a resolution of the parental disagreement about the apology. Having been extended the recognition that she was important to her daughter, this formerly alienating mother became an active and cooperative repairer of the PAS.

I next scheduled a session between the mother and her daughter, first meeting with the girl to obtain her feedback about the first therapeutic visit. She expressed to me, "I am ready to see my father again even though my mother does not think so." This comment gave further credence to the girl's trap. With my support, she agreed to express her readiness to her mother, who then joined us in the session. The mother accepted her feelings and reassured her that she has her support for rebuilding her relationship with her father. I scheduled another session between the girl and the father, and the contrast in the girl's interaction with her father from the first to the second therapeutic visit was as different as night from day. I was convinced this was directly attributable to her mother's

approval. The girl would not leave her father's side, and she hugged and kissed him frequently; she brought him up-to-date about school, friends, activities, and interests. At the end of just the second session, the girl and her father expressed their love for each other, and they cried in each other's arms regarding the loss of each other for the prior several years. Observing this interaction between father and daughter, one would never have suspected that there had been a several year breach in their relationship. This girl is so typical of how quickly PAS children flip their feelings for and interactions with their alienated parent once their alienating parent sanctions that they do so. This girl is the rule and NOT the exception to such a change. And the swiftness in the girl's change of heart further signifies the speciousness of the PAS child's expressed acrimony for the alienated parent.

The therapy on this case lasted for six months. I worked with the family as a whole—which included the mother, father, stepmother, and the girl—and with various subgroups, such as the mother and father; the mother, father, and stepmother; the father, stepmother, and the girl; the father and the girl; the mother and the girl; and the mother alone. In the sessions with the father and the girl, I coached him to correct the misperceptions about himself without blaming the mother. For example, while it is essential for him to inform his daughter that he did not voluntarily withdraw from her life, he must not accuse the mother of facilitating this alienation. I guided him to relive with her the meaningful involvement he had with her before the alienation was initiated. He described for her every way and every activity in which he had participated in her life; he declared that he had always protected her and that he will always do so; he reassured her how he had not willfully abandoned her; he affirmed that he had never stopped trying to have contact with her after he and her mother had separated; and he expressed his love for her. The stepmother was an effective co-therapist by helping her husband to sublimate his anger resulting from the humiliation and grief that his ex-wife had caused him. The co-parenting sessions achieved a number of goals: the mother updated the father on their daughter's educational, medical, and social developments; they made medical decisions together; the three parents agreed on the role for the stepmother to play in the girl's life, including discipline; the mother and father learned to compromise on their parenting differences; the mother agreed to notify the court of her approval for unsupervised visits; the mother requested and received the father's support for her supervision of the girl, who typically attempted to manipulate her; and finally, the parents agreed on the content of the apology the father would give to his daughter. He correctly maintained that giving an apology for something he had not done would create equivalent harm as if it had actually happened. He was able to persuade the mother to accept this position. In the apology session with the girl and her parents, the father stated to his daughter that he is apologetic for not having respected her age that perhaps she had been old enough to handle the situation herself. The girl readily accepted her father's apology stating she wants everyone to move on and forget the incident. The father then expressed to his daughter (what all too commonly occurs in cases of fallacious sex abuse allegations) that he is holding himself back from being affectionate with her for fear of making her upset, and he requested her help in letting him know how he can touch her. With this comment, the girl ran to her father, embraced him, and she exclaimed, "This is how." Her mother's affect conveyed her approval. With the mother's agreement, I recommended to the court

that the father be granted unsupervised visits. The court consented, at which time I closed the case.

I can declare unequivocally that an individual treatment modality would have failed to "reason" the girl out of her irrational fears and beliefs about her father. The successful outcome in this case resulted from an intervention using a structural family therapy modality which capitalized on the face-to-face experience between father and daughter; encouraged the exchange of emotions between them; facilitated the father in re-writing the family's myths; nurtured an environment which supported the unwavering love that parents and children instinctively have for each other; and gained the alienating parent's collaboration in the therapy and willingness to forsake alienating behaviors. It was the father's calm and comforting expressions, his patient listening to his daughter's concerns and beliefs, his nondefensive responses to her misguided accusations, and his reassurance of his love for her that effectuated the healing of their relationship. No therapist can possibly recreate such a therapeutic holding environment via an individual treatment modality. The reversal of the PAS was facilitated by a family systems approach which recognized and supported a collaborative effort between the formally alienating mother with the father and with the therapist.

I began to work with Jennifer, whose heartbreaking saga was previously recounted in detail. She initially requested my help to motivate her very bright son to attend school. He was truant almost 50 percent of the time. During the process of exploring her efforts to solve this problem, it appeared to me that she had become more responsible than was her son for his own education. Her preoccupation with being super-mom aroused my curiosity that there was much more to her story. In response to my curiosity, she burst into tears and revealed her dreadful alienation saga. In a subsequent session, she was looking completely perplexed but simultaneously sanguine. She had received a phone call from her alienated daughter of 14 years, and she suggested having her brother live with her believing that the closeness in their age may give her leverage in motivating him to attend school. For Jennifer, this was a sugarcoated pill. On the one hand, she relished the contact with her daughter; but on the other hand, it meant relinquishing residential care of her son. It was an agonizing déjà vu experience. She scheduled a therapy session with her two children, and I facilitated the development of a plan and the conditions under which Jennifer would consent to a temporary change in living arrangements for her son. The arrangement, of course, would involve regular communication between Jennifer and her daughter concerning her son. Their interaction was palliative; it permitted the girl the opportunity to finally recognize her mother to be the loving and devoted mother whom she always had been throughout the process in which they collaborated together to help her son. The boy returned to his mother's home after residing with his sister for a semester, but Jennifer and her daughter continued to recover their relationship. I continued to work with Jennifer during this time and coached her how to handle her emotions as well as the trauma which this new situation had stimulated. Their saga is still evolving. I suggested that she may wish to belie the revisionist history for her children, but Jennifer has yet to acquire the courage to do so. She hopes that this book will make a difference. I provided her a copy of her video interview detailing her heartbreaking saga, and she someday intends to view it with both of her children so that they realize that she did not abandon her daughter.

I began to work with a divorced mother, her daughter in her early teens, and her son in his mid-teens. She and her ex-husband had been through a very bitter divorce several years earlier, and she remained angry with him for having cheated on her—feelings which she had no compunction about sharing with her children. The mother was requesting counseling for her children because they had refused all contact for five months with their father, and he had petitioned the court to enforce his visitation rights. The mother was not interested in encouraging a relationship between the children and their father. Rather, she was seeking my help, at the suggestion of her attorney, to obtain validation of her defense before the court that the children's feelings regarding their father were uninfluenced by her. She further conveyed to me that the children frequently became annoyed with her and angry at her as a result of her "pleading" with them to visit with their father. She stated that she was exhausted from fighting with them about this, although she acknowledged that issues of adolescence also contributed to their anger. I explored with her about her life as a single working parent who is rearing two teenagers, and she acknowledged that it is quite stressful. I identified with her, having once been a single working mother. She stated that she had little life outside of the children, and in essence, she was revolving around them. I encouraged her to cultivate activities and peer relationships, but she was reluctant to do so. She emphasized that she wished my help only for the presenting problem. I suspected it would be difficult to challenge her enmeshment with her children, but, at her request, I refocused the therapy on them. When she introduced me to the children, they spontaneously announced in unison, "We have no use for our father, and we don't want to ever see him again." Upon exploration of their feelings, all three denied that the father had been abusive or neglectful of them, and the children were further unable to provide any justification for their enmity for him. What they did express was their desire for me to notify the court of the following: "Our feelings are our own; our mother does not interfere with us having a relationship with our father; our father has chosen his mistress over us; our father does not deserve to have a relationship with us; he is wasting his time taking **us** back to court." Nothing the mother or the children stated justified the children's rejection of their father, so I then attempted to help the mother recognize the importance of fathers to their children. I hoped that if I educated her about this, she would come to see the errors of her ways. I met with her and provided her with abundant research and literature about this. She was unmoved. She expressed the typical rationalizations and ineffectual efforts that I repetitively hear from alienating parents as to why they are unable to get their children to comply with the visits. This mother never gave a direct demand that the children attend, always implying that it was their choice and that she was respecting their wishes when they refused to see their father. As my initial efforts failed to convince the mother of the importance of the father to her children, I expressed to her that I would like to meet with him and the children. She readily agreed as she anticipated the children being quite vocal in expressing to him their opposition to a relationship with him. The father immediately scheduled an appointment to meet with me. During the session, he stated that he believed his ex-wife was interfering in his relationships with their children. He further expressed that he was convinced of his children's desire to see him but that they were afraid to antagonize their mother. He agreed to cooperate with any therapy that I thought might be helpful.

I arranged for a session with the children and their father, and I sought the mother's help to assist the process by encouraging her children to work things out with him. I accepted her offer to participate in the initial session. The father initiated the conversation by asking the children about their school, their friends, and extracurricular activities, and the children responded by providing only superficial information. The discussion soon turned to the issue of the visits, and the father requested that the mother take a firm stand with the children by ensuring that they keep their visitation arrangements with him. She insisted that she desires for them to cooperate but is unable to get them to do so even though she has nagged to the point that she was incurring their wrath. The father responded that she would be successful in getting them to attend if she really wished for that to happen. After a few rounds of punch and counterpunch, I turned to the mother and I stated, "I am really quite surprised at how protective you are of your ex-husband, given your anger for him." The family members looked at me in bewilderment as no one would have characterized the mother's treatment of the father as "protective." She adamantly denied that she had intentions of protecting him, and she inquired as to how I had reached this interpretation. I explained the following:

> I realize that you do not intend to be protective, but it is happening nonetheless. It's clear to me that you are sparing the father from getting your children's teenage-related anger as the failure to have visits deprives them of the opportunity to dump on him as they are dumping on you. Furthermore, by having no contact with the children, their father cannot support your authority with them or impose limits and discipline, which consequently makes your life harder as the only "bad" parent. And finally, you are absolving him of any

responsibility for them thereby enabling his fun and relaxation while you remain on duty 24/7.

With these comments, I ended the session, leaving the family perplexed.

When the family arrived for the next session, the mother announced that the children had visited with their father during the previous weekend. I inquired as to how she managed to bring that about, and she responded, "I told them they had to go!" The mother called to cancel the next scheduled appointment stating that the presenting problem had been resolved as the children and their father are speaking with each other regularly on the phone, and the children agreed to keep the visitation schedule as outlined in the divorce agreement. The mother added that the children were inexplicably polite and cooperative with her! She was perplexed as to how she had brought about this change, and I did not offer my thoughts. During a call to the father in subsequent weeks, I verified with him that the children were visiting regularly and were behaving as if there had not been an estrangement. A follow-up phone call several months later confirmed that the children were still visiting with their father and that he had withdrawn his petition requesting enforcement of his parental and visitation rights.

The reader is correct in the recognition that the successful outcome of the therapy with this family resulted primarily from a strategic intervention. Structural family therapy has evolved, and it recognizes that all treatment modalities offer effective and valuable contributions to the treatment process. Structural family therapy will therefore borrow maneuvers and interventions from all the systems therapies and, at times, even from the psychoanalytic method should such interventions further the therapeutic goals. But these maneuvers and interventions are always in service of the philosophical underpinning of structural family therapy that a change in one member will effect changes in the others and that members of families cocreate each other. This case also punctuates that the reunification occurred because of collaboration with the alienating parent and would likely not have resolved out of court without her approval. Systemic and not individual treatment was required. Additionally, this case substantiates how the PAS can be speedily and easily reversed once sanctioned by the alienating parent. It further illustrates how eagerly children will "conquer" their expressed repugnance for their alienated parent—as swiftly as flipping a light switch—once the alienating parent sanctions the rapprochement. The case offers authentication for the superficiality and fakeness of PAS children's expressed enmity for their alienated parent.

A family with a multiple sibling group was referred to me by the children's attorney in order to facilitate a reconciliation between their father and them after visit refusal had been occurring for almost a year. The lawyer suspected an alienation, not only because of the visit refusal, but because of the commonality of the children's expressions of irrational hatred for their father. The case had been lingering in the court for an even longer time due to multiple adjournments. I scheduled the first interview with the mother in order to join with her so that she would become an active participant in effectuating the reunification. I commented to her how it is a reflection on her good parenting that all of her children were well behaved in school, were on the honor roll, and had no behavioral problems in any setting. She expressed her appreciation, maintaining that her estranged husband failed to credit her parental accomplishments. I listened to her story about how controlled she had felt by her husband, but, not wanting to reinforce her self-perception as a victim, I empowered her by refocusing her on how she could achieve the goals to which she aspired for herself. Indeed, she hoped to pursue her Masters degree in education so that she could become financially independent. I also helped her to recognize her role in her marriage, for if she had been victimized, she had permitted it in some way. She conceded that she not only failed to be self-assertive about her needs, wishes, and opinions, but she simultaneously elevated her husband on a pedestal. When a person recognizes that she/he plays a part in how the situation unfolds, then she/he cannot be a victim and further has the power to produce remedy. She was further fearful of losing the affections of her children because her estranged husband controlled the purse strings. She was grateful that I was not judgmental of her nor blamed her for the state of the relationships between her children and their father. Although I did recognize her participation in the children's rejection of their father, I conveyed that my objective was to gain her support for the reconciliation process. I expressed that I was concerned with remedy, not blame. I further reassured her that my intention was to facilitate the rebuilding of the relationships between the children and their father and not to rob her of her children by supporting a transfer of custody or elevating him into the role of sugar daddy. Such reassurance is crucial to facilitating the reversal of the PAS process as, very often, the fear of losing the children—if not physically, then emotionally—is a motivating factor for the alienating parent. Once I had gained her trust and had conveyed compassion for her situation, the mother revealed that she, herself, had been a victim of the PAS and still experiences the detrimental effects. (I previously stated that the PAS is frequently passed down through the generations if its transmission is not interrupted.) As she revealed her painful histo-

ry to me, she relived her childhood trauma, and she decided at that moment that she would not subject her children to the same ordeal. She pledged that she will not make her children endure a tug of war between their parents, as she had felt growing up. She appreciated my compassion in response to her story, and, at that point, I revealed to her my own childhood victimization by the PAS and the consequent detrimental effects that resulted to my sister and to me. At that moment, there was an irreversible joining with her. I then asked her what she would express to her children to encourage their cooperation in the sessions with their father. (Collaboration with the alienating parent makes everything go so much more smoothly. It is ludicrous not to attempt this.) In response to my question, the mother stated she would tell the children that anger is inconsistent with their religious values. She further stated she would convey to them that it is not healthy for them to keep anger and she hoped they would resolve their feelings for their father with him. We scheduled a session for her and the children. She persuasively expressed to them that she believes anger is unhealthy; she stated, "It is like carrying around a 100-pound bowling ball." She encouraged the children to work through their issues with their father because "you need him, and he loves all of you." The third session with the family was scheduled with the father and his children, although I had arranged with him to arrive early so that we could discuss his version of the family's history. He disputed a number of issues of which he had been accused—primarily that he had not been involved in his children's lives and that he had not been supporting them. I stated he should bring all information he has to dispute any untruths about him to the next session. He responded that the children's attorney informed him that by doing so puts the children in the middle of parental battles.

(Alienated parents frequently become victimized by multiple double-binds, which are often created by the professional rescuer: in these situations, when they attempt to clarify the misperceptions and malicious fabrications about themselves, they are accused of putting the children in the middle. But if alienated parents do not correct the lies, then the lies remain alive and well in the minds of their children. (It often seems to escape the logic of some attorneys for the children, of some judges, and of some individual therapists that it was the alienating parent who had initially put the children in the middle by revealing to them information that occurs in the court proceedings and by creating malicious and fallacious accusations about the alienated parent.) I responded to this father that it is imperative that he correct any misperceptions about himself and that this can be accomplished without casting aspersions on the mother.

When his children arrived, they all conveyed their thoughts and feelings through the oldest sibling, the 17-year-old girl, who was the chief complaint officer. The major grievance was their father's alleged failure to support them. He responded that he has provided and continues to provide monthly support for all their needs and that he will produce the supporting canceled checks and other documents at the next session. The younger children were amenable to their father's dispute about the accusation, but his 17-year-old daughter remained antagonistic, dismissive, and disbelieving. The children then accused him of his lack of involvement with them while still living at home and which they alleged continued after he had moved out. The father clarified his children's misperceptions by reminding them of all their activities in which he had participated with them. He further expressed that he was unable to attend everything that their mother had as he was the sole supporter of the

family. He explained that his long work schedule was a result of an agreement between him and their mother, and this agreement enabled her to stay home to take care of them. He expressed that, after he had moved out, he was either not provided with a schedule of their activities or else they had made it clear to him that he was unwelcome at their activities. He sobbed as he conveyed his undying love for them, that he would never turn his back on them, that he misses them terribly, and that the previous year had been the worst year of his life. His two youngest children were soon sobbing with him, upon climbing on his lap. An older boy maintained his distance, but he expressed to his father that he wants him to attend his next game but to watch from afar until he can prove that he had been supporting them. Nevertheless, this boy was soon sobbing along with his father and two younger siblings although still unwilling to physically embrace his father. The 17-year-old girl made no movement during the entire session and insisted, "I don't want a relationship with my father. I have no use for him."

I arranged with the mother for another individual session and requested that she talk to her children about the session that had occurred between them and their father. When she arrived, she reported that the younger children expressed positive feelings about their father but her 17-year-old daughter remains livid with him. She affirmed for me that she had encouraged her daughter to reconcile with her father. The relationship between this girl and her mother was the most enmeshed as she had become the parental child upon her parents' separation. I suspected that the girl risked feeling that she would be betraying her mother if she allowed her father to reenter her life. The mother agreed to reassure her of her fervent desire that she reconnect with her father and recognize that her father is particularly important to her during this developmental stage of her life. Another session was scheduled for the father and his children, and, as he had pledged, he brought to the session the canceled checks of support and other documentation that he had been providing for all of their needs. The children were impatient to review the documents, and they were all, including the 17-year-old girl, won over upon viewing the supporting evidence. The children breathed a sigh of relief, needing a moment to take it all in. They began one by one to update their father about what was transpiring in their current lives. They each provided him a list with all their extracurricular activities, and they enthusiastically requested his attendance. The session was so remarkably positive that the father and the children, upon conferring by phone with the mother, arranged to spend the afternoon together. Subsequent to that outing, the father would return to my office to attend a co-parenting session with the mother. Upon returning, the father elatedly announced, "I have my kids back!!!!!!!!!!!!!!!!!" Additional sessions between the father and his children were unnecessary as he just did his "fatherly thing" with his kids, and they responded positively to him. The parents and I, however, continued to meet for six co-parenting sessions, during which time they resolved their significant parental disagreements. Discussion of finances remained the one unsettled issue, which was to be resolved by their respective attorneys. The parents worked out a flexible and liberal schedule for visits; they mutually agreed about extracurricular activities for the coming year; they developed a plan for mutual involvement in their daughter's college applications and interviews; they arranged for the father to be kept apprised of and involved in the decision-making of all the children's activities, interests, educational and medical developments, and so forth. They arrived at a mutually accept-

able agreement on many of the issues confronting the family and the children. They further agreed to speak to the children together and convey to them that there is no devil or victim in the divorce decision but rather that they had mutually grown apart. (It is important for parents to recognize that how they handle their feelings and what they convey to their children regarding the decision to divorce will impact how their children will cope with the divorce and come to view male-female relationships. For example, if the children believe that wives are victimized by husbands, they will likely repeat this way of relating with their respective spouses by either identifying with the aggressor or else declining that role and becoming weak and servile.) I was able to facilitate a cooperative and civil shared parenting arrangement in which the parents compromised with each other in making decisions for their children. They further accommodated to each other's needs, realizing that they would be treated by the other in kind. For example, the father was supportive of the mother's wish to complete her master's degree in education by rescinding his insistence that she obtain employment in order to help with the finances. In return, the mother agreed to relinquish her sole custody petition in favor of joint legal custody. They met together with the children and expressed to them that this was the best arrangement for them. A follow-up phone call to the family two years later, as of the writing of this book, confirmed that the agreements which were arrived at in therapy remain in place, that the children continue to visit regularly with their father and have meaningful relationships with him, and that the parents continue to have a civil and respectful co-parenting relationship.

The treatment of this family certainly reached a successful conclusion–the total reversal of the PAS and the development of a civil, shared parenting relationship–in less than three months! It is irrefutable that my work with the mother was vital to the positive outcome. I believe, also, that the mother's fear of the authority of the children's lawyer played a significant role in effectuating this outcome as she did not wish to appear as an alienator to the court. And certainly no individual treatment modality could have achieved these results–especially in such short time. Despite the father's delight with the outcome, he posed a question to me that went unanswered then and for which I still have no answer: "Why did it have to take so long?"

The lawyer for two children, a boy in his preteens and a girl in her early teens, referred their family to me to help the parents resolve their visitation disputes. There had been visitation refusal for more than a year, and there was virtually no communication between the children and their father during the entire period of time. The father had been in and out of court for several years requesting redress for the denial of his parental rights to visitation. A prior year-long therapy had failed to effectuate a cooperative co-parenting relationship between the parents, and thus, as a consequence, there was no reconciliation between the children and their father. Visits were still suspended when the case was referred to me. I met first with the children's mother to join with her and gain her cooperation. She insisted that she did not wish to interfere with the relationships between her children and their father; she merely wished to shield them from a father who was too easily angered if the children perceived things differently than he and from a stepmother who was too controlling. I asked for her input as to how I could avoid making the mistakes committed by the previous therapist, and she responded that I needed to be a good listener, and she meant as much to her as to her children. I stated that

she is the expert on her children, so I would need her ongoing feedback as to what was helpful and what was not as the therapy proceeded. She had a favorable response to my taking a one-down position with her when it came to her children. I listened to her exponentially carefully, making note of every concern she raised about life, as she saw it, in the father's home. The father was living with his new wife, her fifteen-year-old daughter by a prior marriage, and their six-year-old daughter. For sure, there were blended family issues that needed to be addressed. It became obvious to me that the mother was a switchboard between her children and their father, and I posed to her the suggestion that she is the messenger who must be getting shot. She agreed this was true and that she and the father are unable to have a civil conversation because he is constantly screaming at her. I contracted with her to help enable her children to have a voice with their father so that they can practice on their father with the skills they will need in order to communicate with peers and future spouses. She acknowledged that she has been somewhat overprotective of her children due to issues resulting from her childhood, but she nevertheless agreed that her children were old enough to advocate for themselves. She was able to arrive at this place only after I made it unambiguously clear to her that I had listened to all her concerns for her children. I met with the father and his wife, and they updated me on the alienation between him and his children dating back to the father's separation from the mother many years earlier. They stated the children have expressed what amounts to frivolous rationalizations as their justification for their visit refusal, and they raise issues but only after their mother broaches her concerns with them.

I scheduled a session between the father and the children. The father was pleasantly surprised by their congenial attitude and cooperative participation, and I stated that I was convinced that this resulted from their mother's encouragement subsequent to my meeting with her. I shared with the children that my sister and I were the products of a bitter divorce at approximately the same age as the older sibling and that I believed that my parents could have handled it better. I then asked them how the past several years had been for them. The girl expressed revulsion regarding the fighting between her parents and held them equally responsible. The boy held the father exclusively culpable for the hostility between his parents. I inquired as to what they hoped to achieve from the therapy, and the girl stated the desire that the three parents would try "to get along and to co-parent." I expressed that I was impressed with the intelligence reflected in that comment, indicating that everyone has to change for things to get better. Their father conveyed his pain at missing them and that he deeply regrets that he is not as involved in their lives as he had always hoped to be. The session ended with a mutual exchange of hurts and regrets and the desire to remedy their estranged relationships. I reiterated that it was evident to me that the children's mother played a key role in the productive outcome of the session as she must have conveyed to the children that she was supportive of the therapy and its goal of reunification between them and their father. The children were appreciative hearing this comment, which they intended to communicate to their mother. In the next session a week later, the children and their father discussed a plan to resume their visits. The boy expressed displeasure about how the father berates him regarding the need for family time and that he easily flies off the handle when they have disagreements. With my help, the father recognized the validity of his son's remark and that he does not always appropriately express his anger; he apolo-

gized to his children, stating that he will work on how he expresses his disagreements to them. He then appropriately shared that his anger is a cover for his pain regarding the loss of his relationships with them. The children accepted his apology, and they joined their father in exchanging emotions regarding their estrangement. After a few moments of nonverbal bonding, they began a discussion about the resumption of the visits. They agreed to begin with day visits, and they planned activities to be undertaken. We met four more times to facilitate effective communication among the members of the father's household, including the stepmother and the other two children in the home before day visits were resumed. I received feedback from the mother that she was relieved that the children had been able to express how they feel without their father "exploding" at them. She supported the resumption of the day visits leading to overnights and weekends shortly thereafter. The three parents agreed to a co-parenting session, but the session did not go well as the mother and stepmother, both of whom admitted to being "firecrackers," engaged in a screaming match with each other, with punch and counterpunch. We decided that future parenting sessions would be limited to the father and the mother, and these were much more productive but not always devoid of hostility. I repeatedly used metaphors with the parents, such as that the children are like the house that was destroyed in the movie, *The War of the Roses;* or that the children are like a rope in a tug-of-war between their parent's, and just like the rope they will unravel. I talked to the parents about the daunting statistics regarding children from divorce whereby two-thirds develop serious emotional and behavioral problems and that it is only a civil co-parenting relationship that accounts for the remaining one-third, who do well. The most effective technique, however, and which I orchestrate whenever possible, was having the children verbalize to their parents how they hate the fighting; how they were being adversely affected by the animosity; how their concentration in their studies was reduced; and how they were becoming fearful of adult relationships. In fact, in one session, the girl astutely exclaimed, "The money for our college education is lining the pockets of your attorneys. Can't you two be sensible and settle this in therapy!" In yet another session, when the parents began to argue, the boy exclaimed to them that they were acting like they were two years old. I supported the children's "chastisement" of their parents for not protecting them from their hostility for each other. The coalition between the children and their mother slowly began to weaken as the children grew closer to their father. One indication of this occurred in a family session in which the girl confronted her mother about her history of demonstrating extreme negativity towards her father. The children expressed to their parents that they had yearned for the day when their parents could routinely talk civilly to each other, as they had accomplished in several of the family sessions. The parents were duly shamed by their children for their past history of incivility with each other. I supported the children when they confronted their mother about how she makes them feel like CIA agents in the father's home by having to report back to her about everything that occurs there. Other sessions between the children and their father reinforced how he can better express his anger, which he occasionally transferred from his ex-wife to his children. Later sessions with both parents and the children were pretty typical of what occurs in lower conflict families who enter therapy: I supported the parents in developing a unified front in guiding the children through the typical adolescent issues. Throughout the course

of the therapy, the visitation was gradually increased to include overnights and weekend visits until the visiting arrangements were in full compliance with the divorce decree. The therapy lasted a little more than a year, initially being one to two times per week for the first several months, gradually becoming one time per week for another several months, and decreasing to every other week for the balance of the therapy. I met with various subgroups including the two parents; the father and his two children; the mother and the two children; the father, stepmother, the two children, their half-sister, and their stepsister; the two children with both parents; the father, stepmother, and the two children. Individual sessions with the mother were interspersed throughout the therapy. During the sessions with the mother, I became a sounding board for her needs as well as for her difficulties at being a single mom. She also sought my aid in helping her to determine what comprises healthy relationships as she doubted that she knew what they looked like. I contacted the family to update this book: several years after termination of the therapy, the children continue to visit their father as per the divorce agreement, and the children are cooperative and pleasant. The parents do not have what I consider to be the model co-parenting relationship, but the children have been detriangled for the most part from any hostility between their parents.

In the case of a young adult girl who had refused all contact with her mother for six months, a very brief treatment resulted in the mitigation of the PAS. The alienation was encouraged and supported by her father, who not only engaged in a brainwashing campaign but who also financially supported her while she was residing with his extended family. The family membership was the mother and the father, who were currently separated and in the middle of a nasty divorce and custody battle; the girl; and her twelve-year-old brother, for whom each parent had filed a sole custody petition. The therapy consisted of several individual sessions with the father, a couple of unsuccessful co-parenting sessions, and a few sessions between the girl and her mother. The first session between the mother and her daughter was quite contentious with the girl regurgitating all of her father's issues with the mother, and the session ended in hopelessness. The girl refused to accept her mother's revisions to the family's myths regarding her. In the second session, the mother again failed in her attempts to correct the girl's revisionist history regarding herself. I contacted the father to arrange a session with him. Although there had been two unsuccessful co-parenting sessions, the one positive result of the session was that my neutrality was unassailable. I had conveyed my empathy for his pain over the loss of his marriage and separation from his son, and I did not sit in judgment of him. I relied on this reservoir of good will to be blunt with him. I stated that I was convinced that he was empowering his daughter to disrespect and demean her mother, although I granted that it may be occurring on an unconscious level. I expressed that his daughter's knowledge of the events in the divorce proceedings–explicitly his side of the issues–indicated that he was inappropriately apprising her of the marital issues. I held him accountable for the girl's unfounded enmity for her mother expressing that is was indicative of a brainwashing. I reminded him of my conversation with his son's attorney in which he had conveyed his concerns about the potential for an alienation with the boy as well. After all, if the father had engaged in an alienation with his daughter, it is logical to conclude he would do so with his son. Shortly after the session with the father, I received a call from the mother stating that her daughter had

dropped by the home to visit with her brother and that she and her daughter held a pleasant conversation. They agreed to return to therapy. As it is my practice in alienation cases, I videoed the session. I do so for many reasons, but in this particular situation I had hoped it would elicit civility with each other. The session was quite ameliorative with the girl listening to her mother's clarification of the family myths as well as of the girl's misconceptions of her. The girl was receptive to her mother's rewrite. The mother again apologized for not always calmly disciplining her and for sometimes stating things in anger which she subsequently regretted. After this session, I called the father and apprised him of the outcome. I thanked him for his efforts to influence his daughter as I was sure that his support and approval must have been a factor in the girl's receptivity. He affirmed that he had spoken to his daughter and strongly encouraged her to reconcile with her mother. In the subsequent session between the mother and the girl, I gave the mother the DVD of the previous session so that she and her daughter could view it together in order to reinforce the progress they had made and to relive the emotions they had exchanged. (It is also my practice to give the family the DVD of a session when it facilitates the therapeutic goal.) Mother and daughter were appreciative of this gesture, and they became teary-eyed, perhaps reliving the emotional moments just by thinking about them. In the current session, the two women made arrangements to spend time together, and they planned activities of mutual interest. The girl shared with her mother her intentions for seeking a more challenging job, and the mother offered her assistance in updating her resume. The mother cancelled the next session stating that things were going very well between her and her daughter and she anticipated her daughter's return to her home. The mother confirmed that they had watched the session together and, as I had expected, the girl rediscovered what her mother means to her. Shortly thereafter, she did move back home with her mother. They decided in the short term to attempt to resolve their remaining difficulties on their own.

I spoke to the mother to obtain an update for this book. She stated that her daughter recently moved in with her father, who had manipulated her allegiance in his custody battle regarding their son and that, to her regret, the adversarial nature of the legal proceedings were prohibiting further progress in reversing the PAS. Nevertheless, she believed that the adversarial relationship between her and her daughter was mitigated: her daughter had failed to appear in court to testify against her in the father's frivolous petition for an order of protection against her. The mother does not believe that this positive development could have occurred were it not for the therapy. She is also hopeful that their relationship will improve once the legal issues are settled. She is optimistic that estrangement from her daughter will not again rear its ugly head.

The initial mitigation of the PAS was accomplished as a result of working with all family members as well as with the son's attorney. There would not likely have been any progress without this systemic approach—and by systemic, I am referring not only to the family system but also to the judicial system. The alienating father was crucial to influencing the girl—both positively at first and then negatively. The leverage I had with him derived from the support of his son's attorney. Clearly, an individual treatment modality could not have afforded the environment in which occurred the exchange of the palliative emotions between the mother and daughter. Those meaningful emotional moments released in the therapy will likely have a lasting palliative impact on the girl

and may yet lead to the resumption of a meaningful mother/daughter relationship. At least this is the mother's expectation.

I began to treat a family consisting of three children (two latency age boys and one girl in her late teens) and their two parents who had a contentious divorce. I initially met the parents a number of years earlier when they initiated treatment for marriage counseling. Treatment terminated after a few sessions because they concluded they had irreconcilable differences. Neither parent left with the belief that I had judged or had blamed either of them. Several years later the father contacted me, alleging that his former wife was attempting to alienate him from his three children. He stated that none of his children return his phone calls, text messages, or e-mails and that his 17-year-old daughter has not visited in three months. He further stated that his sons visit only sporadically and it is frequently an argument with his former wife to send them out for the visits. He alleged that his former wife does nothing to encourage the visits, and when the boys do visit, they are frequently silly, uncooperative, and sometimes disrespectful. He petitioned the court to have his visitation rights enforced, and he alleged alienation as grounds for the petition. The children's lawyer recommended family therapy, and both parties approved my assignment as the family therapist. I am confident that the mother had consented to my appointment because of my neutrality in the marital therapy. I met with her for an individual session to explore what she perceived was happening in the family and particularly with the relationships between the children and their father. She began the session by expressing to me about her deep commitment to her children and that she did not doubt the father's love for them. She declared she had been the primary caretaker during their marriage: she was the parent who arranged her work schedule around the children's needs so that she was available for all school activities, supervising homework, making lunches, keeping all routine and emergency medical appointments, arranging for family photos, chauffeuring the children to and from their extracurricular activities. She was the parent who arose at night with the sick child and assumed responsibility for helping their oldest child apply to colleges and complete scholarship applications. Regarding her former husband, she expressed her fears that he might try to gain their children's allegiances with his superior financial resources. She expressed further concerns that he does not set appropriate limits and discipline for the children. It was apparent that she was fearful that the father would be perceived by the children to be a sugar daddy while she was viewed as the disciplinary grinch. She acknowledged that she has no life outside of motherhood. In her desperation not to lose the affections of her children, out of her fear that she is unable to compete with her former husband's resources in providing for the children, out of smarting from the rejection, and because of her perception of having been discarded like an old shoe, she embarked on a campaign of alienation. I listened intently and empathetically to her concerns and to her underlying feelings, and I believe that I was able to gain her trust that I would be as objective in the co-parenting and family counseling as I had been in the prior marital therapy. I surmised the alienation could be reversed if the father was able to convince her that he did not wish to minimize her to the children or use his superior resources to influence them to prefer him. I then met with the father and encouraged empathy for his former wife's plight so as to minimize her sense of worthlessness and dependency. He, too, needed to know I understood the validity of his anger due to the alienation. It was not easy to get him to empathize with her for

her new position as a consequence of their divorce than it was for her to recognize that the new situation required more of a shared parenting arrangement.

I scheduled the session between the father and the children, and I joined with the children about how they would like their family to change during this difficult time. The children were quite verbal about wishing for an end to the parental hostility, for which they held their mother only minimally responsible while placing most of the blame on their father. I was impressed that they did not completely exonerate their mother; this was hopeful. I asked them a question, which is also my typical routine in these cases—to rate their parents on a scale of one to ten regarding how effectively they are co-parenting, with number one being terrible. The consensus was a "three." Nothing to write home about! Their father acknowledged their observation, apologized to them, and committed to rectify the situation. The children shared these same feelings with their mother in the session with her. Each parent was duly shamed by their children for their immaturity regarding how they treat each other. (Challenging people about their own misbehaviors is an intervention of systems therapy, and it is particularly effective when family members accept this task so that the therapist can remain above the sparring.) Sessions between the father and the children were also utilized to support the father's efforts at setting appropriate limits on the children in response to their disrespect and defiance of him. He also shared his pain regarding their refusal to have a meaningful relationship with him. He further used the sessions to clarify the misperceptions they held about him and about his lack of involvement with them. As per my agreement with the mother, she encouraged the children to discuss with their father any issues they had with him so that she could resign as their messenger. As the therapy progressed, I was able to help the mother acknowledge that she unwittingly burdened her children with her emotional baggage so that they felt obliged to be her emotional support—a very typical dynamic in single parent families and particularly applicable in families with an alienation. Using me as a sounding board became an intermediary step for her so that the children could be freed from this responsibility. But I also encouraged her strengths. For one thing, she developed the confidence to return to school to complete her master's degree. After six months of therapy, the hostility between the parents was greatly reduced. As of this writing, the father reported that the visits with his children have improved greatly: all three children visit regularly and their behavior is greatly improved. He recently exclaimed to me, "I have my kids back!" (This seems to be a common refrain from alienated parents when they are reconnected with their kids.)

I attribute the reversal of the PAS in this case to the philosophical underpinnings of structural family therapy: that the family members heal each other out of love for each other—in this case, the love that the parents have for their children superceded their enmity for each other. The other critical factor was early court-ordered intervention for family therapy before the PAS had progressed too far and before a professional rescuer was able to embolden the residential parent.

Upon the recommendation of the children's attorney, I was assigned by the judge as the family therapist for two latency age children and their father to provide therapeutic visits and make recommendations to the court as to when the father should have his unsupervised visits restored. The father and his estranged wife were engaged in a nasty divorce and battle for custody. The father had been prohibited from any contact with his children for four months as a result of an order of protection. Upon the advice of the mother's attorney, she declined to participate in co-parenting counseling. (Heaven forbid there should be attempts to transform the adversarial nature of custody proceedings into one of cooperation and collaboration. What could have possibly been the attorney's motivation?) I met with the father, and he related to me the circumstances under which the order of protection had been granted. At the time, he was still residing in the marital residence but his wife was scheming to get him out. Had he voluntarily moved out, he would have been accused of abandoning his children. The order of protection "resolved" this marital dispute. The father related how his wife would frequently disappear with their children, sometimes for weeks at a time, and refused to inform him of their whereabouts. Unwilling to remain in the dark, he decided to follow them, but his wife sped away. Driving above the speed limit, she was stopped by a policeman to whom she reported she was escaping her physically abusive husband. An order of protection was thus granted, not only in reference to his wife, but which also included his children, on the basis that the father had put his children at risk by "forcing his wife to drive recklessly" in order to escape him. Talk about blaming the victim! I confirmed with the children's attorney that there were no allegations of neglect or abuse against the father. The father conveyed to me that the attorneys had informed him that it will likely take the children's therapist a minimum of six months to ready them to see him again. I responded to the father that he is the only one in a position to accomplish this "readying." I informed him that therapeutic visits between him and his children will immediately commence with the goal of reunification as soon as possible. The father broke down and sobbed and expressed that no other words could bring him more pleasure and relief. Upon seeing their father during the first therapeutic session, the children ran to him and fought to sit on his lap. His older child exclaimed, "We finally got to see you!" They expressed, "Mommy told us that the judge thought that we'd be upset to see you. That's not true!" (Gee, I wonder how the judge got this idea.) The children pleaded for things to go back to the way it was before when they could see him every day. Upon my recommendation, the father was granted a weekend visit with them, and I scheduled the second session between the children and their father subsequent to the weekend visit. I inquired how the visit had transpired, and the children were gleeful about it. I terminated the therapy by recommending to the children's attorney that the father's full parental rights be immediately restored. I added the caveat that the parents should be mandated into co-parent counseling, which the father was willing to do. I conveyed to the father to feel free to call me at any time should he need my services again. I was not again contacted by the family or by the lawyer, which I interpreted to mean that two things had occurred: the father and the children continued to have meaningful relationships, and the mother, upon the counsel of her attorney, continued to reject the suggestion for co-parent counseling. I contacted the father many months later, and he confirmed that his relationships with his children have continued unfettered but that his former wife refuses to engage in a co-parenting relationship.

I cringe to conjecture about a very different outcome that likely would have materialized had an individually oriented therapist been instead assigned. Such a therapist would have required protracted time to join with the children and then to reach an "interpretation" about their readiness for a relationship with their father. Of course, the children

would have been escorted to this therapist under the auspices of their alienating mother, thereby almost guaranteeing that they would have parroted their mother's hostile feelings and attitudes towards their father. The time required for the joining process might well have afforded the mother the opportunity to succeed in brainwashing them against their father. (The reader has already discovered the typical developments in these situations. It is exemplified by the latency age girl who, in just a few months, changed from a child who lovingly and affectionately interacted with her father to a denigrating puppet who verbalized visit refusal.) My major issue, however, in this case was the conduct of the mother's attorney. I refrain from using the characterization as professional rescuer; I do not believe the lawyer's motivations were even misguidedly noble. I suspect that this attorney falls into Mr. Previto's designated category as a "ravager." Without establishing any just cause to alienate the father, this attorney served to embolden the mother's alienating efforts. The attorney did not behave in a manner consistent with the best interest of the children or, for that matter, in the best interest of the client: not counseling the client in accordance with the previously referenced case law requiring the residential parent to facilitate a relationship with the other parent. In fact, the attorney did quite the opposite by filing a petition for an order of protection based on spurious allegations. This exactly exemplifies my assertion that the alienator alone cannot victimize the targeted parent but requires professional support to do so.

When I began working with an alienated father and his two children, one a preteen and the other in early teens, the level of the PAS was relatively mild. There had been no visits for more than five months due to—you guessed it—a child abuse finding. In my opinion, the case was mishandled by PAS-unaware CPS staff, who had indicated the father based on a single, highly embellished, suspicious abuse allegation: the younger child had sustained a tiny mark as a result of the father's efforts to restrain her from a violent, physically aggressive temper tantrum. CPS had been further co-opted by the alienating mother, who buttressed the abuse case by asserting that the father had a long history of physically abusing the family. The mother "documented" this purely specious history, which was corroborated by the brainwashed children, with an order of protection, that had been obtained on completely fabricated domestic violence allegations, but which had also been corroborated by the children. By not fully exploring the specious abuse and domestic violence allegations, the police, the judiciary, and CPS instead accepted the mother's and children's accounting of the family history. They acted to condemn the father on such flimsy grounds, which could not be substantiated by disinterested parties. The professionals thereby emboldened the alienating mother, disempowered the father, and validated for the children the myth that their father was an abuser.

In the initial therapy sessions, the children were only mildly to moderately disrespectful and deprecating, but this soon diminished as the father reminded them about his far-reaching involvement with them–information I certainly did not possess–using pictures and videos as well as exhaustive discussions about the family history. Being careful not to criticize their mother, he debunked the myth that he is an abuser. The children, in just a few sessions, responded positively to him: they updated him about their lives; they informed him about school, their friends, and about their activities; expressed to him in and out of session that they looked forward to the visits with him; they were affectionate with him; and both children shared

with him many maudlin moments as they went down memory lane together. The indication of the presence of the PAS was reflected primarily in the children's precautions to "safeguard" their mother from ascertaining how positively they felt towards him. With each new therapeutic visit between them, the mutual bonding intensified. Their mother, however, had traveled much further along the PAS continuum, and she was determined not to go it alone. She continued to engage in alienating behaviors, but the children initially resisted the brainwashing. They became severely ensnared in the PAS process, however, at the precise moment when the court reduced the mother's maintenance award. She then capitalized on this opportunity to yank the children along with her into the severe category. Alleging that their father was no longer meeting his child support obligations, she withheld necessities and extras from them. She asserted to them that he had hoodwinked the court into believing that his income had drastically dropped, which it indeed had. The children's maltreatment of their father commenced at the precise moment of their mother's escalating deprecation of him. When she arrived at my office to pick them up at the end of the first visit subsequent to having received the court ruling, she exploded at her ex-husband like a volcano. It was amazing how quickly the children reverted to the deprecation of their father. After having witnessed their mother's blistering harangue of him, they never resumed being loving, affectionate, and joyful with him. During every succeeding session and visit, they harangued him about failing to support them. The campaign of vilification and denigration had been introjected as they regurgitated their mother's demeaning epithets and then contributed their own condemnations. They began to physically attack him as well. Ultimately, the alienating mother's goal of "parentectomy" was achieved.

There has been a complete severing of all contact between the father and his children. Several years subsequent to the therapy, there are no visits; the children do not respond to their father's e-mails, phone calls, or text messages. The father knows nothing about their current medical, psychological, educational, and social lives.

This case was obviously not a treatment success. I have included it here to make two important points: (1) to exemplify that facilitating corrective interactions between the alienated parent and the child can have an immediate palliative result, and (2) to emphasize that there would have likely been a very different outcome were it not for all the professional rescuers.

I was assigned to provide therapeutic visits between a previously discussed latency age boy and his father. The father had been denied all contact with his son for five months resulting from a flimsy CPS finding of neglect, which would have likely been reversed had the father possessed the funds to go to trial. The mother refused to participate in the therapy beyond the initial **if only** session. The boy was initially verbally and physically abusive to his father, which lasted for several sessions. There was a gradual improvement during a one-year period until they attained a healthy father/son relationship and a reunification. Four years subsequent to the therapy, they are today very bonded to each other. The success can be attributed to a structural family therapy modality which empowered the father in the sessions to facilitate a deprogramming of his son. The therapy supported the perseverance of the father, who refused to submit to his despair after the initial painful sessions of abuse and humiliation and who did not allow himself to be manipulated by his estranged wife into being excluded from his son's life. The father demonstrated his love for his son by remaining involved and persistent. He developed the skills to avoid transferring his anger for his former wife to his son when the boy assumed the role of the puppet of his ventriloquist alienating mother. Throughout the initial therapy, the father continually weighed the options between remaining in his son's life—thereby contributing to the stress on his son from being caught like a rope in a tug of war between his parents—and dropping out of his life—thereby eliminating the stress of the tug of war. In the end, he instinctually fought for a role in his son's life.

But the positive reversal of the PAS was also a result of my collaboration with the court, which was willing to exercise its authority to mandate the alienating mother to comply with the therapy and with the unsupervised visits. The judge served notice on her that he would impose severe consequences—including the possibility of awarding the father sole custody—if she continued to sabotage the relationship between her son and his father.

The attorney for a boy in his mid-teens referred him to me to facilitate a reunification with his father due to an estrangement fostered by the boy's mother. The court had informed the mother that she will lose custody if she sabotages the therapy and the reunification process. The family had been in and out of court for several years, the father having to fight for his parental rights and visitation at every turn. Long periods would transpire during which time the father's visits with his son were unfettered. But on the mother's whim, she arbitrarily refused to permit contact for extended periods, and the father sometimes reacted to these alienating maneuvers by withdrawing instead of fighting. In keeping with my customary practice, I met first with the mother, the residential parent. She conveyed that she does not trust her former husband's motivations, alleging that he waltzes in and out of their son's life. I surmised that she also felt abandoned, and

I also suspected that she feared that the father would become a more significant parental figure than she because her son was now a teenager. She further expressed that the father has an "anger management issue" and that her son is silenced by him for that reason. She was convinced that her son feared his "controlling" father and that this fear would prevent him from expressing his feelings and opinions openly. I listened to her concerns and fears, and I reassured her that I had no intentions to undermine her relationship with her son as I helped him to rebuild the relationship with his father. I further stated that facilitating healthy communication between her son and his father could certainly be one focus of the therapy. She declined my suggestion to participate in counseling beyond the **if only** session, but she pledged not to demean the father to her son. She and I agreed that she should feel free to contact me about any concern as the therapy developed. My suspicion was that she had been duly chastened by the real possibility of losing custody should she be a saboteur, and I was counting on this fear for assurance that she would not undermine the therapy. The therapy lasted for a year and a half, beginning with weekly sessions between the boy and his father for a period of a year and then decreasing to biweekly sessions during the final six months. I remained in periodic phone contact with the mother throughout the treatment. The sessions for the first six weeks were difficult, awkward, and painful. The boy entered the first session addressing his father by his first name and declined his father's request to use a term indicative of their relationship. The father expressed his pain because the boy had labeled him an "absentee father," among other degrading epithets. The boy was unmoved and unapologetic. He tenaciously held firm that his father had "abandoned" him, and he expressed that his father had surreptitious ra-

ther than genuine motives for seeking a relationship with him. The father apologized profusely for the periods when he had withdrawn from his life and expressed that he would do it very differently, if he had it to do again. He clarified for his son that, while he was responsible for some of their estrangement, he was not at fault the majority of the time when he had fought tenaciously to have contact with him. The father began to sob about the events in their lives that had brought them to the current sad state of affairs. The boy was not at all gracious in response to his father's vulnerability and humility. He declined to accept his father's apology, regrets, or his efforts to rebuild their relationship. He stated that his mother told him that his father will see him only if another obligation brings him to their neighborhood and that his mother reiterated to him that he should not trust that his father will remain in his life. My optimism that the mother would not sabotage the reunification was fading. It was clear to me that the boy felt caught between his parents out of loyalty to his mother and to the efforts being put forth by his father. In conversations with me, the mother had made comments that the father was insincere and manipulative. I responded by sharing the detrimental effects on her son of being caught between his parents, like a rope in a tug of war. At some point she became reassured that her relationship with her son was not being threatened, and she did eventually mask from her son the negative feelings she held for his father. The father did not give up, despite his son's anger, resistance, and challenge at almost every turn. He kept showing up–to every degrading therapy session; he shared his pain regarding the state of their relationship, at times sobbing about his fear of losing his son permanently; he expressed to his son that he is the most important person in his life and that he gets depressed at the thought that they will not overcome their estrangement; and without casting aspersions on the boy's mother, he recounted all his legal efforts to enforce his parental rights and visitation. The boy began to soften in about six weeks, and the father asked him for suggestions as to how they can move forward. The boy agreed to meeting outside of the sessions for brief planned activities, and the mother supported these arrangements. Therapy helped the father to avoid transferring his anger for his former wife to his son when he became his mother's puppet. I coached the father to relinquish his defensiveness when hearing his son's concerns, and I helped him to distinguish legitimate concerns–such as how he silences his son by interrupting him– from spurious allegations. The limited outside activities were so successful that all day visits began after two months of the therapy's commencement, and weekend sleepovers commenced after three months. And, oh yes, by the end of the second month, the boy began calling his father, "dad." When the extended weekend visits were initiated, I suggested to the mother that being "off-duty" had been well-earned, and I explored with her in what ways she might use the time to take care of herself. She did appreciate my concern for her emotional needs. Shortly thereafter, the boy reported that he had informed his mother that he does not like it when she demeans his father to him or that she puts him in the middle of their parental disputes. Ten months into the therapy, the boy and his father were spontaneously sharing their respective fears of being hurt, and they developed a metaphor for their pain that they each carry a "shield" behind which they can hide in self-protection. The father helped his son with this issue by using self-disclosure about his own difficulties relating to peers when he was his son's age. The father encouraged his son to engage in peer activities, such as sports, as the boy was so-cially withdrawn. (I contend that healthy self-esteem develops as a result of how our parents relate to us and to each other and by subsequent engagement in positive peer relationships. It is therefore the parents' job– and not the job of the therapist–to develop a child's self-esteem.)

The boy eventually accomplished what I had been unable to do: get his parents to communicate with each other on his behalf. He did so by failing some subjects. The mother initiated contact with the father, and the two of them met on their own to implement a plan to set limits and consequences on their son and to put an end to his ability to manipulate them. I am convinced that this development was facilitated by the father, who overcame any temptation to demean the mother to the boy and because he did not blame the mother for their son's problems or threaten to seek residential custody. The parents collaborated together, and gradually the boy's behavior was brought under control. The therapy reached a pinnacle when the boy and the father shared with each other in session their respective short-story writings. This experience opened up a deeper and more meaningful exchange of feelings. The boy's fear of relationships was revealed in his writings, and his father guided him through this process, acknowledging that his role models have not been the best. The father then added that he and his mother are working conscientiously together to model the relationship which they would like him to eventually develop with a partner. The father read one of his short stories about a boy and his father who had been estranged but who eventually found each other. The two of them, along with this therapist, became particularly maudlin at that moment. When we summed up the therapy, the boy and his father agreed that their relationship is meaningful and that the boy is maturing age-appropriately. A telephone call to the family for an update for this book confirmed that the father remains very much in the boy's life.

It must be obvious that the emotions which were shared between the father and his son were the basis for the reversal of a severe case of the PAS and that such emotional connection could not have been created in a therapy between only the boy and a therapist. It was also the result of the firm position by the court that alienation would not be tolerated. The modest input from the mother was also a factor.

A latency age boy was verbally and physically abusive to his father, but the father did not give up despite the maltreatment and despite the mother's ongoing alienating maneuvers, which included the filing of fallacious reports of child abuse and domestic violence. The therapy, in which the mother refused to participate, consisted of the boy and his father. In my role as catalyst, I facilitated the father's deprogramming efforts to dispel his son of the malicious family myths about him, helped the father to set appropriate limits and consequences on his son for the maltreatment, assisted the father to sublimate his anger, encouraged their relationship through interesting activities outside of the therapy sessions, and supported the father's multiple petitions for legal remedy. The boy soon began to treat his father with respect. The therapy lasted a year, principally because the mother was emboldened to continue her alienating maneuvers as a result of support from co-opted, PAS-unaware professionals, including a matrimonial attorney, an individual therapist, and CPS personnel. As of the writing of this book five years later, however, the father and the boy maintain a meaningful and healthy relationship with each other in spite of the mother's persistent alienating maneuvers—her refusal to co-parent, and her unabated child abuse allegations.

I was referred a case for therapeutic visits by the lawyer of a preteen child who lived with both parents but did not acknowledge the father's existence, not even to say "hello" when entering or leaving the family home. I was in continual contact with the child's attorney to whom I reported all the events occurring in the therapeutic sessions, and I updated him on my assessment that the mother was engaging in an alienation. During the sessions, the boy repeatedly lambasted his father with humiliating but frivolous rationalizations; he revealed no ambivalence or guilt; and he reflexively supported his alienating mother. I helped the father to avoid transferring his anger for his estranged wife to her puppet son, and I coached the father in efforts to dispel for the boy the numerous malicious family myths about him. There was little movement in the therapy, however. I expressed my serious concerns to the child's attorney as to the abusive effects on the child due to the alienation. The child's obnoxious and disrespectful behaviors did not bode well for the prospects for handling authority relationships. The normalization of lies and deceit was also not in the child's best interests. I further registered my strong objections to the mother's petition requesting to move with the child across the country, believing that the result would be "parentectomy." The attorney registered credible opposition to the mother's petition, and the judge was persuaded to deny the petition. The mother moved without the child, and the child meaningfully reconnected with the father overnight.

My collaboration with the child's lawyer on another case also enabled significant progress in reversing the PAS, although treatment is still occurring as of the writing of this book. The lawyer had referred to me his preteen client for therapeutic visits, who had refused all contact with the mother for 14 months. As is my practice, I offered co-parenting counseling. The father initially participated for a number of sessions, and then the child began to interact positively with the mother during the therapeutic visits. The father unilaterally and inexplicably withdrew from the counseling, and the child again disengaged from the mother, becoming verbally and physically abusive of her. I was in continual contact with the child's attorney, and he kept the judge apprised of the developments in the case. I conveyed to the attorney my unequivocal professional opinion—supported by observable events—regarding the negative effects of the PAS on the child, and I strongly and persuasively documented in a court report that alienation is a form of child abuse. At the hearing subsequent to the submission of my report, the judge affirmatively used his authority to convey to the father that he will not tolerate the continuation of the alienation, and he threatened a change in custodial custody as a penalty. From that hearing date forward, the PAS began to reverse. The mother arrived with her child for the subsequent therapeutic session announcing that their visits had resumed and that, "My affectionate and loving child is back." When I asked the child what accounted for the turnaround, I was apprised that the father had insisted upon it. And just like that, instantaneously, 14 months of reproach, estrangement, aggression, and disdain were reversed. This case is further evidence of how specious the PAS rejection actually is.

A father contacted me to provide court-ordered therapeutic visits between him and his two teenage children. From the time his children were preschoolers, his former wife ran interference in his relationships with them, and she had permitted only a few visits each year for a decade. He had been in court this entire time, and multiple therapists were assigned to facilitate a reunification, but to no avail. Either the individually oriented

therapists accepted the children's verbalized abhorrence for their father and declined to effectuate the reunification; or else the therapists were quickly fired by the alienating mother when they declined to be co-opted by her. The mother never received more than a verbal admonition from the judge for obstructing the relationships between the father and his children. I do not understand how the system allowed this travesty to occur. At the time I was hired, there had been no contact whatsoever between the father and his children for more than a year. The children did not respond to the father's phone calls and text messages except to express that they did not wish to visit with him. After my initial meeting with the father, I scheduled a session with the mother, who feigned cooperation: she permitted only two therapeutic sessions, which went so well that the father's expectations were far exceeded. In those sessions, the father went down memory lane with his children, having brought pictures at my suggestion, and reminded them of his involvement with them before he and their mother had separated. He sobbed about how much he misses them and how hurt he is because of their estrangement. The three were soon sobbing together and went through an entire box of tissues as they expressed their love for each other. Both children confirmed that they desire that the visits immediately resume. But when their mother arrived for the children at the conclusion of the second session, she declined to schedule another appointment, and she subsequently informed me that the children had lied about everything expressed in the two sessions. She stated that they have no desire to see their father, and she refused to schedule any additional therapeutic visits. I contacted the father for an update for this book, and he informed me that he had again initiated court action subsequent to the therapy with me, and yet another therapist was assigned. When the new therapist supported the reunification, the mother again withdrew from the therapy. Having exhausted his funds, the father returned to court pro se. The judge, perhaps appalled by the history of this case, ordered full compliance with the father's visitation rights with his children. And guess what? Several more months have transpired since the court hearing, and the mother has yet to comply with the visits. The father will again be returning to court to file a violation. He believes that his older child is lost to him at this point.

I am sure it does not escape the reader why I cited this case as a treatment example: the two sessions will likely be unforgettably memorable for the children; and, of course, it is just one additional illustration of the speciousness of the PAS child's claims of animosity as well as exposing the receptiveness of these children to contact with their loving, alienated parent. It further exemplifies the injustice in our current systems that a father must spend more than a decade in court and still has received no justice.

A father of a preschool boy contacted me to help the child "get over feeling rejected by his mother." The father, who is the residential parent, expressed to me that his son had returned from a visit with his mother and sobbed that his mother had told him that she does not love him. The father reacted by discontinuing the mother's visits and initiated legal action to have the court sanction his action. I talked to the father about how the cessation of visits will only confirm his son's fantasy. He agreed to co-parent counseling, and I arranged for a session with the mother. There are always two sides to every story, and why individual therapists do not recognize this is beyond me. I met with the parents a few times to address their unresolved marital issues, which were contaminating their parental roles, and I helped them resolve their significant parenting differences. I

shared the alarming statistics on children from divorce when the parents fail to maintain a civil and respectful co-parenting relationship. The parents had a rude awakening from this information. The father immediately restored the mother's visits, and he withdrew his petition. They continued in co-parenting counseling for a brief period to maintain their progress.

This last case, in particular, exemplifies the life-altering, differing approaches to treatment between an individually oriented therapist versus a family systems therapist. The individual therapist rarely contacts the nonpresenting parent while the family therapist would not proceed to treat without reaching out to the other parent. The former intervention generally sets off a chain reaction which emboldens the alienating parent, further disempowers and eventually victimizes the targeted parent, and deprives the child of one of the two most important people in her/his life.

I have presented a small fraction of my cases at all stages of the PAS. The improvements and outcomes provide substantiation that family systems therapy is highly effective in treating the PAS family and should therefore be the treatment of choice. This book would have been too lengthy to include additional treatment summaries–some equally successful in reversing the PAS, some failures, and some in which the seedlings of the PAS had been planted but did not germinate because a systems intervention was initiated in the early stages of the family's dissolution.

Two factors account for the successful treatments. One factor was the stage in which the PAS was at the time family therapy was initiated. But the more probable factor can be attributed to a collaborative relationship between the family therapist and the judicial system–a judicial system when it used its authority to take a firm stand against the PAS and guaranteed a level playing field between the alienating and alienated parents.

I must make one last point that is an essential quality of my therapy as a structural family therapist, and it may come as a surprise to some readers. This factor is how I use myself as a therapist. More important than any intervention technique–and to call it a technique is a misnomer as per Minuchin–is the human element which I bring to my therapy. As the reader may recall from my treatment summaries, I judiciously disclosed in the sessions my personal experiences. I think perhaps that I did not emphasize strongly enough just how important self-disclosure is to my therapy. Having been a child victim of the PAS, I believe it has given me a unique capacity to empathize with each family member and with each role the member plays in this crazy family dance called the PAS. I share with the family the feelings I have endured from my personal experience with it. I share the detrimental effects on my sister and me resulting from the perverse triangle; I share how being brain-washed to hate my father affected my intimate peer relationships; I share what it was like to be a rope in a tug-of-war with each parent pulling on the separate ends; I share how my mother felt in an emotionally barren marriage due to my father's workaholism. I share how my mother's mother, who lived with us until my parent's divorce, engaged in a perverse triangle with my mother to scapegoat my father. But I also convey hope and possibilities in that the triangle was not repeated in the next generation when my son's father and I divorced. The families change because of the human experiences which I bring to the sessions and my willingness to share it with them. And then I expect that they will respond by changing each other in the best interests of their children.

So I will close this chapter where it began, with the wisdom and compassion from my mentor, Sal Minuchin (1981), who expressed the following about how the therapist's **emotional** as well as intellectual presence assists in the healing, "When techniques are guided by such wisdom, then therapy becomes healing" (p. 290).

Chapter 24

PARENTAL ALIENTATION SYNDROME: A FORM OF CHILD ABUSE AND MORE

Who are the true victims of the PAS? What price is being paid for the damages it inflicts on family functioning? I have heard it expressed by more than one judge, by more than one attorney for the child, and by more than one therapist that only the alienated parent suffers abuse resulting from the PAS; and because they are "big boys and big girls," they are expected to, "Just get over it and move on." The difficulty in acknowledging the PAS as a form of child abuse is a consequence of society's failure to have reached a consensus on what constitutes emotional abuse. Emotional abuse is not so easily recognizable because it does not leave physical bruises or scars, and the PAS child does not confirm the brainwashing but instead refutes it.

I take an unequivocal position that the PAS is a form of emotional child abuse, as do those who were interviewed for this book. What is the support for this position? Gardner (1998) stated, "A parent who inculcates a PAS in a child is indeed perpetrating a form of emotional abuse in that such programming may not only produce lifelong alienation from a loving parent, but lifelong psychiatric disturbance in a child" (p. xxi). Gar-

barino and Scott (1992) labeled the PAS child as being "psychologically battered." Clawar and Rivlin (1991) asserted:

The effects of losing not only the intact family, but also a parent, hang heavily over children, touching them in ways that can wreak havoc in many realms of life both in the present and future. As adults, many victims of bitter custody battles who had been permanently removed from a target parent . . . still long to be reunited with the lost parent. The loss cannot be undone. Childhood cannot be recaptured. Gone forever is that sense of history, intimacy, lost input of values and morals, self-awareness through knowing one's beginnings, love, contact with extended family, and much more. Virtually no child possesses the ability to protect him or herself against such an undignified and total loss. (p. 105)

Major (2006) declared the following:

Because PAS is among the most severe kinds of abuse of a child's emotions, there will be scars and lost opportunities for normal development. The child is at risk of growing up and being an alienator also, because the alienating parent has been the primary role model. (p. 285)

The resistance to recognizing this syndrome as a form of emotional child abuse must be understood in the context of the alienating parent's ultimate goal, which is to permanently sever the relationship between the other parent and their child. Cartwright (2006) elaborated about this point:

> The awful outcome of PAS is the complete separation of a child or children from a parent. Even more dreadful is that it is deliberately caused, maliciously done, and entirely preventable. This terrible form of child abuse has long-lasting effects for all concerned. (p. 286)

The detrimental and abusive affects on children resulting from the loss of a parental relationship is aptly characterized by Everett (2006) when he defined PAS as "a destructive family pathology because it attributes a quality of 'evil,' without cause or foundation, to a parent who once nurtured and protected the same child that has now turned against her or him" (p. 228). And Frank Williams (1990) coined the phrase "parentectomy" to describe the ultimate goal of the PAS, which is to sever the relationship with the child and the targeted parent.

In her book, *Adult Children of Parental Alienation Syndrome,* Baker (2007) concluded from her research on this population that the PAS is a form of emotional child abuse. Some of her core findings I paraphrase here as follows, but I refer the reader to her book for a complete accounting:

1. Damage to the child's self-esteem resulting from the pain of being "enlightened" that the targeted parent does not love and has rejected her/him;
2. Feeling bad about herself/himself resulting from the introjected negative view of a parent, with whom children instinctively identify;
3. Being ignored by the alienating parent for association with the targeted parent;
4. Terrorizing the child, who is criticized and/or punished for expressing normal feelings and opinions;
5. Corruption of the child whereby the alienating parent tolerates extreme acting out behaviors in exchange for the child's allegiance and also because the child's maltreatment of the targeted parent is normalized;
6. Exploiting the child's dependency as a captive audience of the alienating parent, who chooses to expose the child to adult information that exceed the child's cognitive and emotional capabilities to handle;
7. Formation of shame and guilt resulting from the child's inability to fulfill the alienating parent's expectation as her/his problem solver; and
8. Subjecting the child to the fear of abandonment as a punishment for the child's desire for contact with the targeted parent (pp. 84–99).

Baker (2007) summarized the research of her book as follows: 65 percent of the study's participants were afflicted with low self-esteem; 70 percent suffered episodes of depression due to the belief of being unloved by the targeted parent and from extended separation from that parent; 35 percent engaged in substance abuse as a means to mask their feelings of pain and loss; 40 percent lacked trust in themselves as well as in meaningful relationships because the trust was broken with their parents; 50 percent suffered the heartbreaking repetition of the alienation by becoming alienated from their own children; and 57.5 percent were beset by divorce, higher than the national average of 52 percent (pp. 180–191).

Robert Hiltzik labeled the PAS a form of child abuse when he described what he has witnessed in his 22 years of family law practice:

> The alienating parent is not enforcing discipline. The crucial dynamic is that the alienating parent strives to be the child's best friend while the other parent is left with the responsibility of being the disciplinarian. The children then run amok, and the alienating parent is sanctioning this because they are saying to their child, "I won't enforce the rules as long as you do what I say and give your other parent a hard time. Make him miserable." I think the damage is pervasive. If you allow a child to conduct himself/herself in such a conflicted way, the child carries that throughout life. If the child can be so disrespectful to a parent without any justification whatsoever, then there is no doubt the child will exhibit similar conduct before other authority figures. Even the most amicable divorces have a negative impact on children. And with the PAS, the conflict is so heightened that the child becomes a victim of war. How healthy is it to turn feelings on and off? If you hate one of your parents and you don't know why, you can't love yourself and you can't love others.

Mr. Hiltzik asserted that, although there are therapists and attorneys who understand the negative ramifications to children of parental alienation, many judges do not recognize that it is a form of child abuse. He stated this problem as follows, "When the courts look at alienation, whom do they see is the victim? They see the victim to be the alienated parent. The courts don't see that it damages children."

Mr. Previto graphically described what he has encountered in his 17 years of practice as a marital attorney as to the damage done to children by the PAS when he stated, "If a child is walking across the train tracks, gets an electrical shock from the third rail but is not killed, the scars will be there for the rest of his life. The emotional scars resulting from an alienation are not going away either." Mr. Previto described some of these injuries to children as having to live with tremendous guilt for having allowed themselves to be manipulated by the custodial parent to be so abusive to their other parent.

Ms. Saltz stated in her interview that alienation is a form of child abuse. She expressed it this way, "Alienated children do not form healthy relationships as adults. And very often as adults, they don't have healthy relationships with their own children." Ms. Saltz added, "It's not healthy for these children not to see the noncustodial parent. I think children need to know where they come from, and if they are missing a parent, they are missing a part of themselves. If they miss out on one of their parents, there is a hole inside of them. And they don't fill that hole with good stuff." Ms. Saltz agreed that these children tend to hate themselves as a result of hating a parent. She commented, "And when you hate yourself, you are likely to act out."

Mr. Hecht believes that the negative effects of parental alienation are "impactful and severe" and agrees that children are susceptible to brainwashing by the residential parent because they are generally so impressionable. He expressed, however, that the courts face an acute dilemma in recognizing instances of parental alienation because there is only circumstantial evidence. He expressed the dilemma as follows: "There are no bruises and there are no scars with alienation. It's all under the surface. That's perhaps the biggest problem."

In my interview with Dr. Burkhard, I inquired as to her opinion as to whether she considers the PAS to be a form of child abuse and how it can be readily identified when observed. She replied the following, "This is maltreatment of children in the most profound way." She continued to explain that they are seeing children years subsequent to their initial evaluation so that her agency is in a position to observe the outcomes. She is concerned that PAS children are empowered when asked to join with the alienating parent as an ally. As a result, Dr. Burkhard affirmed the following:

These children do not follow rules; they are out of control; they are basically naughty and lack limits. These children behave as if they have license to do whatever they want. It may have begun as a breakdown in not having to respond to the authority of and respect for the other parent. In the cases of treatment or court failure to reunite, we have seen the lack of respect for authority figures including the favored parent, school, and the law. Among the cases where reunification efforts have failed are children who have dropped out of school, become addicted to drugs, born children out of wedlock addicted to drugs, and engaged in other antisocial behaviors. This is not a good outcome.

Dr. Burkhard became maudlin upon reporting these developments, and she expressed her chagrin by explaining, "They initially came in as high functioning kids from seemingly high functioning, involved parents."

To provide a clearer picture for the reader about how disturbed these children become, Dr. Burkhard compared them to another group of kids whom she treats on a regular basis. This other group of children have been raped, burned, beaten, sexually abused, and victims of crime. "If they are in the newspapers, the children are likely to wind up in this office because we specialize in traumatized children. And yet, they don't hold a candle in terms of symptoms and prognosis to the PAS children. PAS kids are

a mess." Dr. Burkhard continued to express how PAS children suffer emotional abuse:

Childhood is a time to develop a sense of responsibility. It is a time to develop a conscience. Children who become alienated have this fundamental aspect of their development derailed. They are not only not held accountable for their mistakes and misdeeds, they may be encouraged to tell lies or exaggerate the truth and otherwise act in ways that are disrespectful of others. That these behaviors are reinforced by a trusted parent further undermines normal moral development as well as the development of their ability to develop normal relationships.

Dr. Kelly asserted that children who become victims of the PAS suffer lifetime damage. She expressed, "They do not learn interpersonal problem solving because they are often prevented from working out realistic everyday conflicts with a parent. This is simply not healthy in the long run. This affects them in a very negative way." In addressing the damage of the PAS on adolescents, who are generally not receptive to confrontation, Dr. Kelly stated the following, "Adolescents are very difficult to disabuse of the PAS. Having permission or a sanction from a parent to treat the other parent so badly is going to, at some point, have a very deleterious effect on their ability to interact with others." Dr. Kelly is also concerned about the serious damage to children from false sex abuse allegations. She stated, "It confirms damage to the child as if the abuse really happened." She further commented:

The PAS undermines healthy family functioning, such as family hierarchy in that the boundaries between the parental and child subsystems breakdown when the child is elevated by the alienating parent to an adult level as a result of their coalition. This explains why PAS children often do not respond appropriately to authority figures, such as school principals, teachers, etc.

Dr. Kelly cited an example from her practice to concretize this message. She began working with a girl when she was nine years old, and Dr. Kelly was convinced that "the mom was determined to surgically remove the father from the girl's life." Dr. Kelly cautioned the mother that she was setting the girl up for "all sorts of authority problems because, when you teach a child to disrespect one authority, it will be transferred to other authorities." Dr. Kelly was reintroduced to the girl again when she was 15 years old, and, as she had predicted, the girl was exhibiting serious behavioral issues. The mother was unable to control her; the girl was not listening to any of her teachers or to any other adults, for that matter, and she had a problem with truancy. According to Dr. Kelly:

> Another lifelong penalty is that PAS children often pay results from the guilt that they bear for having abused their targeted parent, because, on some level they know that this treatment was unacceptable. And should the targeted parent no longer be available to them when they come to the realization of what has occurred in their family, there is no possibility for atonement.

In response to my question as to whether all children who are victims of the PAS are damaged, Dr. Kelly responded, "There are always resilient children, just as you see with physically abused children. But they are the exception!"

Ms. Zarkadas confirmed for me that she has witnessed during her 20 years of practice severe detrimental effects to the child as a result of parental alienation. She stated that

these difficulties run the gamut from problems in education, difficulties in peer relationships, illegal substance use, engaging in criminal activities, development of mental health disturbances. Ms. Zarkadas expressed, "These children are being asked to deal with adult situations that even adults don't know how to handle." She believes that when a parent engages in alienating practices, the child will walk away with the idea, "What did I do wrong?" Ms. Zarkadas elaborated by stating, "These kids walk away from these messes feeling that they are to blame."

I inquired of Ms. Zarkadas why the courts do not deem alienation to be a form of child abuse given the severity of the conditions which she had just described. She responded that it has not met the criteria of Article 10 of the Family Court Act, which defines abuse. But she insisted, "It should be criminalized. The pain these children suffer because of the decision by one parent to erase the other parent out of their life–is criminal!"

Ms. Courten stands with the others interviewed for this book in considering parental alienation to be a form of child abuse. She described what she sees happening to these children:

> In terms of showing disrespect for authority, it is absolutely there. These children get so convoluted in their thinking because mom tells them she loves them and says do this. And dad tells them he loves them and says do that. You get really mixed up little kids out of it. Because these kids lack control over what is happening to them by finding themselves in an upside down world–a world in which they are manipulated into believing that love is hate; that disrespect, defiance and maltreatment are acceptable; that their feelings must be denied–I do not see a good outcome for them. They become self-destructive. They attempt to take back con-

trol by adopting behaviors over which they do have control, such as bedwetting, drug use, eating disorders, drinking, and stealing. They become violent people.

Dr. Havlicek declared to me, "There is no question that PAS is a form of child abuse. It is a horror show. The damage to children is enormous. When a child loses a parent, they are killing off a part of themselves because there is an identity between the child and both parents. The result is that they become self injurious." Dr. Havlicek confirmed:

I see all the warning signs and all the red flags of this self-hatred: nightmares, anxiety, oppositional behaviors in school, presence of gastrointestinal syndromes, falling school grades, more susceptibility to peers with oppositional behaviors, juvenile delinquency, substance abuse, depression.

He asserted that he has much anecdotal evidence for the abuse from his practice in that he sees symptomatic adults who were child victims of the PAS.

Dr. Havlicek concluded that, in his professional opinion, most psychological problems and problematical behaviors do not have a primarily biological basis. Instead, he asserted, "the basis is rooted in a combination of disordered family circumstances and biological factors." Dr. Havlicek's extraordinary observation confirms what I had argued in the last chapter: that the mental health profession is rushing to medicate for a chemical imbalance before undertaking a comprehensive assessment of the IP's family situation in order to determine its impact on the patient's symptoms. By locating the site of pathology within the dysfunctional family transactions rather than within the individual has very different implications for treatment.

In his article, "Father? What father? Parental Alienation and its Effect on Children," appearing in the *Law Guardian Reporter,* Chaim Steinberger, Esq., (2006) painstakingly summarizes the literature which addresses the detrimental effects on children of the PAS. These effects include but are not limited to anxiety, self-loathing, rigidity, hopelessness, powerlessness, confusion, withdrawal, isolation, and hypocrisy. This exhaustive summary can be read in completion on Dr. Havlicek's website, www.drhavlicek .com.

The preceding chapter discussed the pathological implications for children who are caught in the perverse triangle. In the worst-case scenario, a psychosis is the result. In the least-case scenario, it was shown that the PAS inflicts on its young victims various degrees of chronic emotional disabilities, ongoing circumscription of potentials, and vulnerability to antisocial behaviors and to interpersonal difficulties. These damages accrue because of: a programming which distorts reality testing, perception, and judgment; a cognitive distortion resulting from the belief that the targeted parent's love and nurturing is instead maltreatment and rejection; the normalizing of deceit and cruelty; the fostering of a dependency upon a manipulative parent; the suppression of the superego, or conscience; the self-alienation from the repression of one's true feelings; a chronic state of anxiety that a slip of behavior will expose the true positive feelings and longing for the alienated parent; the loss of self as a result of the rejection of the alienated parent.

There is, additionally, the issue of damages to society from the PAS: it exacerbates the deleterious effects from divorce on the institution of the family–the building block of our culture. Given that 52 percent of marriages end in divorce, massive numbers of families and children are affected by the inevitable emotional turmoil that results from even the most amicable family break-up.

Divorcing parents who are mature and who therefore subjugate their needs to those of their children are able to minimize the damage to their children. But much of the research and anecdotal evidence indicate that children usually become triangulated into at least some of their parents' sparring even in the least adversarial divorce proceedings. Triangulation resulting from divorce is a cancer on our society, and it is metastasizing. It can no longer be swept under the rug. As concerned citizens, we must address the effects on culture when the family fails in its responsibility to keep children protected. Society ignores this circumstance to its own peril because there are inevitable costs attached to the psychological treatment of the conditions that result from the PAS. Society at large must ultimately bear these expenditures through higher health care costs, through incarceration expenses, and through social services and income maintenance when these children's handicaps prevent them from functioning as contributing members to society. These costs are particularly devastating at this time when public budgets are under economic stress. But the greater tragedy is that the PAS is preventable.

The following chapter makes recommendations to all the systems which intervene in families and child custody decisions so as to prevent and/or remedy the PAS.

Chapter 25

JUDICIOUS INTERVENTION

Nothing can come of nothing.
–Shakespeare, *Much Ado About Nothing*

Wrong rules the land, and waiting Justice sleeps!
–J. G. Holland

It is so often spoken that the following axiom is virtually a cliché: "The wheels of justice grind slow, but the wheels of justice grind fine." When it comes to the PAS, however, there is the "slow" but there is seldom the "fine." This unfortunate outcome is because the application of the PAS to the law is as baffling as is the mysterious identity of the axiom's author. Without a doubt, there is a de facto sanctioning for "justice to sleep" in the case of the PAS, and this sanctioning rests at the feet of the mental health, child protection, law enforcement communities as well as the judicial systems. It seems that nothing good is frequently the outcome from the typical approach of these systems to the parental alienation syndrome.

Jeannemarie Massetti, R-L/ACSW, Supreme Court Principal Court Analyst/Court Evaluator, Suffolk County, New York, was interviewed for this book on 3/16/11. (Written comments are in the possession of the author.) She is highly respected among the lawyers who know her as well as many of the lawyers whom I interviewed for this book.

Many have described her as being highly dedicated, knowledgeable, and extremely hard-working. Several lawyers expressed about her, "I wish she could be cloned." This has also been my experience with Ms. Massetti, with whom I have collaborated on a number of cases during a multiyear period. She stated,

> The judges in both Supreme and Family Courts are dedicated, caring justices whose responsibility is to render a decision in the best interest of the child. The decision is based on both the evidence and testimonial documentary that is introduced during the course of the trial and within the confines of the law.

Regarding this testimony, Ms. Massetti declared, "The mental health professional is an integral component of the parties' case in which aspects of alienation can be presented. Therefore, in order to better serve the court, it is the responsibility of the mental health professional to be knowledgeable and well versed in all aspects of alienation."

217

Mr. Hiltzik expressed the quandary confronted by many attorneys with whom I have collaborated when their clients are being alienated and their children's therapist does not have a clue about what it is. He expressed it as follows: "If the mental health professional is unaware of what the PAS is, then how is the attorney for the child and the judge going to be made aware of its presence in a particular case?" Mr. Hiltzik continued, "A lot of judges don't know about alienation because it is a term without a firm definition. Alienation is a dirty word to many because it is so reprehensible–reprehensible not because of what it does but because the authorities mistrust its use." Mr. Previto corroborated Mr. Hiltzik's opinion about the difficulty of convincing the judge about the existence of the PAS in a particular case as reflected in his following comment, "Judges view alienation with skepticism. It's very hard to prove."

Mr. Hecht agrees with his colleagues as to the need for further education among members of the bench and bar, and he expressed it this way:

> Judges are too often left in the unenviable position of trying to assess what transpired between the four walls of the parties' home, and they are left with little more than the parties' two diametrically opposing renditions of what had occurred. While the courts can, and often do, rely on forensic psychologists, judges themselves are left with the undesirable task of discerning fact from fiction.

Chaim Steinberger, Esq., graduated Magna Cum Laude from Brooklyn Law School in 1994 and practices exclusively as a marital and family law attorney. He clerked for a federal judge in New York. He authored the previously referenced paper entitled, "Father? What Father? Parental Alienation and its Effects on Children." I urge the reader to

obtain a copy of this article, which is a meticulous summary of the professional literature that documents the damages accruing to children who are the victims of an alienation. Of equal importance is his summary of the alienation cases adjudicated in New York which cite the state's recognition of the importance of both parents to the child and the requirement of case law for the custodial parent to assure, as a primary responsibility, the meaningful contact between the other parent and their child. It is therefore not necessary for me to reference in this book his acknowledgment that parental alienation exists and that it is a harsh, prevalent occurrence in divorce situations—even if it is very difficult to demonstrate its presence in any one particular case before the court. I surmised that Mr. Steinberger's contributions to this book would be invaluable after I had learned about him from Dr. Havlicek and having subsequently read his article to which I just referred. Mr. Steinberger was interviewed on 6/15/11. (A video recording and written comments are in the possession of the author.) He agrees with his colleagues that the mental health professional must do a better job educating judges about the existence and telltale signs of alienation: how to identify it and how it should be treated. He further concurred with the other attorneys who were interviewed who declared that many mental health professionals are unable to accomplish this because they, themselves, are unaware of its prevalence and its insidious effects. When a mental health professional does recognize its presence in a particular case, Mr. Steinberger asserts, "They should not be mealy-mouthed about declaring it." He makes the point that the judge cannot be expected to make a hard call if the mental health professional is unwilling, ambivalent, and equivocal. That is because judges see great risk not only to the child but also to their own reputation and good name. "No judge wants to see himself/herself named in a headline story of a daily newspaper about a child who committed a suicide because he/she was ordered to visit or live with the alienated parent," Mr. Steinberger asserted.

Conceding that lawyers and judges do not typically have a grounding in psychological issues, the attorneys interviewed here affirmed that they must depend upon the mental health professional to testify about healthy family functioning and about any deviation from the norm that is occurring in the particular case before the court—and they hope that the therapist is PAS aware in cases of alienation. The attorneys further asserted that any ambivalence by the mental health professional in providing professional opinion as to whether alienation is present and its detrimental effects on the particular child would make it almost impossible for the court to change the course.

Dr. Havlicek also recognizes the legal barriers to establishing the presence of the PAS in case before the court. He stated in his interview:

Sadly, the courts have washed their hands of these gut-wrenching, heartbreaking cases that are well known to be so damaging to the mental health of the child, who is the victim. Judges are not trained in this. They learn only from the testimony in the court room. Alienated children don't express their sentiments to the judges that there will be a chronic mental health disorder that is going to emanate from parental alienation. Judges have a knowledge of justice but don't know the psychological background to understanding the PAS. So when the child testifies, "I hate my father, I want to live with my mother," it's hard for judges not to be affected by hearing this. So they resolve the case by giving sole custody to the alienator.

Ms. Zarkadas—in her capacity as a geneticist as well as an attorney—offered as an explanation for the resistance to accepting the PAS as that it is a relatively new syndrome, and human culture evolves incrementally. She commented, "Human evolution as a whole takes a long time." She elaborated that the situation is complicated further by the fact that it is difficult to prove with credible evidence and there are not many experts on it who can provide such evidence to the satisfaction of the court.

This issue is punctuated by Richard Sauber, Ph.D., who holds Diplomats in Clinical and Family Psychology, ABPP. He was professor of psychology in the departments of psychiatry at the medical schools of Brown, Penn, and Columbia. He trained at Harvard, and he has written or edited 16 books. He is the current editor of *The American Journal of Family Therapy*. Dr. Sauber (2006) stated:

When the judge first hears the term PAS presented, the first major factor is whether he or she is familiar or unfamiliar with the concept. . . . If the judge is familiar with the concept, then the next question is how knowledgeable and acquainted he or she is with determining the implications of PAS, it's case implications, and his or her willingness to utilize his or her judicial powers. (p. 12)

Even more problematical than the pervasive ignorance about the PAS among mental health professionals and consequently among the professionals in the judicial community whom they are yet to educate, is the issue that the PAS does not garner uniform legal standing among the 50 states. For example, some states, according to Sauber (2006), deem the PAS to have passed the Frye Test, meaning that it has satisfied the criteria of scientific evidence and is therefore an unchallenged, admissible condition in a court of law (p. 12). But what happens in the majority of states in which the PAS has not been accorded legal standing–primarily because of the wide-spread ignorance in the mental health community about its existence–about how to identify it and about its effects on children.

In my professional opinion, there is no longer a rationale for the ignorance of the mental health professional about the PAS. Countless highly respected therapists and matrimonial attorneys worldwide have validated from the observations in their practices and from long terms studies, such a consistency of symptoms present in PAS children that they remarkably resemble each other. The PAS-aware community has simultaneously observed the alienating parent's repeated, predictable patterns of behavior which interfere with and eschew the role of the targeted parent to their child. Leona Kopetski, M.S.S.W., (2006) summed up the significant observations of the PAS-aware professionals when she stated:

> Science refers to a systematic process for investigating reality in a way which is as clear, comprehensive and undistorted as possible. The fact that the observations of PAS described by different contributors over the past 20 years have been remarkably consistent is scientifically significant, indicating that PAS is a valid concept which can be reliably identified. (p. 385)

Attorney and psychologist, Demosthenes Lorandos, Ph.D., J.D, (2006) acknowledged the painstaking scientific rigor to which Gardner subjected his observations when he stated the following:

> Is this science? Certainly it is. Gardner's process over the years has been qualitative research, whereby he has systematically and cumulatively described a type of divorce-specific, familial interaction, which he properly labeled a syndrome. As a qualitative researcher, Gardner's goal was to understand and elaborate the phenomena of interest, rather than to reduce and simplify them to laboratory vari-

ables. To augment this work, he decided at the end of his life to try his hand at quantitative research, producing a follow-up study of 99 PAS children (which was the first of its kind) designed to address the question, "Should courts order PAS children to visit/reside with the alienated parent?" (p. 409)

R. Christopher Barden, Ph.D., J.D., LP, (2006) psychologist and attorney, having received two national research awards in psychology and a law degree with honors from Harvard Law School, states that his professional experience confirms the existence of the PAS, if not by name then by the cluster of characteristic symptoms identified by Gardner. He commented:

> More importantly, the basic, psychological processes underlying the PAS have been well documented in the peer reviewed professional literature over many decades. Reliable research on the processes underlying PAS has been published in the highest quality peer-reviewed journals. In sum, the theoretical foundations of PAS are, in fact, built upon some of the most reliable and best documented of all psychological processes–parental influences on children. (p. 420)

Barden (2006) convincingly reaffirmed in the following words what those who went before him had affirmed about a parent's immeasurable and unrivaled influence over their children:

> There can be no credible controversy about the power of parents to influence children. It is unfortunate that in reviewing PAS-type issues, courts have often stumbled over the meaning of technical terms such as "syndrome," the inclusion of specific labels in official diagnostic manuals, and other largely irrelevant minutia–thus missing the critical obligation to carefully review the influence of parents, therapists or other adults on the attitudes, beliefs and memories of children. (p. 420)

Ms. Zarkadas additionally postulated that cultural bias explains why the PAS is not readily accepted for what it is, and this bias is the reverence that is attributed to motherhood, "which is placed on a pedestal." She portrayed society's perception of motherhood as, "Nothing can touch it. We hold it in such high regard that it's very hard to believe that such venomous, vitriolic behavior could ensue from a person who produces life." Mr. Previto observed the same phenomenon referring to it as, "the power of the mother." Mr. Steinberger (2006) stated:

> In today's climate as a culture, we don't generally send mothers to jail, and we don't generally order mothers to pay fathers maintenance and child support. There is a doublestandard: a father will go to jail for not paying child support. But, as one judge of the supreme court told me, "We don't send mothers to jail."

Mr. Steinberger cited the case of *John A. v. Bridget M.* (2004, 2005) in which the trial court ordered the transfer of custody of two three-year-old girls to the alienated father after testimony and evidence substantiated that the mother had knowingly made multiple false allegations of sex abuse which resulted in these young toddlers being subjected to several unnecessary vaginal examinations. But the Appellate Division, First Department, (2005) reversed the ruling essentially holding that, "The mother has learned her lesson," according to Mr. Steinberger. While affirming the trial court's determination that the mother had engaged in alienation, the Appellate Court deemed that such grounds alone were not sufficient to conclude that transfer of custody was in the best interests of the children. The Appellate Division, First Department (2005) decreed:

> Despite the finding that the mother was attempting to undermine the relationship be-

tween the father and the children, the relationship was, in fact, a healthy one, one that even yielded affection and fondness between the children and the father's wife. Moreover, Dr. Billick also found that the mother is a "good enough mother" who demonstrates general day-to-day competency in that regard. . . . It was not in the children's best interests to award the father custody and to subject them to the trauma of being separated from their primary caretaker since birth and removal from the only home they have ever known. The appropriate response to the mother's unacceptable conduct, that is, using the children as pawns in her battle with the father is, as Dr. Blumenthal opined, not removal from the mother's custody, but treatment of her condition. (p. 4)

Mr. Steinberger fears that this ruling does not bode well for future appeals involving alienation.

Mr. Levitt confirmed that the bias in favor of the mother was the roadblock he had encountered in *Young v. Young* (1994, 1995). He stated, "We had a traditional, old time judge who, in his heart allowed his personal views to translate into his decision—this view being that the best caretaker is the mother. It was the judge's 'tender years' doctrine.'" Mr. Levitt believes that no matter what evidence he had introduced, it would not have dissuaded the judge from his preconceived beliefs about the family.

My practice has encountered at least two hundred children—and I am still counting—who incontrovertibly replicated the symptoms which Gardner identified as being characteristic of the PAS child along with the recurring pattern of behaviors that he attributed to the alienating parent. Regardless of whether we attach a syndrome label to this condition or not attach a label, it must be acknowledged that a condition of alienation exists when one parent engages in either an unconscious or a calculated and malicious effort to obstruct the other parent's relationship with their child and which all too frequently produces a severing of that relationship.

In addition to the dissension of the nonbelievers or of the ill-informed who deny the PAS or the family interactional pattern known as the perverse triangle, the professionals whom I interviewed for this book underscored other variables which interfere with the application of swift and fine justice to the PAS.

Dr. Havlicek addressed one of these variables when he commented on the fundamentally incompatible mix occurring when the law is inappropriately interjected into family matters. He stated, "There is the additional complication when judges apply a legal principle to resolve a family dispute. Judges see it as an adversarial system which needs remedies by applying the law. But judges must be made aware of the full set of intervening circumstances–psychological, psychosocial, educational, relational, and emotional–that pertain to the family. Applying the law in isolation of competent psychosocial analysis to family matters is too narrow and circumscribed."

Mr. Previto commented on other variables that delay justice, and he laid responsibility at the feet of the matrimonial attorney. He stated, "Attorneys may fear the 'educated judge' because it may not redound to the benefit of their clients." He confirmed a pecuniary incentive for attorneys to engage in protracted proceedings:

Matrimonial attorneys fall into two categories: "ravagers" and "redeemers," and the ravagers are clearly the issue. Except for a bankruptcy proceeding, divorce is the only legal matter in which the lawyer knows exactly what the client is worth. This information then affords the lawyer the opportunity to know just how far the

client can be pushed economically.

The dilemma for Mr. Previto, who classified himself as a redeemer, is that, "If your opponent is a ravager, you get dragged down to their level because you have no choice but to continually counter and defend against dubious allegations and frivolous motions."

Mr. Previto explicitly informs his clients that they cannot engage in an alienation campaign. He expressed it as follows:

You can't allow the client to drive you. They make the fundamental decisions but you have to give them the information to make the best decision. I tell my alienating clients, "You have to get your child to the visit. Stop talking to your child about their other parent. I can't represent you if you don't follow my advice. You might as well do surgery on yourself."

Mr. Levitt agreed with Mr. Previto in that he was of the opinion that some matrimonial attorneys make the proceeding much more adversarial and contentious than it needs to be to reach an amicable settlement for both parties and which is in the best interests of the children. He stated, "I never looked to make tremendous amounts of money by taking every case to the brink." He placed less emphasis on monetary motivations than did Mr. Previto, and an apt metaphor for Mr. Levitt's point of view is that of the tail wagging the dog in that many prospective clients are looking for the pit bull attorney expecting to maximize their advantage in the settlement. He characterized what happens as follows:

Some attorneys feel that going to war is what their client wants, and they're going to live up to their client's wishes; this is what they believe they are supposed to do. Because "going to war" is the attitude of so many divorcing parties, they seek attorneys who have a reputation for being fierce. And this is how many matrimonial attorneys market themselves. Many people going through a divorce want the lawyer who says they will fight to the bitter end. This is what encourages it. I got the sense that some attorneys would actually encourage their clients to starve the other parent out. And if they feared being starved out, they use the children.

Mr. Levitt therefore believes that the system is partly responsible for the nastiness and adversarial nature of divorce and custody proceedings. It was just this kind of adversarial approach to matrimonial law that hastened his departure from the field.

So how does Mr. Levitt recommend that his profession be changed? He suggests that the matrimonial bar declare that they are not going to allow this to happen any further; it must place greater emphasis on mediation. He urges matrimonial attorneys to control the combativeness by advising their clients that it is time for them to settle; and when they see the nastiness and vitriol resulting, especially with the negative consequences to children, Mr. Levitt asserted, "We need to contact the other side and agree that, just because we have a bunch of crazy clients, it does not mean we, as the attorneys, must accept it." The reticence of some attorneys to do this is a result of the fear of losing their client, according to Mr. Levitt, so this rarely happens. He maintains that this can be overcome by taking the time to develop a strong enough relationship with their clients to tell them when they are doing something wrong. Here, Here! Relationship is what it is all about. This reinforces the sentiments of many of his colleagues, namely that attorneys have the responsibility to counsel their clients as to what they believe to be wise and sensible procedure. By doing this, they will have great impact in preventing the case

from dragging on needlessly and generally to the detriment of the children. Mr. Levitt told his clients when he believed that the other side was making a valid point. For example, he counseled his nonmoneyed spouse as follows, "Make sure you develop a relationship with your ex-partner so that you can co-parent the kids. Have your kids not be harmed by this; you get more with honey than you do with vinegar." He counseled his moneyed spouse as follows, "You will only hurt your children by threatening your former partner with withholding support." He encouraged his clients to settle things as quickly and fairly as possible so that their lives would not be destroyed. Mr. Levitt stated, "The attorneys who don't do any of this are at fault here. This is the part of the profession which requires some kind of social work."

Mr. Levitt declared that he had a real problem with people who put their own interests ahead of those of their children. He stated that he would apprise his clients of this when he saw it. He expressed his incredulity about how some parents could so selfishly behave to the detriment of their own children when he stated, "What is the point of damaging the relationship with your ex knowing it is going to affect the kids? I would try to have people see it that way. I would ask them if they really wanted to spend the next 10 years dealing with these issues. I would ask them if it was worth spending upwards of $100,000 when it just might be in everyone's best interest to settle." Mr. Levitt agreed with Mr. Previto that when the other side refused to settle, there was no alternative but to go to trial.

Ms. Courten concurred that the adversarial nature of matrimonial and custody proceedings are unnecessarily exacerbated by the attorneys when, according to Ms. Courten, "They try to showboat for their angry client who wants a pound of flesh. The lawyers acquiesce to this request." She stated that she frequently observes the parties engage in a highly-charged situation during the four-way conference or in the halls of the courthouse. She commented, "There some jaded attorneys who are just doing it for the money. And this is a heartache." She made the same comment about some judges. When Ms. Courten's clients engage in parental alienation, she admonishes them, "Cut the crap. You could lose your children. It is the parent who is more open to the other parent's input who should get custody and probably will get custody."

As with many of the other attorneys interviewed for this book, Ms. Courten takes her role as attorney and counselor at law meaningfully. She stated,

> I want to see people leave here with their money intact as well as their souls intact. We are in a branch of law in which we are dealing with human beings with all the value that human beings can have. You have to give them the time. I sit down and listen and ask the right questions. If you ask the right questions, it will lead to the right answer. You might be able to fix it before it gets to court.

Mr. Hiltzik expressed comparable sentiments about situations in which he discovers his clients engaging in parental alienation. He also conveys to them the requirement of case law for the residential parent to facilitate a meaningful and substantial relationship with the other parent. His policy is to caution all of his divorcing clients, "I will not tolerate the weapon of alienation to be used in this arena." Should he subsequently encounter alienating behaviors by his client, he tells them, "Cut it out!"

Ms. Saltz stated that if the alienator is her client, she admonishes them that they must "stop engaging in alienation. You have to stop talking about the other parent to your family and best friends when the kids are in

the house. You have to stop showing them the paperwork. And you have to encourage the visits!"

Mr. Hecht stated that he counsels his clients to protect their children by keeping them insulated from the divorce and custody proceedings and from issues related to finances. He advises his clients to tell their children the following, "Mommy and daddy are doing the best they can for you, and we both love you. Mommy and daddy may have their differences, but we will work together for your benefit; you are our greatest concern."

Mr. Steinberger, has, in actuality, adopted into his matrimonial practice a collaborative model, which is philosophically aligned with the nonadversarial principles that are advocated by his colleagues who were interviewed for this book. What intrigued me about Mr. Steinberger and what he contributed most notably to the rationale for this book, is this implementation. Mr. Steinberger, until recently, co-chaired the Collaborative Law Committee of the New York State Bar Association Dispute Resolution Section and chaired the ADR committee of the ABA Family Law Section. He described the collaborative approach as:

> A nonadversarial, facilitative method of teaching parties to resolve their disputes using mental health professionals. The mental health professional also sometimes advocates for the children. Neutral financial professionals are also used if needed. We negotiate a resolution that is good for the mother, for the father, and for the children. It is perhaps the first time that people who are getting a divorce can do so in a way that is not destructive to the relationship with their former partner so that it does not inhibit their ability to co-parent their children in the future. It is a rehabilitative process which helps them to heal in a safe environment so that they

can move on and hopefully co-parent their children. It is truly a magical approach.

I share Mr. Steinberger's feeling of exhilaration as I, too, experience that magical process whenever I am able to help divorcing parents retain their dignity while simultaneously recognizing the value of the other to their children. The underlying philosophical principles of the collaborative model as described by Mr. Steinberger are the very principles that underlie the family systems modality I employ in treatment. As I had discussed in a previous chapter, family therapists bring opposing parties together in a safe, neutral environment in which the therapist can elicit the underlying incentives, concerns and interests of each one's position; an environment in which each party is encouraged to hear as well as be heard; an environment which does not generate defensiveness. According to Mr. Steinberger, "The collaborative environment provides a platform that all parties can buy into because it does not push hot buttons but, instead, it makes proposals in such a way that the other side can hear." He further explained that the collaborative process addresses not only the legalities but also the psychosocial aspects of the opposing parties. Taken together, this approach "builds the basis for goodwill which can then lead to resolution." Mr. Steinberger, who ingeniously employs metaphors to exemplify his positions, offered one to punctuate the effectiveness of the collaborative approach. He orated about the rabbi commissioned by his king to rid the king of a particular enemy who unabashedly proclaimed his distaste for the king. Shortly thereafter, the king spots the enemy, who could be heard from afar singing the praises of the king. The rabbi is summoned to the king, who admonishes him for not complying with his dictate. The rabbi retorts, "But I

have complied. I killed off your enemy by converting him into a supporter." Mr. Steinberger similarly characterizes the success of the collaborative method because it "takes the venom out" thereby negating the need or desire to destroy the opposing side.

Mr. Steinberger acknowledged that the collaborative approach is "somewhat new and controversial" being around for only about 20 years and has not yet garnered widespread appeal. My mentor, Dr. Minuchin, is unquestionably familiar with the effects of resistance. He still feels like a salmon swimming upstream when attempting to proselytize his colleagues into adapting a systems treatment modality—even though family systems therapy had its birth more than 60 years ago. Mr. Steinberger credibly argues, however, that most cases settle—many later rather than sooner. He proposes that it is more beneficial for children, and certainly less stressful for litigants, to settle sooner rather than later and embark on a process that is geared toward settlement. Should collaboration fail, there is always the opportunity to litigate at that time. Mr. Steinberger summed-up the benefits of the collaborative model as follows:

It is not always best to start with the adversarial approach. It often makes more sense to start with a collaborative process, which is a much healthier way for all parties, and it is not destructive for the children and then switch to an adversarial approach only after the nonadversarial options have been exhausted.

In addition to the power of resistance in preventing a greater use of the collaborative method, it can be an expensive process, being compounded by the fees of the mental health professional and sometimes financial advisors. The less-than-privileged, therefore, are likely closed out of this model.

I do agree fully with Mr. Steinberger that the collaborative model is the preferable system for resolving divorce situations when children are involved. It indisputably serves the best interests of children as it minimizes destruction–given that divorce by definition inescapably entails the destruction of a marriage, of the family as the child has always known it, and of the relationship with the nonresidential parent. But, regrettably, in our present state of divorce, a huge percentage of cases "linger" in the adversarial system either by choice, coercion, ignorance, or indigence. Given the overwhelming numbers who consequently pursue divorce through the adversarial model, it is incumbent upon those who wish to mitigate the damage to children to reform this model while simultaneously pursuing efforts to make the collaborative model more universal. Each attorney who interviewed for this book expressed the preference for a nonadversarial approach, and each make diligent efforts to counsel the client to refrain from engaging in alienation. But the thorn arises when the opposing attorney is intent upon getting down and dirty in the mud. It has sadly been my predominate experience in talking with alienating parents, they have **NOT** been advised by their attorneys of the requirements of case law for the residential parent to facilitate a relationship between the other parent and their child. They have not been informed by their attorneys that engaging in alienation is grounds to transfer custody. I am incredulous that I am frequently the one who advises them about case law. And amazingly, once I have done so, their cooperation frequently improves exponentially! I wonder how much consternation, resources, and loss of valuable time for the court calendar could be avoided if only (this being an "if only" of which I endorse) attorneys recognized their obligation to inform their clients about this. I presume they advise their clients that they can-

not perjure themselves at deposition and that they cannot pilfer the marital assets and that they cannot lock their spouse out of the marital home, and so forth.

My esteemed colleagues in both the matrimonial and mental health communities who were interviewed for the book were quite troubled about the recent ruling by the New York State Appellate Division which redefined the role of the child's attorney. Ms. Zarkadas is most unhappy with the new guidelines which took effect on 4/1/10 because she is denied the flexibility of being able to advocate for what she believes is in the best interest of her minor client. According to the new directive, she must, instead, advocate for the wishes of her client–as if her client were an adult–regardless of how astonishing, irrational, and influenced that those wishes might be. She commented on this setback as follows:

We had the right to impose our own vision. But a year and a half ago on 4/10, the Appellate Division changed my title from Law Guardian to Attorney for the Child. Our role now is no different than if we were representing an adult. I no longer have the flexibility to say "wait, that's not in my client's best interests." So when a 12-year-old tells me where they want to sleep or not sleep, I have to advocate for that position. How do you decide that? If a four-year-old is logically telling me my dad's house is not safe, I have to represent his wishes not to go there. If my client is not old enough to drive, vote, buy a beer or cigarettes, or enter into a contractual arrangement, what makes my client knowledgeable as to what they want? The revised law makes it very difficult.

When I asked Ms. Zarkadas if there were any circumstances under which she had the option to substitute her judgment and advocate for what is in her client's best interests when in opposition to her client's wishes, Ms. Zarkadas explained that there is "a very high standard" in order for her to do that. She explained that she must go on the record and establish that her client is suffering a physical or mental disability or emotional distress and that her client, consequently, does not realize the severity of the circumstances she/he is requesting. Or if, upon investigation she discovered that her client would be in harms way, such as the custodial parent having a drug problem, she would be able to oppose the wishes of her client.

Nevertheless, Ms. Zarkadas goes above and beyond to seek a remedy that is in the best interests of her client. She stated:

> I take my role as Lawyer for the Child very seriously. I have to get to the bottom of what is happening to my client. I can't accept doing what my client asks without making an effort to influence all players, such as the parents. It would be no different if my client were an adult and he asked me to do something illegal or immoral. I need to investigate my client's life, which is comprised of parents, friends, grandparents, school, church, the coach, the therapist, the pediatrician. It would be the same as if I were exploring my adult client's finances.

In recognition of the child's typically immature emotional life and limited cognitive abilities, Ms. Zarkadas recognizes that she cannot rely exclusively on client/child self-reporting to obtain the total picture about her client's life. To remedy the limitation of self-reporting, she requests input from all the aforementioned influences on her client so that she is able to receive more than "the fragmented picture that the child is giving me." Ms. Zarkadas elaborated, "My client can give me only what they possess and that is the life of a child."

It is accurate to conclude that Ms. Zarkadas places heavy emphasis on her license that identifies her as a Counselor at Law, meaning that she invests time and energy in persuading all the parties who have influence over her minor/client to work together and reach a settlement in the child's best interests, and she is not afraid to use her authority to broker a settlement. When she encounters an alienation situation, she will confront the custodial parent by saying to them: "What gives you the right to say the child is mine? The child did not come from a sperm bank. Is the child your property? It took two parents to create the child, and it will take two parents to raise the child."

Ms. Zarkadas acknowledged that it is very difficult to make such statements without being accused of being biased towards the other side. Sometimes she is told that she does not know what she is talking about, that she is off-base, and that it is unbelievable that she believes the child over the adult parents. But she asserts that her successful settlements have far outnumbered her failures. This outcome, in my professional opinion, is due to Ms.'s Zarkadas' commitment to fairness, objectivity, the best interests of her client, and, significantly, having knowledge of the child's entire world at her fingertips.

Ms. Saltz expressed apprehension about the ramifications resulting from the change in her title to lawyer for the children and how it consequently impacts her role. She, too, would like to be able to resume her prior function as law guardian and represent her client's best interests and not necessarily what they say they want. She expressed her concerns as follows:

> Under existing law, I have the obligation to say what my client wants. I have to represent my clients expressed wishes. I can no longer substitute myself, my own judgment. In chambers, I can say to the judge,

this is what my client wants. But I am suspicious. This is what my client wants; I have an obligation to tell you this as well. But I cannot do that on the record.

Ms. Saltz nevertheless stated that the judges continue to rely on the Attorney for the Child in order to make a decision based on the best interest of the child, which is the judge's obligation. So in order to attain this goal, Ms. Saltz has concluded:

Even though our role has changed, the judges still want our opinions, as in the past. I can cite one case in particular in which my preteen client expressed that he did not want to see his father, and the judge sent me a message that conveyed to me, "Well I hope you disabused him of this feeling." I think the judge is still reliant on us to do the investigations we used to do. They rely on us to protect our clients if we suspect something. You can still substitute your own judgment with a very young child because a five-year-old, for example, doesn't understand what's really going on. If your client is a mature and articulate child, you're supposed to counsel the child to come to your way of thinking. But that doesn't always happen, especially with alienation. It has become a very difficult situation. You will have to take the pretty bold step to disagree on the record and you have to be really sure of your facts and circumstances.

Ms. Moss is most "unhappy and frustrated" with the redefinition of her role as Attorney for the Child. She expressed her chagrin this way:

To some extent, the system is working in the wrong direction when they changed the title from Law Guardian to Attorney for the Children. Under the governing rules of the Law Guardian, I could go into court, inform the judge what I actually saw was happening and what was needed to get these people help and what I thought served my client's best interests. Under new rules, even if I don't agree with my young client's position, unless what the child desires places the child in danger or in harms way, I must go to court and advocate for their position. I have nothing to hang my hat on as an Attorney for the Child when I suspect that there is alienation going on because I can't take a position that it is contrary to the child's position. I don't know how helpful this is going forward. I would like to go back to my old job."

Ms. Moss illustrated the absurdity of the potential implementation of her new role when she postulated the following scenario:

I can actually foresee a day when there is going to be a table for the husband, a table for the wife and the counsel table for the Attorney for the Child, which means that the child would be sitting there alongside me, exposed to the proceedings. There is great potential for devastation to the children: namely that they need to be protected from exposure to adult issues. The children are being slowly but surely pulled into this. It's problematic. If I'm Attorney for the Child, how am I supposed to represent them if they're not sitting right next to me hearing the testimony?

Ms. Moss feared another possible unintended consequence: "One of the great unanswered questions is what to do if mom and dad come to a settlement, and my minor client objects to the stipulations and requests a hearing? I cannot then sign off on it. I am no longer involved in this to speak to the child's best interests."

Ms. Moss futhermore bemoaned how the revision empowers the child: "We have certainly given all this power to the child. And that's the person who really shouldn't have any power. Divorce alone makes children powerful. My new title grants them even more!"

When Ms. Moss concludes that her minor clients' wishes are not in their best interests, she enacts her role as "counselor" and attempts to counsel them to decide on the basis of their own best interests. She informs her clients that their choices about with whom they want to live may be more than two: "They can tell me mom or dad or they can tell me I don't want to choose." Maintaining the conviction that children do best when they have a relationship with both parents, she counsels her clients as follows: "You have the right to love both your parents. You have the right to have both parents love you. You have a right to a relationship with both parents."

Recognizing that alienated children resist counsel and in cases when she suspects an alienation is present, Ms. Moss will attempt to have a forensic evaluation ordered. She is hopeful that the evaluation will reveal what is occurring, and, if alienation is established, she hopes that the long-term negative effects are also documented. She then feels it may be possible to take a position that is contrary to her client on the basis that her client's wishes will put her/him in a harmful and/or dangerous situation.

Ms. Courten echoed a similar refrain regarding the change. She expressed, "You have empowered children! They should not have been in power in the first place." Ms. Courten worries that this power will be capitalized on by alienating parents, who can manipulate a weak child into becoming their puppet and mouth their positions to the child's lawyer. She cited one of her cases in which the alienating father gave his child his lawyer's number, orchestrated the call to his attorney, and then coached him what to articulate. Ms. Courten declared:

I don't think the change is really helpful. The Law Guardian was a better description of their duties and obligations as to what that person should do. Now that they are not allowed to give an opinion, why are they needed? You don't need someone just to mouth the child's words; most judges will talk to the child anyway and ascertain what they want, and most judges do a pretty good job talking to the children. When it comes to alienation, it's the worst possible change. You have empowered parents to wrongfully empower children to fight the parent's agenda.

Mr. Hecht jumped on the bandwagon of incredulity regarding the change in the role of the Attorney for the Child. In his view:

Asking the Attorney for the Child to advocate for their clients' best interests based solely on their client's stated preference is a bit like asking someone to swim with hands tied behind their back and a cinderblock attached to their waist. It reduces the Attorney for the Child from their previously important role to that of messenger. The child's preference is but one of many factors that have to be considered. In my view, the children's attorneys need to be able to take into consideration the biases and motivations of the parties and the reasons behind the child's wishes. Is the child choosing a particular parent because that parent does not set any limits or boundaries? Is the child rejecting the parent who provides structure and guidelines in that child's best interest? Is the child's attorney to simply rearticulate their client's stated preference to live with one parent in instances where that child has fallen victim to the other parent's manipulation in deciding with whom to live, such that they are just mimicking what that parent is telling them?

With this change, Mr. Hecht fears that the prospects are infinitesimally increased that the parent who manipulates the child is the parent likely to be awarded custody. As with his colleagues, he is concerned that the change provides the potential for exposure of the child to the divorce proceedings and the unhappy circumstances between the parents.

Mr. Previto was equally perturbed by the change, and he expressed it this way, "The entire concept of a child having a lawyer is insane. By definition, a child is a minor, lacks legal competence, and is not empowered to contract with a lawyer. To afford the child's wishes more standing than what's in their best interests defies rationality." Given the revised role, Mr. Previto believes that the role of the lawyer for the child is superfluous and should be eliminated. But Mr. Previto had an issue with the Law Guardian role even prior to the revision. He believed that they had too much power, which was the basis for the appellate division's revision to their role. His concern was that they could be easily seduced by an alienating parent if they are PAS-unaware. In that situation, they could do much damage as a result of an alliance with the alienator.

Mr. Previto stated:

The children's lawyer can either work against the alienated parent's attorney or they can corroborate the alienation allegations. And the judge being persuaded as to the presence of an alienation often depends upon whom the child's lawyer is, how knowledgeable he/she is about the PAS, and how the PAS applies to the particular case in question.

Mr. Previto suggested that a mental health professional trained in family dynamics replace the lawyer for the child in all high conflict custody cases so as to assess for the facts regarding alienation. He would also grant the family therapist the authority to make nonbinding recommendations to the court. Hmm! Somehow I like the suggestion for an expanded role for the family therapist! But, as Mr. Previto specified, the case must be assigned to a therapist who is trained in family dynamics. As the reader discovered from my case examples, therapists who work in the traditional individual models have been quite destructive and only serve to solidify the PAS as a result of being co-opted by the alienating parent. But I also still see a role for a lawyer who represents the child's best interests; that is, functioning under the Law Guardian description.

Ms. DeNatale also places a high value on therapeutic intervention, judging it and parental education to be the only effective methods for resolving alienation. She expressed her opinions this way:

A rational person not going through a family crisis could probably figure out how to problem solve with the other parent. However, going through a life change such as divorce tends to cloud one's judgment. Thus, I believe that therapy and education of the parents going through a divorce is the only way parental alienation syndrome could be ameliorated.

Mr. Hiltzik expressed a similar fear if the child's lawyer is PAS unaware. He is appreciative of their importance in providing the necessary corroboration of the alienation when they are PAS aware. He affirmed, "When the Attorney for the Child is convinced about the alienation, their corroboration is gold!" He affirmed that he recently experienced harmful outcomes as a result of the revision to the title of the child's lawyer. "If you are not old or mature enough to drink, drive, smoke, or vote, why are you old enough to determine whether you see a parent or to choose one parent over the other? It is nonsense! The inmates are now in charge of the asylum," Mr. Hiltzik declared.

I interviewed two lawyers who practice primarily as the Attorney for the Child and who both requested that their names be withheld. One practices in Nassau County, New York and the other in Suffolk County, New York. Both of them were extremely troubled by the change in their role and wished to return to the job description of Law Guardian. They each agreed with the suggestion to give cases of alienation or alleged alienation priority and a speedy trial date. One of the lawyers stated:

> It is a real bind when I strongly suspect or even am sure that my client is being unduly influenced by their custodial parent; but unless I can establish that my client's wishes to remain with that parent will put them at risk, I must advocate for their position. It would really be helpful if a forensic evaluator could testify about the harm that will be done to the child by remaining with the alienating parent.

The other off-the-record attorney for the child expressed identical sentiments.

In his interview, Dr. Havlicek made the following comments regarding the revision,

> The law is part of the problem and making it worse. If there is even the slightest indication of parental alienation, it must be immediately evaluated by a mental health professional who will then advise the lawyer for the child as to what is in the child's best interests. This should then be what the children's lawyer advocates for.

Expressing his incredulity as to the rights that are bestowed upon the child under the revised law, Dr. Havlicek stated:

> The law assumes that a child is an adult and can act in an equivalent manner in seeking legal consultation as does an adult. That is absurd! Moreover, alienation is a deep mental state; and if a seven-year-old has been brainwashed, then what? The law must be changed to recognize that a child can be manipulated to hate a parent because the other parent has an agenda. The system is broken when it comes to the children's lawyer handling family reunification resulting from parental alienation. It's terrible. There must be circumstances where it is imperative that the children's lawyer act in the best interest of the child.

Based on my previously cited, reprehensibly mishandled alienation cases, the mental health system has much to reform regarding its all too frequent "treatment" of family issues. It is most disconcerting when therapists attempt treatment and make recommendations to the court based on a one-sided evaluation that did not include input from the nonresidential parent when accessible. In his interview, Dr. Havlicek addressed the recurrent indefensible conduct among our mental health colleagues when he commented:

> All mental health professionals, pediatricians, social workers, forensic evaluators have an obligation to thoroughly interview and test both parents and the child, including questioning all collateral sources and to be neutral with both before providing an analysis and recommendations. They must establish an appropriately professional relationship with both parents before making any recommendations and diagnoses. But to my regret in too many cases this is not done.

Dr. Kelly commented on how easily mental health professionals may be seduced by the alienating parent into furthering the alienation process. She commented:

It is important that our profession not be emotionally drawn in by believing the sometimes absurd statements made by the alienator and the children, who come in with an agenda. How some therapists who have never met the other parent testify and make recommendations is beyond me.

Dr. Burkhard recognizes that therapists and forensic evaluators carry an enormous responsibility for educating those who are making the decisions for children in the judicial system. Her regret is that all too many of our colleagues are PAS-unaware and that results in further damage to children when these mental health professionals are seduced by the favored parent and/or the child into furthering the alienation by aligning with them. Dr. Burkhard commented:

We often find that the mental health profession is feeding the alienation because many child therapists deal only with the child or the parent who brings the child to therapy. The targeted parent is rarely involved on an equal basis. It is not uncommon for the therapist to take the child's word when he or she expresses fear of or maltreatment by a targeted parent. And, without corroboration, they may reinforce a false sense of victimization thinking they are treating the child for trauma or anxiety. In our practice, we always contact the other parent.

Dr. Baker expressed concerns that there are not nearly enough therapists, forensic evaluators, or parent coordinators trained in understanding the dynamics of alienation.

She expressed her concerns about those who are PAS-unaware as follows, "They get drawn into the alienation to side with the alienating parent. If they don't know what they're doing, they can do a lot of harm. And things will get a lot worse."

Dr. Baker is working with Dr. Sauber in developing standards to recommend the licensing of the title of "PAS specialist." I agree wholeheartedly with this. Dr. Havlicek would surely support this as well. He commented that effective treatment of the PAS requires a therapist whose training is steeped in family dynamics theory. The supportive, empathetic, nonconfrontational approach of the traditional individually oriented therapies, according to Dr. Havlicek and to me, is not effective in mediating the PAS–and may actually woresen it.

Mr. Hecht stated his concerns as follows, "The expertise and professionalism of the therapist is a major issue." He expressed that all too frequently he has encountered situations in which the therapist never contacts the alienated parent. He cited a case of his in which the mother brought the children to the therapist alleging that they have issues with their father, yet the therapist permitted the mother to remain in the session with the children while the therapist was supposed to be discussing how to rebuild the relationship with the alienated father. Even more astonishing, the therapist never contacted the father. Mr. Hecht expressed his incredulity about the therapist's actions when he commented, "You would think that since the father is on the outs with the children, the therapist would want to contact him." The contact between the father and the therapist occurred only because the father contacted the therapist and insisted upon a meeting. After this one meeting and without any HIPAA authorization, the therapist wrote a letter to the court diagnosing the father as an "alcoholic who was unfit to see the children."

Incredibly, as well, the therapist never discussed with the father the issue of alcoholism, which had been alleged by the children's mother. Mr. Hecht queried of me as did many of his colleagues, "So if this is the expertise of the therapist, how can the court actually gauge and discern fact from fiction?"

I am unable to dispute Mr. Hecht's concern that "there are therapists out there who are willing to play the role of the hired gun." And doing so only further exacerbates the problem. Just as any of his many colleagues commented on the willingness of lawyers to accept the role of the hired gun, the mental health profession is not squeaky clean when it comes to accepting this mission. Monetary gain is not necessarily the prime motivation for doing so, although it applies to some in my profession. Very frequently the motivation is the "rescue fantasy," which is typically the original incentive for entering a field in one of the helping professions but which should be relinquished as we learn from our training to control for countertransference. The rescue fantasy is sustained by a general lack of awareness about the PAS in the mental health field.

I asked each of the attorneys what they believed to be the reason that the court so frequently permits justice to grind so slowly in the face of allegations of alienation–even when there has been strong expert testimony provided to support the assertion.

Ms. Zarkadas expressed that the courts are unwittingly seduced by the alienating parent: "The courts are very hesitant at times to take a strong position and tell the alienating parent that they cannot engage in this destructive behavior or else there will be consequences. The result is that the alienators become emboldened." This sentiment was echoed by many of her other colleagues who were interviewed.

Mr. Levitt, who lived and litigated the most famous, or perhaps infamous, alien-

ation case discussed in this book, offered the following remark about how the court, out of ignorance, exacerbates the alienation. He stated: "When I was practicing matrimonial law, there was a lack of training and understanding by some supreme court justices about parental alienation. At that time, I don't think they were familiar with this type of allegation." Referring again to the Young case, particularly regarding the sex abuse allegations which the four children had allegedly reported to their mother, Mr. Levitt stated:

The judge in the case could not understand why small children would lie. Taking seriously the allegations of sex abuse and not comprehending the parental alienation, the judge purposely made the case linger, granting adjournment after adjournment, never having continuous hearings, and never setting it down for an emergency hearing. To compound matters, the case was never put on the fast track whenever a new sex abuse allegation–every one having been unfounded–was claimed, thereby resulting in another long suspension of visits.

The divorce proceeding commenced in 12/88, took two years and several months for receipt of the lower court ruling denying the father's petition for custody, and then was appealed to the appellate division in 2/95, where it was reversed in 6/95. Mr. Levitt views this case to have been a travesty of justice, stating, "Justice delayed is Justice denied."

Mr. Hecht could not agree more with Mr. Levitt's assertion that it is imperative to move swiftly in such situations. He stated, "When it comes to parental alienation, time is not on the child's side. Time is not on the alienated parent's side. The delay creates as much damage because the underlying alienation progresses. He expressed how he perceives

that there is a tremendous disconnect between the bench and the bar. He expounded
further that, in instances where other forms
of abuse are alleged, the court is very quick
to act, but not, in his view, the case when
instances of parental alienation are alleged.
The time expensed by the parties' lawyers in
thoroughly preparing the application, who
want it to be impactful and hard-hitting,
results in further delay. According to Mr.
Hecht:

> It is a frustrating process when applica-
> tions are filed and then you get a decision,
> and then the alienating parent is probably
> not going to abide by that decision. So
> you go back to court, and you file an ap-
> plication to enforce that decision. The de-
> lays can extend eight or nine months, at
> least, before the issues are ultimately ad-
> dressed. The alienating parent only be-
> comes further emboldened by the delay.
> They view the court's inaction as a rubber
> stamp to continue the alienating behavior,
> which often becomes worse and more
> pervasive.

Mr. Hecht described a number of situations in which he filed an emergency application for a hearing on that day. But without
the facts before it, the courts rarely grant
emergency relief.

Mr. Hiltzik is also concerned about the
many judicial delays in situations of parental
alienation, and he laments, "Effective remedy is often applied too late to make a difference." He expressed that the importance for
cooperation between the mental health professional, the lawyer for the child, and the attorney for the alienated parent cannot be
overstated. He commented, "It's very difficult to get a judge to make a decision about
parenting. They need corroboration." But
again, the previously discussed issue arises
when there are so many PAS unaware ther-

apists and lawyers for the child. According to
Mr. Hiltzik:

> The next line of defense is cooperation
> from the forensic evaluator. But that can
> be quite costly, and many parties do not
> have the funds to pay for this. In addition,
> it can take many, many months to com-
> plete. And all the while, the alienation
> progresses. The other drawback is whe-
> ther the evaluator is PAS aware.

I inquired of my colleagues about their
experiences with and recommendations for
the situation that occurs when visits between
the targeted parent and the children are suspended because of abuse and/or neglect allegations. They were all concerned with the
message that this sends the children–that it
confirms for the child that the targeted parent must indeed have done something horrible to them. This is particularly harmful to
the relationship between the child and targeted parent because it furthers the alienation. Most evidence actually confirms that
the occurrence of abuse in custody situations
is quite negligible. I discussed with Dr. Havlicek his experience and his position on visitation when abuse is alleged. He has concluded, as a result of his professional experience, that the number of true incidents of
physical/sex abuse is "miniscule in comparison to the total number of cases, though adequate assessments should always be immediately undertaken to enable appropriate visitation to resume as quickly as possible." Dr.
Havlicek further stated:

> The number of false allegations promoted
> by the complaining parent compared to
> the relatively small percentage of valid
> complaints, does not justify the suspen-
> sion of visits without an immediate, thor-
> ough assessment by a qualified mental
> health professional. My belief is that you

don't suddenly stop visitation. If you stop visitation, nine times out of ten, it is for the wrong reasons. The damage that this causes to the child's beliefs is immense. The child then thinks, "Oh, now the judge is saying it about my father (mother). My mother (father) must be right about him (her)." There is really a problem with this approach. The system must be changed.

Dr. Kelly is also concerned that the suspension of visits is very destructive to the relationship between the child and the alienated parent. She stated:

Alienators seem to utilize the courts, sometimes with frivolous action in order to delay or suspend the visits. They may even intimate the existence of abuse or suicidal behavior. Judges are obviously concerned when they hear from the child, "I'll kill myself if I have to see my father. I'll throw myself out of the car." In the vast majority of cases there is no reason to stop the visits.

Dr. Kelly described inconsistency when it comes to parents whose children were removed from their care due to adjudicated cases of abuse and/or neglect. She stated, "Federal and state laws scrupulously protect the visitation rights of parents whose children are placed in foster care in that visits are mandated to occur on a regular recurring basis. No such protection is accorded the targeted parent who is falsely accused of abuse or neglect."

Given his experience with the multiple unfounded sex abuse allegations in the Young case, Mr. Levitt's opinion on the suspension and resumption of visits was quite relevant and instructive. He stated:

When allegations are unfounded, it should not be a question of slowly rein-

troducing the alienated parent to his child. It should be a question of removing the child from the parent who prompted the child to make these allegations. Was the other parent encouraging the false reporting? If that's the case, then you're looking at it in the wrong way. It shouldn't be how slowly the father should again develop his relationship with his child but rather how quickly we can remove mom from the relationship that she has with the child.

Mr. Levitt believes that such situations, and particularly what had happened in the Young case, was "a classic case of blaming and penalizing the victim." Mr. Levitt further confirmed the concerns which were expressed by my professional colleagues, namely that if the child thinks that the abuse was true, then withholding visits only reinforces the belief. But if the judge permits the visits, the child will likely be disabused of the belief of having been sexually abused. Mr. Levitt affirmed, "When visits are suspended, it seems suspicious to the child. The child thinks that something must have happened, and the suspension makes it true."

Ms. Zarkadas expressed great concern about the suspension of visits between the children and the noncustodial parent whether due to CPS allegations or due to the children themselves refusing visits with the sanctioning of the residential parent. Ms. Zarkades stated:

Children can no longer be driving the visitation bus. The residential parent has to lead the way. Children will take their cue from the residential parent. If the residential parent shows interest and is an instrumental force encouraging the relationship with the other parent, the visitation happens; it is never a problem!

I discussed with Mr. Hiltzik the dilemma he confronts when arguing before the court for the reinstatement of the alienated parent's visits. He responded that he is in a box because he must request what is practical even if it is not the full reinstatement of the visitation plan. He finds the concept of the old theory of "reintroduction therapy" a sexy solution. He stated:

Intuitively, it makes sense. As the attorney for the alienated parent, I have to go slowly or it all gets thrown out right away before I get started. I may have to suggest supervised visits. I have to make the decision easy for the court. Yet I know, when this is done, it validates that something is wrong with the father by going slowly. But I'm not dealing in a vacuum. In order to get something accomplished for my client, that's what I have to do.

I shared with Mr. Hiltzik that the research and evidence based practice does not support the concept of "reintroduction therapy" and certainly does not apply to the parent/child relationship; that in fact, it is actually contradicted by knowledge about effective treatment for anxiety and resistance issues. Mr. Hiltzik responded to this point by saying that the mental health professional must be more proactive in making this opinion known to the court.

Ms. Saltz acknowledged the importance of maintaining contact even when abuse and neglect are alleged. She affirmed: "I never recommend suspension of visits. They should be supervised and therapeutic but not suspended. Because the kids will then start believing in the false allegations. Even if they didn't initially think something happened, they will then tell themselves, 'Well, maybe I'm not remembering it.'"

Ms. Saltz did not agree with a slow reinstatement of visits when they are suspended

due to false accusations of abuse. She responded this way:

You can't give the full rights immediately? I would say that's another way of depriving the children and the alienated parent of getting their relationship on the right track. You can't shoot your parents dead and then throw yourself on the mercy of the court because you are an orphan. The alienator is the one who caused the separation, and then they have the audacity to demand that things proceed at a snail's pace?

Mr. Hecht agreed with the consensus that false and trumped up allegations of sex abuse are used all too frequently by the alienating parent to have parental access suspended. In his experience, many of these cases result in unwarranted "indicated" findings by CPS, while cases of blatant alienation are deemed "unfounded." He cited one of his cases in which the CPS caseworker made a finding of neglect but could not so much as define "neglect" as set forth in the statute. He affirmed, "CPS is too often overzealous as the alienating parent's unwitting accomplice in severing the relationship between the child and the other parent." Mr. Hecht further joined many of his colleagues in his ire at how fathers must defend themselves and lose time with their children as a result of completely fabricated sex abuse allegations. He questions how a father, who never had a single allegation of domestic violence, abuse or neglect of his children ever leveled against him in all of his years of marriage, suddenly finds himself in a CPS investigation, which conveniently is commenced during the pendency of the divorce proceeding. According to Mr. Hecht, one would think that if a father had done such terrible things, the allegations would have been made during the marriage. The reader will likely not be surprised that

Mr. Hecht strenuously disagreed with the prevailing philosophy of going slowly in restoring visits. His response was, "More is better because when the child is not with the alienated parent they are under the influence of the alienating parent so it has to be counteracted as much as possible."

Dr. Burkhard reflected about the dilemma for the mental health professional and for the court regarding enforcement of the visits when she stated the following:

> An overwhelming problem for many cases is that the children are very believable in their assertions of fear and distrust of the targeted parent. Mental health and legal professionals are torn in weighing the impact of forcing a child to spend time with the targeted parent against his or her wishes. In some cases the child makes suicidal threats or allegations of inappropriate touching or sexual discomfort. These types of allegations and threats give even the toughest judicial representative and certainly a mental health professional pause. As professionals serving children, it is critical that we put aside our biases and observe and assess the outcomes going forward in an attempt to improve our knowledge base to determine the best practice for these very troubled families.

To this end, Dr. Burkhard and Dr. Kelly have developed a treatment protocol to facilitate reunification for children who have refused all contact with a targeted parent. Dr. Burkhard described the program as follows:

> The treatment model that has evolved over many years of working with estranged children and parents is an integrated approach. The integration is between the court and the clinic. The basic premise of the treatment model is that the choice to spend time with a targeted par-

ent must be removed from the child. Only if the choice is removed is the child free to resolve whatever real issues may be present and to move forward with that parent. Although the therapist may be successful in some instances in working with the favored or alienating parent in freeing the child, this is generally not a likely pattern. Parents who alienate are generally fairly locked into the patterns of vilifying the other parent. The patterns of thinking and behaving are very difficult, if not impossible, to change. Unlike the clinic, the court holds the power to free the child. The child may be freed via orders for visits, extended vacations with the targeted parent, and in extreme cases, a change in custody. The court's role is to free the child from having the power to choose to avoid the targeted parent. Once the child no longer has the power to choose, the therapist can apply techniques for dealing with anxiety and conflict resolution including gradual exposure between the parent and the child and discussion of ways to move forward.

This treatment protocol is consistent with the emphasis that a family therapist places on the healing which occurs specifically as a result of the corrective experiences among family members. Dr. Burkhard elaborated about this: "In general, the treatment involves exposure and the generation of new and normal experiences with the targeted parent as well as finding ways to help the child 'save face' given the past allegations and disrespectful behaviors."

In countering the presumption by the PAS-unaware professional that children will not accept a relationship with the other parent should visits be enforced over their resistance or should custody be transferred, Dr. Burkhard completely disagreed. She stated, "Many children will turn on a dime if the freedom to choose to reject a parent is fully removed." She cited an example observed recently in her office:

> The children behaved horribly, totally rejecting the father's overtures. They claimed they feared their father; and they repeatedly called him as well as me a "fucking asshole." They broke toys, and they threw things at the ceiling. They turned the lights out in the office so that I could not see them, thereby indicating the fallacious nature of their fear.

In conjunction with the conditions of the integrated treatment, Dr. Burkhard suggested to the judge that he reverse the order prohibiting unsupervised visits between the father and the children. The judge agreed with her recommendation and so ordered unsupervised visits. Subsequent to the first unsupervised visit, the children came into her office, bouncing with excitement and eager to play with their father before they were to return to their mother. They danced and sang for her, who provided the following psychological explanation for the children's jubilation: "The judge relieved them of feeling that they betrayed their mother."

I could not agree more with the importance of maintaining the relationship between the child and alienated parent and providing the therapeutic environment which facilitates the healing process. Nothing good can arise from the suspension of visits. What this does is to embolden the alienator, confirms for the child that their wicked perceptions about their targeted parent are valid, and allows for the opportunity of the poisonous brainwashing to continue unabated and undisputed. It is a classic case of penalizing the victim.

The treatment protocol developed by Dr. Burkhard and Dr. Kelly further confirms the positive impact when there is collaboration between the judiciary and the therapist who works with the family system orientation to facilitate healthy family interactional patterns.

Now, to the recommendations suggested by the matrimonial attorneys and my mental health colleagues to address the systems changes necessary to achieve the best interests of the child in divorce and custody situations.

Given Mr. Levitt's several year litigation of the precedent-setting Young case, I shall begin with his recommendations for proceeding were he to be the presiding judge of divorce cases when children are involved. As the judge, he would call the opposing parties together, and he would make this **announcement to the litigants**:

> I expect the following. You will follow all court orders, such as for support and visitation; if you play a game, I will bring you back here and have you explain to me why you did it. And if you did it without reason or justification, I might just change custody right on the spot. You might lose custody right then and there. I intend to be more part of the process. I will not be speaking just to the attorneys. I will be speaking directly to you, the litigants. If you start violating the things that I think are important, you are going to suffer certain consequences. It's not just parental alienation. I will put you in jail for not paying child support. I want to be very clear about this: we are sitting in judgment of children's lives. We are dealing with children in important stages in their lives with their relationships with their parents. It translates into how they will see their spouse and themselves and to all their relationships.

And when the judge concludes this, he would then make the following **announcement to the respective attorneys**:

If alienation is being alleged, I intend to give the case priority to go forward immediately. I intend to take hold of this. If I recognize that alienation is taking place, I'm going to speed up the case, wrap it up quickly. I'm going to stop the damage that was already done from the alienation. You better be ready when I set it for trial. I will not tolerate frivolous requests for adjournments. In parental alienation, you're talking about a parent who is doing harm to a child. When those allegations are made, they must be given top priority. You need to explain the ramifications to your respective client.

I am sure Mr. Levitt's point is crystal clear: cases of alleged alienation must be given priority. In fact he suggested that cases for divorce should be triaged as follows:

Equitable distribution issues should go into one category; custody cases that are simply concerned with determining who is the better parent go into a second category, and the cases in each of those categories don't get touched until you have completed the cases where there are either allegations of abuse or neglect or cases that involve allegations of parental alienation.

I asked Mr. Levitt about how to handle the difficulty in making the case for alienation, and he responded:

Alienation just doesn't develop once the matrimonial case is filed. The relationships may have been going on for some time before that. So there may be a history with the father or mother being degraded in front of the kids. You should have enough evidence to go forward. You can still apply for a forensic on the family. If necessary, provide all the services that are provided by family court. Alienation is abuse. How is that different than what occurs in family court? Perhaps the parent making false allegations should then bear the cost of the investigation.

Mr. Previto agreed with the suggestions offered by Mr. Levitt. He suggested that, as soon as a case for divorce is filed when children are involved, the judge should schedule a conference with the litigants and their respective lawyers. Any history of abuse **prior** to the decision to divorce should be assessed. (Mr. Previto also recognizes that fallacious allegations of abuse are common after the petition for divorce is filed.) Having ruled out such prior history, Mr. Previto recommends that the judge should make it clear that parental alienation will not be tolerated and that the consequence of such behavior will be the loss of custody. Mr. Previto would impose justice in this manner:

Emphasize alienation as grounds for change of custody in appropriate cases and be willing to enforce it. It is a legal tactic to get people to cooperate with each other. Kids want to love both parents. Mandate court intervention immediately if there is suspicion of alienation in the form of a speedy trial. An early trial is good because it is a quick remedy before the alienation gets worse.

Mr. Previto suggests initially imposing heavy fines and threatening incarceration for the custodial parent's failure to support visits, but he ultimately recommends the transfer of custody if the custodial continues to engage in the alienation. He indicated that at least part of the problems occurring in the matrimonial division stems from the fact that it often attracts more neophyte jurists because, "divorce and family court proceedings are viewed by much of the legal profession as existing at the lower end of the legal spectrum." He articulated his incredulity about this, however: "Yet there is nothing more important to the fabric of our society and the health of our culture than the health of family relations."

Mr. Hiltzik also expressed his concern for the future of our children because he views alienation as a severe form of child abuse which must be taken seriously by the courts. He believes that admonitions against alienation by the courts warrant back-up with penalties such as the imposition of heavy fines, incarceration, and ultimately transfer of custody if the custodial parent cannot be deterred from pursuing the crusade of alienation. He explained it this way:

> If you can't get your child to go on the visits, then you can't be the residential parent. Part of being a parent is that you tell the kids what to do. What happens when the child doesn't want to go to school? Or to trumpet practice? Or to soccer practice? Or to Girl Scouts? Or to the after-school program? So, if the child doesn't want to do something, they don't have to do it? We are making decisions for children all the time. Why are they allowed to decide whether or not to see the parent? If the residential parent can't get the child to do what he/she wants, then he/she shouldn't have custody.

Mr. Hiltzik affirmed that this message must be conveyed by the judge to the residential parent: "Judges must be unyielding and serious when it comes to upholding the relationship between children and their non-custodial parent."

Ms. Zarkadas suggested the following, "The judiciary must work swiftly in all cases of visitation violation. Set a trial date for ten days. Stop all other negotiations and adjournments. And once the violation is estab-

lished, be forewarned that the penalty will be incarceration." According to Ms. Zarkadas, this remedy would have the double effect of having the child live with the alienated parent during the incarceration period. And if the alienator, after serving time, continues to engage in alienation, Ms. Zarkadas offers the following remedy, "Threaten a change in custody which you are prepared to enact. I see more and more that just the threat of loss of custody is having an impact." She cited a case of long-standing visit refusal in which the judge ordered the exchange for visitation in front of her. The judge informed the mother that she risks losing custody if she did not effectuate that visit and all future visits. Guess what? The transition occurred without a hitch!"

Ms. Zarkadas affirmed:

> There can never be a presumption that one parent is superior to the other. Once that presumption is adopted by one side it must be quashed immediately to safeguard the mental health of the child, the development of the child, and the child's right to have access to two loving parents.

Ms. Saltz concurred, "The threat of transfer of custody is good right up front. That is the law right now if alienation can be proven, although transfer of custody rarely happens." She agreed with the others who were interviewed that the failure to follow through with the threat has the effect of emboldening the alienator. She is concerned, however, that the alienating parent may portray themselves as a martyr to the children if subjected to heavy fines and incarceration. She agreed with the idea for a speedy trial in ten days when alienation is alleged, and she acknowledged that certain situations, such as removals, take priority and precedence over all other issues. She concurred that alienation is a form of child abuse and should be given priority, perhaps according to the standard of "time is of the essence," when it is alleged. "That is a very good point, and a very good idea," she declared.

Ms. Saltz strongly supports increasing the time with the alienated parent and informing the alienating parent this will be a remedy, "Just add on more and more time to the alienated parent's visits!" Ms. Saltz considered the extension of the visits to be an excellent remedy because she believes that children welcome an excuse to have time and a relationship with their alienated parent. She agreed that when a parent is deemed to have knowingly filed false allegations of abuse and neglect, that parent should be responsible for the legal fees which the other parent incurrs to defend herself/himself. She also supported the suggestion that any parent who is found culpable of engaging in an alienation be levied 100 percent of the forensic evaluation fee.

Ms. DeNatale also feared that monetary sanctions or court admonishments would not be effective, and she expressed her concerns, "Many times punishments such as these only serve to solidify the parent's perceived injustices in the system. The parent is now a martyr fighting for their child. I place more confidence in the mental health professional to help the parents resolve their issues collaboratively."

Mr. Hecht posits that in instances where parental alienation can be established, the courts should allow the alienated parent to reenter the family residence and have the alienating parent removed from the residence. According to him, such a remedy would have dramatic consequences for the abusing parent, would restrict his or her ability to further manipulate the child or children, and would maximize the child's exposure to the other parent to restore the relationship. "This would be a tremendous step forward," according to Mr. Hecht, who is also not averse to hitting the offending parent in the pocketbook either. He postulated, "If they don't enforce the relationship with the visits, why should they be entitled to child support? This would ratchet up the pressure. I think that's tremendously important." In the end, however, Mr. Hecht affirms that transfer of custody is likely the only effective remedy in the most severe cases of alienation. He was also enthusiastically supportive of the idea for the judge to conference the case with the litigants and their respective attorneys from the bench at the very beginning and then to schedule a speedy trial if there is a whiff of alienation. He stated, "These are fantastic recommendations. I think they would move the ball forward."

Ms. Courten was another passenger on the bandwagon to encourage more judicial activism, to be operationalized as follows, "As soon as there is a whimper of alienation, the judge must come out on the bench and hear it. Immediate hearings, immediate exposure of the problem." She particularly liked Mr. Previto's and Mr. Levitt's suggestion to bring all parties together in all filings of divorce when children are involved. She commented on it this way, "Absolutely that's a good idea. Make a ruling and then enforce it! Do something. Don't put me off for two years waiting." If she had her druthers, she would encourage the judge to be willing to listen to all the parties because they all want to be heard. She cited Judge Liese, who would take the bench every morning promptly at nine o'clock and used that time to hear everyone who wished to appear with their client to express their point of view. Ms. Courten summarized his procedure, "He would put everyone right up at the counsel table, and they would meet the judge. We could have a motion for temporary relief for visitation or custody or spousal maintenance or counsel fees, or exclusive use of the home, and so on."

Ms. Courten also supports Mr. Levitt's suggestion to grant priority to custody cases, particularly when alienation is alleged. She stated that this is already occurring in the appellate division where custody matters are heard before other civil matters. "I applaud this approach," exclaimed Ms. Courten, who further acknowledged that there are some judges in supreme court who are savvy enough to give custody matters a priority in their high case load of some 400 cases. But, Ms. Courten continued, "There is no rule that puts custody ahead of anything. That's unfortunate. I support the point of your book making that a rule. Excellent, excellent. It should be a priority." According to Ms. Courten, there is also a practical side of resolving custody first because, she stated, "Typically when custody gets resolved, most everything else is resolved."

Ms. Courten also conveyed similar concerns as did some of her colleagues that there is a segment of judges, just as with a segment of attorneys and with a segment of mental health professionals, who "don't know which end is up and may not care." Although some jurists are "absolutely brilliant and passionate about what they do," according to Ms. Courten, other judges in the matrimonial division, she believes, "cannot wait to be reassigned to the civil division." She characterized the matrimonial division as "the training wheels of the judicial system." Remedy, she suggested, is to perhaps have judges run for the position as matrimonial judge for the matrimonial court.

As in any profession, Ms. Courten recognizes that judges come with their own personal baggage, biases, and beliefs. She asserted, "Some judges are extremely sexist and believe that the mother should have the children, no matter what. These judges have not transitioned from the tender years doctrine to that of the best interests of the child doctrine," which Ms. Levitt believes applied to

the judge in the Young case.

As with her other colleagues discussed here, Ms. Courten has no compunction about recommending the immediate transfer of custody when alienation is founded. She declared, "It's not negotiable. It's a big kick in the head to the alienator. They have just lost all their fuel." She also believes incarceration should be a remedy, and she expressed it as follows: "Any deterrent must be a stern warning with a bite. Back it up with action. For the love of God, back it up. There are no consequences when there is only a threat but no action."

On a more practical and less controversial level, Ms. Courten recommended a fix to probation. She suggested there be a lawyer to review every petition so that it is done correctly. When filing for custody, orders of protection, orders to produce a child who had been taken away–many petitions are jurisdictionally defective because they are not completed properly. If an attorney is present to review the petition to be sure it is legally sufficient, it will cut down on time before the judge and will minimize the humiliation to the parent who had brought the dismissed petition. The result is a loss of time, no relief, and a parent who loses face with the child. Ms. Courten expressed belief that: "You have to help these people. Petitions get dismissed and you wait so long to get them before the judge. Most of the time, the petitioner doesn't even know why the case was dismissed. They just told him that there was no prima fascia case."

Although Ms. Courten asserted that the "time is of the essence" clause is a contractual term which requires specific performance by a certain date, its philosophical underpinnings of the requirement for imposed finality appears, to her, to be the standard that must be applied to cases of parental alienation.

Dr. Havlicek expressed, "Impose jail time and heavy fines. Offending parents have gotten away with this for too long."

Dr. Baker's research makes a strong case for acting on the principal that time is of the essence. In a survey that she had completed on targeted parents, she found that the alienating parent fails to comply with the judicial plan in 99 percent of the cases. And the targeted parent was enormously resentful given all the money and effort that went into obtaining the order for enforcement of her/his parental rights. Dr. Baker expressed her incredulity about the unjustness of the justice system when she articulated, "It seems grossly unfair to me that there is a system in place to make child support enforceable but there is no system in place to see that the visits are enforced."

With regard to the present system of delay and delay and delay, Dr. Baker deemed that it ultimately enables the alienator, and she expressed her chagrin:

The psychological makeup of parents who are alienating is such that they will not follow the court order for co-parenting. They are impervious to feedback. They have a single-minded mission to keep the children for themselves. They have not ended up in jail for violations of the court orders and refusal to follow the guidelines. Something has to be done to enforce the parenting plan with the visits. Orders are not enforced. In fact they are unenforceable. There is nothing in place to make sure that it happens.

Dr. Baker portrayed the current system as one which rewards the alienator for being an alienator. Because the courts are reluctant to make changes, she asserts that every action supports the violation of the targeted parent's rights. She affirmed that the system must find a way "to make the alienator behave." An ounce of prevention is worth a pound of cure is an admonition that has

much relevancy to the PAS." This is the primary point that Dr. Baker wished to impart in her interview. Dr. Baker, therefore, recommends that early judicial remedy and intervention have the greatest prognosis for positive outcome. The remedy which she supports is taking time away from the alienating parent and giving it to the alienated parent. Although Dr. Baker is focusing her efforts now on prevention, she acknowledged that most alienators are likely workable at least from the initial point of view of educating them if intervention is taken early in the process. She stated, "The longer it goes on, the harder it is to undo. And we don't know who is going to evolve from the naïve to the active to the obsessed," which are the categories that Dr. Baker uses for the continuum on which the alienator travels.

I agree with Dr. Baker: Human behavior is highly resistant to change and is generally not responsive to reasoning, begging, cajoling, persuading, and talking, to expressions of sympathy and empathy, or to other forms of "encouragement" in the absence of a meaningful threat of consequences. It is likely that the reader has had a lasting impression from some resonating remark that was made by a respected authority, and one such remark for me was made by my Sociology 101 Professor, Edward Sagarin. It was 1965, and the class was debating the implementation of the voting and civil rights acts. One of my fellow students expressed his belief that the legislation will fail to be successfully implemented as morality cannot be legislated. Professor Sagarin acknowledged that the student was correct in the way he had framed the issue; but Dr. Sagarin further argued that implementation is not about morality; it is about behavior. The good professor then retorted, "You can legislate behavior–by imposing significant penalties."

My colleagues in both the mental health and legal professions also recommended the need for both professions to become fully educated about the PAS through continuing education.

Ms. Courten stated that the number of judges who participate in continuing education "is not what it should be. And they may not pay attention." She also believes that lawyers should be subject to reprimand when they do not perform an adequate job of informing their clients of a principal responsibility as the custodial parent to foster a relationship with the other parent.

Educating the judiciary was a common refrain among the lawyers and mental health professionals who were interviewed for this book. Ms. Moss expressed that judges need to be educated about alienation:

I think the judges would be receptive to suggestions because they struggle with what to do in these situations. I have never met a judge who did not support the notion that both parents should, as a rule, be involved in their children's lives. However, how to handle the situation when a child is refusing contact with one parent, particularly when the judge believes that the child's behavior is a result of the actions of the other parent, presents problems that seem unsolvable.

Her preference would be for seminars by professionals who would describe what symptoms are indicative of the alienation, what the ramifications are, and what treatment approaches are available. Mr. Hecht highly supports continuing education about alienation for the judiciary and for matrimonial attorneys.

Mr. Levitt asserted the following in regards to his thinking about raising awareness of parental alienation:

The judge has to get down and dirty when it comes to custody and matrimonial law.

And they need special training as well. Some do not come out of the matrimonial field. They need to be reading up on psychology; they have to be more than the judge. They have to be more than just a fact finder. They need to be more intricately involved in the case. When it comes to issues of custody and visitation, they need to be more knowledgeable about PAS. Nobody knew about Gardner back then, and it was very difficult to overcome. I had a judge who didn't even believe that a child could be subject to brainwashing. We are sitting in judgment of children and what to do for them. Maybe you need to assign cases involving children to judge specialists who know about psychology, and let other judges deal with equitable distribution.

Dr. Havlicek recommended a requirement for continuing education for judges. He stated, "We as mental health professionals have to pay for our continuing education. Why should judges be exempt from doing so?" Ms. Zarkadas stated, "Continuing education is necessary. Application of the law is ever-changing." She expressed her concerns that neither the mental health nor the legal/judicial systems are well-educated even today about the presence of alienation or its ultimate future effects on children. She strongly urged continuing education for each profession, as well as developing programs to educate each other—as well the parents—about how best to work together to identify and reverse the PAS. She expressed it this way:

The legal profession, the litigants, and the mental health experts have obligations to work together for the benefit of the child. If they all work together as an entity and have an open mind, the resolution will be pretty good and in the child's best interests because that is the ultimate test: what is in the child's best interests.

Dr. Havlicek concurred and expressed his chagrin that so many of our professional colleagues mishandle these cases when we eschew the noncustodial parent. He takes a very strong position about treatment in high-conflict divorce cases when he stated, "Mandate family therapy with both parents and educate them about the detrimental effects of the PAS on their children. Every effort should be made to involve both parents in the treatment process to ensure that unhealthy circumstances are ameliorated." Dr. Havlicek places "the cause of childhood psychological dysfunction" unequivocally at the feet of having been placed in the middle of their parents' war. He urges, consequently, early intervention as the best hope for stemming the tide of the alienation process. He agrees the culmination of the alienation can have no good outcome for children because, "even if the children figure out the truth that their alienated parent is okay, then they have to think of their alienating parent in a very negative way. This inescapably undermines their mental health."

Each of the lawyers and each of the forensic evaluators recommended that a system be in place for follow-up by a PAS aware therapist/parent coordinator after the case settles. As Ms. Saltz queried:

How do you know the alienation goes away just because everyone has signed on the dotted line? Very often the case settles but the alienation continues. Something needs to be in place for follow-up. A parent coordinator could try to help the parents solve a problem. They need to work out their differences as parents even though they are divorced. There would have to be an obligation for both parents to attend the counseling if one side brings

it back to the parent coordinator. If the counseling fails to resolve the differences, then the coordinator will be in a position to report to the judge who may be sabotaging; this will avoid the "he said/she said" dilemma because the coordinator hopefully will be able to clarify what is happening.

Much has been argued about the presumed but unsubstantiated "devastation" to children should custody be transferred. And much of what is believed is based on fantasy, old wives tales, and wishful thinking. It has no more reality than the old adage, "Step on a crack, break my mother's back." When we make this presumption as adults, we are projecting onto children our own resistance to change. Children are much more flexible and open to new ideas. They will respond to the transfer if the significant people upon whom they are dependent and who love send them the message that they will be taken care of and will be okay. We are not, after all, talking about transfer of custody to a stranger. We are talking about transfer to the other parent, one of only two people in the child's entire lifetime who will love her/him unconditionally. (Even children who are placed with strangers in foster care somehow manage to adjust to a loving and supportive family. And there are rarely any threats, let alone acts, of suicide in these cases.) The relative ease of transfer which I have experienced in my practice is substantiated by the experiences of my mental health colleagues in their practices. I have established in prior chapters that the resistance of the PAS children to a relationship with their alienated parent is not genuine but instead a response to the requirements of their alienating parent. It is only out of the child's dependency on their alienating parent that they so readily acquiesce to and engage in the alienation process. When the choice about having a relationship with the other parent is taken away, these children generally adjust quite satisfactorily. Nevertheless, the important caveat is that the sooner the PAS is addressed, the better for a less problematical adjustment.

I have experienced the same affirmative, swift reversal on many of my cases when ordered by the judge. To cite just one of many examples, I had been assigned to reunite children with their father in a case of visit refusal for more than a year, and I was empowered to confer directly with the judge if the mother interfered with the reunification. Indeed, both the judge and the children's attorney conveyed their support for transfer of custody if the mother did not facilitate the relationships between the father and their children. The children's response to their father flipped as quickly as turning a light switch once their mother supported the visits; and the mother flipped from alienating to supportive behaviors as soon as she understood that she risked losing custody. The dramatic shift occurred in less an hour! The children had arrived with their mother and exclaimed to their father, "Forget about us Move on with your life without us. We cannot have a relationship with you." The mother, nonetheless, expressed to the father that she wanted to settle and end the adversarial court proceedings. The children were sent to the playroom so that the parents and I could develop a framework for settlement to be finalized by the respective attorneys. The children again joined us, and, as the parents and I had agreed, the mother explained to them that the battle was over; they will begin to visit with their father immediately after the session. The children, who a mere hour earlier had denounced their father and refused any contact with him, happily exclaimed, "Great, mommy." It was as simple as that! From that point two years ago until the writing of this book, the father and the children

have had regular, meaningful, and enjoyable contact with each other. This case outcome was not the exception in my practice either. It is the **NORM**, but only if the larger systems have maintained a level playing field between the parents for the therapy to play out.

Dr. Havlicek related analogous positive outcomes in his practice as a therapist and as a forensic evaluator. He affirmed that a competently trained family therapist can produce quite successful outcomes in reversing the PAS by working with the entire family together and with its various subgroups. He supports meaningful, significant and frequent contact between the child and the alienated parent both in therapy sessions and with visits because it has been his experience that this contact is positive for the relationship.

Mr. Levitt offered the Young case as an example of how readily transfer is accepted by children and how their subsequent adjustment is unproblematic. Even though the father had had very little visitation and assumed care overnight of his four children, ages five, eight, nine, and ten, the transfer and adjustment occurred without incident. I am not all surprised. We are talking about going to live with a parent! Mr. Levitt stated:

> Adjustment to their father was not a problem at all. They all adjusted very well, got along with their stepmother, and were happy to be with them. They were much healthier human beings and reached their potential living with their father. As they got older, however, they understood what had happened, and they became angry with their mother.

Mr. Hecht referenced the following case, which is not atypical for what he has encountered in situations: "When the courts are proactive, take a position on alienation, draw

ficulties. We must capitalize on this opportunity to impart our knowledge and expertise about how children are adversely affected when they are triangulated into the marital/parental dysfunction and become like the rope in a tug of war between their parents. We are therefore in a uniquely influential position for preventing children from becoming entrapped in the perverse triangle or freeing them from it when this dysfunctional cross-generational interactional family pattern is most likely still in its nascent stage–at which time it has the greatest potentional for reversal.

6. The universities of higher education which provide mental health training and degrees must expand their curriculum to place a greater emphasis on the teaching and understanding of family dynamics and the PAS and the effective intervention strategies for amelioration of triangles, particularly as it relates to divorce and custody situations.

7. A family systems approach must be recognized as the treatment of choice for these very difficult situations of divorce and custody. Triangles cannot be undone working individually with the child. Individual treatment modalities often deepen the PAS. Divorce and custody are family matters; the remedy must be provided by a family therapist. (One does not seek medical attention from a brain surgeon when the issue is heart disease.) We must recognize the PAS for what it is–a dysfunctional family interactional pattern, and it must be treated as such. Family therapists are experts on this as they have been treating triangles since the 1950s. They are the experts on its diagnosis and have developed the expertise for intervention. The courts must be educated to understand that all therapies are not created equal. Family therapy, with its understanding of and expertise in family dynamics and effective intervention strategies to promote healthy family functioning, is as different

from every individual treatment modality as matrimonial law is from international law or from tax law or from personal injury law or from real estate law or from SEC law or from any other type of law. The court must be educated to understand that family systems therapy is the most effective treatment of family dysfunction, particularly when resulting from divorce and custody animosities. If the PAS dynamic is treated early, then amelioration has the greatest potential for complete reversal.

8. In recognition that intervention is most successful before opinions become entrenched, emotions solidify, and lines are drawn in the sand, the mental health professional must bring the divorcing parents into co-parent counseling as soon as possible, preferably immediately after the initial consultation with each parent.

9. The licensing of the title of the PAS specialist, who will assess for the presence of parental alienation, is now being pursued by Dr. Richard Sauber and a committee of his colleagues, which he leads. This licensing must be given top priority.

10. Preventive efforts, such as those being undertaken by Dr. Amy Baker to educate children about this family dynamic, must be given universal support. Her book, *I Don't Want to Choose,* written in conjunction with Katherine Andre, Ph.D. (2009), is a good beginning point. With the PAS, an ounce of prevention is worth a ton of cure.

11. Before a rush to judgment is made that a child has ADHD or bipolar disorder, a complete family assessment, which includes input from both parents, must be undertaken. The prescribing doctor must first rule out a "bipolar" and/or "ADHD" family interactional situation before making an interpretation as to the causes of the child's symptoms. I am incredulous to believe that such a huge percentage of our childhood population suddenly became afflicted with one or both of

these disorders. The mental health community must recognize that treating only the child's symptoms is as ludicrous as treating a patient for an infection by giving antibiotics and then returning the patient to the untreated environment with the germ that had caused the infection. Without correcting the dysfunctional family interactional patterns and treating the child alone–perhaps with strong psychotropic medications that have side effects–is isomorphic with the patient being returned to the germ infested environment.

Judicial Recommendations

1. The American Bar Association and The Matrimonial Bar must recognize that a parent turning a child against the other parent is a form of child abuse. The adoption of a collaborative approach to the issues of custody and parenting time, versus the adversarial environment prevalent today, must be the preference in advocating for the "best interests of the child." It is imperative that Bar members notify their clients that to alienate a child from the other parent does nothing but put the child in harm's way. The concept of a shared parenting relationship with joint legal custody–except in cases of serious social deviation by a parent–must be the norm, rather than the exception. Attorneys who turn a "blind eye" to the alienating conduct of their client should face disciplinary action just as they would for any other ethical violation. Just like the mental health professional, the matrimonial attorney is in a unique position to "nip" this destructive family interactional pattern "in the bud." Doing so will spare children from much heartache and potential pathology. A collaborative methodology will further have the practical benefit of not clogging the court calendars. These directives must be made clear and enforceable across the matrimonial spectrum so that it applies to every practitioner, the

message conveyed that there is a "no toleration" policy for engaging in alienation, as there is with regard to other conduct in these actions, such as dissipating and concealing marital assets.

2. Attorneys need to be more proactive in preventing alienating conduct during matrimonial proceedings. Parents should be apprised of the current state of New York law:

> A custodial parent's interference with the relationship between child and the noncustodial parent has been said to be an act so inconsistent with the best interests of the child as to per se raise a strong probability that the offending party is unfit to act as a custodial parent. (*Maloney v. Maloney; Young v. Young*)

Sudden allegations of abuse by the other parent, where there was no prior history, should be met with skepticism, as well as a "warning" to the party making those claims.

3. If the nonresidential parent is the attorney's client, the attorney will inform the client of the obligation to pay child support in a timely manner and that it cannot be withheld as a means of control over the residential parent or for any other reason.

4. Priority must be given to high-conflict custody cases–especially those in which there is the slightest indication of alienation. All other matters, such as equitable distribution and other civil matters will be relegated to secondary or tertiary status until this issue is resolved, lest we risk permanent emotional harm to the children.

5. Completion of co-parent education by a family systems therapist must be compulsory. Parents must be educated about the adverse effects on children of a hostile, adversarial divorce. Programs like the Peace Program in Suffolk County, New York is a model but should be expanded to sufficiently achieve an understanding of the effects on children of an alienation. Other states, such as California, have enacted legislation man-

dating more extensive parent education in these areas. Various other forms of parent education are already official policy in many states, but the programs generally do not go far enough. One factor to be given substantial weight to obtaining residential custody is the demonstration of a capacity to appreciate the importance of the other parent to their child and to promote that relationship. "Custody" should be a "responsibility," not a "right," which includes the responsibility to promote and foster the relationship the children have with the noncustodial parent. Of course, without judicial enforcement, such a factor will have no "teeth."

The courts should develop a list of family therapists who are qualified to provide this service. The court can begin by obtaining from their respective State Mental Health Licensing Authority a list of licensed marriage and family therapists in their jurisdiction who can be offered the opportunity to work collaboratively with the matrimonial court to provide this service. Obtaining the lists and identifying interested family therapists should not incur huge expenses. The cost savings to the jurisdictions as a result of minimizing an adversarial approach should more than compensate. Provision of the therapy is not an expensive proposition as co-parent counseling is a covered service by most insurance plans. Licensed mental health therapists who have completed training at family therapy institutes, such as the Minuchin Center for the Family or the Ackerman Institute of Family Therapy in New York City, will be appropriate therapists for this service as well.

6. Immediately upon receiving a petition for an action involving children, the judge from the bench will meet with the litigants and their respective attorneys and announce the judiciary's expectation that the parents work together to develop a shared parenting relationship because that is in "the best inter-

ests of the child." The judge will convey a "no toleration" policy for parental alienation and for failure to pay child support. The judge will assert judicial authority to impose penalties for these behaviors. Should either party allege difficulties regarding parenting issues, an unwillingness to co-parent, or a refusal to mutually support the other parent's relationship with the children, the judge will immediately refer the family to one of its collaborative family therapists to provide more intensive family therapy. Contrary to popular perception, co-parent counseling does not have to be an expensive proposition. I am about to reveal a whisper: collateral parental counseling is a covered service by virtually all insurance plans. Every family therapist knows this! When the parental subsystem is functioning appropriately, children are symptom free. Yes! That's true. And family systems therapists have the empirical evidence to support this claim. But when the parental dyad is dysfunctional, it creates and maintains symptomatology in the child. Symptom reduction can be achieved **only** by treating the parental dyad, and the insurance companies understand this. If the therapist accepts the family's insurance coverage, then the therapy can be billed to the insurance company. Co-parenting counseling, is, therefore, the **necessary medical remedy**, and failure to obtain the therapy is, therefore, **medical neglect**. It would be no different than a parent who refused to give their diabetic child insulin or a DPT shot, and so forth. Need I say more? The judges need to be educated by the family therapy community about this form of medical neglect. The lawyers for the children who were interviewed for this book are currently using their position to persuade the parents of their clients to cooperate with all recommended services. This role as counselor must be adopted by every lawyer for the child and by all matrimonial attorneys for this "vicious cycle" to end, all for the benefit of the children. The alternative is to continue with the expense of psychological forensics NOT COVERED BY INSURANCE that will run into the tens of thousands of dollars. Additionally, many parents who are victims of alienation do not have the financial resources to pursue such forensics and have to "surrender" to the alienator and lose their relationships with their children. Additionally, the legislatures of the 50 states must be lobbied to pass legislation to make this service mandated.

The family therapist will be empowered to communicate with the judge and the children's lawyer on an as-needed basis to discuss progress and/or resistances. While the therapy is proceeding, the custodial parent will cooperate in facilitating the visits between the children and the noncustodial parent. Should there be an open CPS case, the family therapist will be in contact with the CPS worker to expedite the investigation and to implement the least restrictive visitation arrangement with the alleged perpetrator that will assure that the child's safety is guarded. The fact that a CPS investigation is "open" should not be accepted as grounds for suspending visitation without consulting with the family therapist currently administering the case.

7. Should the collaborative family therapist accept a case from the court for treatment, she/he must be willing to give the family priority attention so that the case does not linger. All efforts must be undertaken to help the parents resolve their respective emotional issues and conflicts with each other and which are likely hindering their willingness to develop a shared parenting relationship. The parents will have the commitment from the collaborative family therapist that she/he will be objective, fair, dependable and supportive to arrive at the appropriate parenting schedule and co-parenting arrangement.

But, the parents must also understand that the therapist's authority derives from the court, and penalties can and will be imposed for behaviors that are destructive to the children.

8. The judiciary must guarantee a level playing field and forsake its double standard/bipolar approach to mothers and fathers. This requires two significant changes:

a. There must be equal penalties imposed on mothers that are recurrently imposed on fathers for similar infractions of family law and of specific court orders pertaining to the family. Although the laws profess to be "gender-neutral," reality says it is not.

b. There must be an end to the bifurcated systems between the family and divorce courts. It is a two tiered system in which the parental rights of parents whose children were placed in foster care due to adjudications of abuse and/or neglect, are scrupulously protected by state and federal mandates. These parents are guaranteed a meaningful weekly visitation schedule for their children. Written approval for their children's medical care, educational plans, and engagement in extracurricular activities must first be sought from the parents before an agency official is empowered to sign the necessary consent. This same status in divorce situations must be accorded nonresidential parents, particularly as they have done nothing harmful to their children.

Although it disappoints me in knowing that not every treatment will be successful, I am nonetheless a realist. Based on the contributions from those who were interviewed for this book, coupled with my 40 years experience working with Family and Supreme (matrimonial) Courts in New York, I make the following recommendations, should the collaborative process between the family therapist and the judiciary not be successful in reaching a settlement between the parents regarding custody and visitation and in support of a shared parenting relationship.

9. The collaborative family therapist will share with the judge the barriers for arriving at a resolution and settlement. The judge will calendar the case for a speedy trial–within ten days if possible–to hear testimony regarding the issues conveyed by the collaborative family therapist.

10. Should the evidence that is presented establish that one of the parents is unwilling or unable to encourage and facilitate the relationship between the children and the other parent, the judge will advise that such behavior will result in the loss of custody and/or parenting time with the children. The courts should not be so reluctant to change temporary custody upon receiving reports from the family therapist of the alienating conduct. At that point, that parent will be "educated" as to the consequences of this abusive behavior.

11. Should the collaborative family therapist give testimony that one of the parties is engaging in alienating behaviors or is sabotaging the establishment of a shared co-parenting relationship, that party may request a second opinion. A forensic evaluation shall be ordered and will be conducted by another collaborative family therapist or by anyone who has become licensed as a PAS specialist. If the allegations are substantiated, the alienating party should be burdened with the full expense of the forensic evaluation.

12. Should the residential parent be judged as engaging in alienating behaviors, transfer of custody or loss of time with the child could be the penalty for refusing to cease those behaviors, and the judge must make this explicit. Should transfer occur, the new residential parent will cooperate with therapy provided by the collaborative family therapist to help repair the damaged fam-

ily relationships and to continue efforts to facilitate a shared parenting relationship. Should the prior residential parent be judged to continue engaging in alienating behaviors, that parent will have only supervised visits until such time that a collaborative family therapist submits a report to the court that the parent understands the damage being done to her/his child and is willing and able to cease the alienating behaviors.

13. In all cases in which alienation has been established, a collaborative family therapist will be assigned to follow the case after it is adjudicated and be available to address future difficulties and refer it back to court if necessary. Any state which does not have such a law on the books, must pass one immediately.

14. The Attorney for the Child must become familiar with the phenomenon of alienation and its detrimental effects on children. Recognizing that it is a form of child abuse provides the attorney with the justification to decline support of the child's wishes, which are, in essence, the words of the ventriloquist alienating parent.

15. Each parent will be accorded the professional standards of being treated with respect, with recognition of her/his importance to the child, with neutrality, and with an open-mindedness.

16. Judges, matrimonial lawyers, and the Attorney for the Child must be required to complete continuing education courses on family dynamics and on the PAS. They must be educated to recognize symptoms and how it is a form of child abuse. Just as therapists are required to take periodic continuing education, so should the other professions which make such momentous decisions affecting the lives of children.

17. Children are our greatest national resource, and the family is the foundation of our culture. Matrimonial judges should therefore receive a meaningful pay differen-

tial should they voluntarily take continuing education about family matters, dynamics, psychology, and so forth.

In acknowledging that our economic times prohibit the implementation of costly programs, I assert that these recommendations will save money by not clogging the court calendars with needless motions, counter-motions, and violations but will instead be addressed in the co-parent counseling. As my case summaries documented, it is amazing how quickly the sparring parents came to agreement when I had a level playing field upon which to treat the PAS family because I had the backing of judicial authority as a result of my collaborative work with the lawyer for the child and the court. And follow-up calls to the families to provide an update for this book confirmed that the progress achieved in therapy was maintained. Of course, the families were aware that I would be available to them as additional issues arose. Some of the families requested this service, and with a very brief course of therapy, the progress again resumed.

The collaborative approach between the courts and Child and Family Psychological Services in Suffolk County, New York is the model for the collaborative approach and should be expanded.

Recommendations to the Police

Please, enforce court orders for visitation when you are called to the moment of transition. The crying child is going with a loving parent whose parental right to visitation was upheld by the court. You have never experienced a child crying for the wrong reasons? Do you rush in to take a tantruming child from a parent who has refused to buy her/him a toy? Of course not! Well, you should no more rush in and use your authority to keep the child from the court ordered visits

with her/his nonresidential parent. Please, instead, support the transition.

Recommendations to CPS

Learn about the perverse triangle and that it is a form of child abuse. Learn how to identify it and understand that the child who is a victim of the PAS has become the puppet of the alienating ventriloquist parent and they are therefore mouthing that parent's words and wishes. Obtain a full picture of the family by according the other parent equal time. Do not empower children by anointing them with the authority to refuse to visit with the nonresidential parent. If they express fear of that parent, ask for the reasons for the feeling and do not be co-opted when there are only frivolous rationalizations for their feelings. If they express hatred, be suspicious. Hatred for a parent is anti-instinctual.

Recommendations to the Federal Government

We assert it so frequently that it has become a cliché: children are our greatest national resource. Being that this is so, we must establish a national policy on custody and visitation that is the least injurious to children, acknowledging that some injury is an unavoidable consequence of the circumstance in which the parents are no longer living together. Washington must therefore lead the way and establish a commission comprised of professionals from mental health, matrimonial law, law enforcement, and child protection in order to determine the least detrimental effects to children resulting from parental break-up. The 50 states currently have 50 separate laws and official policies regarding this issue. A panel of experts needs to explore what is beneficial and what is unhelpful in each state's policy. For example, some states have already passed statutes requiring parent education before a legal case for divorce is allowed to go forward. The best of the state programs should be identified and then adapted by each of the individual states to meet their idiosyncratic needs.

Oh, yes, I hear the moans that tough economic times do not allow for the budgeting of such a commission. Well, if the Washington lawmakers are so concerned with the sanctity of every child's life, then they must put the money where their mouths are and budget for this commission.

The failure to apply the concept of "time is of the essence" to the PAS was best expressed by Shakespeare in *King Henry VI:* "Delays have dangerous ends."

Chapter 26

CLOSING COMMENTS

Professional rescuers are not malevolent, but they harm children. They are misguided do-gooders. Other professionals who intervene in the lives of children are not so magnanimous; they are motivated by their bottom line to make a living, a big living. They will eventually discover that living with oneself has a higher value.

The PAS is real: I lived it as a child, and I am living it now in my role as a family therapist, treating an endless number of families afflicted with this syndrome–a family interactional pattern which family therapists labeled the perverse triangle and have been treating since the 1950s. The families keep coming and coming and coming as a result of the high divorce rate. As long as child custody cases continue to be adjudicated in an adversarial system, the best interests of the child will be compromised by this system in which attorneys for the litigating parents seek to maximize their advantage and fail to admonish their clients from engaging in alienating behaviors; by PAS-unaware therapists who fail to involve both parents in diagnosis and treatment, which can be accurately obtained only by assessing the family's interactional patterns through firsthand observation of the entire family system as well as its various subgroups; and by PAS-unaware forensic evaluators who are appoint-ed by the court to make recommendations regarding custody and visitation. Divorce inevitably involves some degree of distress for the child, and some degree of disruption to the parent/child relationship is unavoidable. But the distress and disruption can be minimized when the professionals work together to help the parents help each other allay each other's respective fears and anxieties in order to then develop of a shared parenting relationship in the best interests of their children.

Because of procrastination, incompetence, rescue-fantasy, ignorance, or sometimes self-interest, the professionals within the aforementioned larger systems which are supposed to support and protect children, instead maintain a dysfunctional family system, known as the perverse triangle/PAS. The therapists who diagnose and treat it, the forensic evaluators who assess for it, the lawyers who quarrel about it, the child protection workers who investigate it, the law enforcement personnel who become ensnared in it, and the judges who adjudicate it must be more proactive in protecting the right of the child to have a meaningful and enduring relationship with each parent. Each profession which has influence over custody and visitation decisions must guard against becoming co-opted by the alienating parent and by their puppet child, who mimics the ventriloquist parent's words. These professions must further recognize that the concept of "time is of the essence" has the greatest relevancy to the PAS.

As I was completing this book during the course of a couple of weeks, I received referrals to treat nine children whose respective families were in the beginning stage of divorce. In each of these families, the perverse triangle was present to some degree. In each case, I immediately contacted the nonpresenting parent, and amelioration was initiated. I also received an update from an alienated father who was not discussed in this book but whose children had refused all contact with him for several years and with whom I had been advising as to how to present to the judge a case for alienation. His case serves to no better exemplify how the professional rescuer deepens the alienation: a PAS-unaware forensic evaluator was court appointed to make recommendations on custody and visitation. The evaluator accepted as incontrovertible truth the alienating mother's assertion that one of her children was threatening suicide if forced to attend an interview with the father. The evaluator accommodated to the mother's manipulation, and, without assessing the children in interaction with their father, the evaluator recommended to the court that the father have only therapeutic visits with his children. Supervised visits and unsupervised visits were each out of the question. Imagine that! Making such momentous recommendations based on hearsay, client self-interest, and client-subjectivity. Aside from these grave concerns, if the evaluator truly took seriously the child's suicidal threat, what was the logic in recommending the therapeutic visits? After two years of being alienated from his children as a result of professional support, this father called to apprise me of a hopeful development. He informed me that the judge

had been persuaded as to the alienation and then informed the mother that transfer of custody would be considered as a remedy. The mother immediately offered to settle and assured the father that she will guarantee his visits and meaningful relationships with their children. And just as quickly as it took to write these few sentences, that is how quickly the children flipped from denigration and rejection of their father to approval and acceptance of him. Two other alienated parents, however, who had also contacted me during this time were not so fortunate. The first was a father whose divorce had occurred years before, and the alienation with his three children was in the severe stage. He sobbed to me about how he was denigrated at his son's high school graduation after his son's mother had given his reserved, preferential tickets to her extended family. When the father conveyed his pain to his son, he haughtily replied, "Well, that's the advantage of being the custodial parent." The other parent who contacted me was a mother of three teenagers, and she and her husband have been going through a malicious divorce and custody battle. I had worked with the family previously before the decision to divorce was made. She related how her husband had since succeeded in turning the children against her by sharing with them his court documents containing fabricated and malicious allegations against her, by using his superior financial position to buy off the children to do his bidding in rejecting and deprecating her; and by brainwashing them into believing that their mother is the one who is breaking up the family, although they were quite aware of their father's mistress. What is most reprehensible about this case were the adversarial actions taken by the father's attorney, who failed to caution him against engaging in alienating behaviors and thereby emboldened him. Out of desperation and situational depression due to her children's denunciation of her, the mother considered committing suicide by overdosing on the father's prescription medication. She reconsidered this thought, but her husband nevertheless had her arrested and jailed on the very rare charge of "tampering with prescription medication." He further succeeded in obtaining–while she was still in jail and not present to defend herself–an order of protection which prohibited her from returning to the family home. What was the foundation for the order of protection? The father brought a petition on behalf of their teenage daughter based on an unconfirmed claim that the girl was fearful of her mother. This cowardly father did not have the "moral fiber" to obtain the order on an allegation related to him. Instead, he used his daughter as ammunition in his war with his wife, and this action will require that the girl either testify against her mother or else risk receiving her father's opprobrium if she declines. How about that for a double-bind!

I have documented in this book the sagas of 56 children from 32 families, most of whom were seriously suffering from the perverse triangle at the time they had been referred to me. Treatment was the most successful when implemented in the earliest stages of the divorce proceedings, when it was respectful of both parents and recognized the need of both parents to their children, and when there were no professional saboteurs from the mental health, judicial, child welfare, and law enforcement systems. My preventive work was implemented ac-

cording to the principles underlying a family systems treatment modality, which promoted a power equalization between the sparring parents. Nineteen alienating parents participated to some degree in the therapy, and many participated considerably. The 13 who did not participate were accounted for as follows: one was deceased; one was living overseas; and, more notably and indefensibly, the remaining 11 refused to return after the initial session because they were emboldened by at least one professional saboteur. Not included in this book were my treatments of hundreds of children of divorcing parents who were spared entrapment in the perverse triangle because family treatment was implemented when the families were in their nascent stages of family dysfunction. Also not included were a number of cases in which the claim of alienation was specious. That situation received the same treatment response from me as did the situation of the PAS: I worked with the entire family system, with particular emphasis on the parental subsystem, to redistribute the power between the parents in order to promote healthy family functioning and a homeostasis that was in the best interests of the children.

Until the professionals in mental health, judicial, law enforcement, and child protection systems affirmatively implement measures in their respective systems which guarantee to the family therapist a treatment environment of a level playing field between the parents, they will be enabling the PAS to victimize the family.

Appendix

STATUS OF THE CHILDREN AND FAMILIES DISCUSSED IN THIS BOOK AT THE BEGINNING AND AT THE CONCLUSION OF THERAPY

Total number of PAS children/families discussed in this book.	56/32
Number of children who were not visiting at time therapy was initiated/ serious alienation.	49
Mild alienation at end of therapy.	13
Moderate alienation at end of therapy	5
Severe alienation (parentectomy) at end of therapy.	15
PAS resolved as a result of the therapy.	27
Number of families in which the alienating and alienated parents both participated in the therapy.	19

Number of families in which the alienated parent only participated in the therapy.	12
Number of children in the therapy with court involvement and back-up.	49
Number of children whose noncustodial parent was the alienator.	5
Number of children who were verbally abusive to alienated parent.	49
Number of children who were physically abusive to alienated parent.	18

Number of children who deprecated their alienated parent.	50
Number of children who used frivilous rationalization.	49
Number of children who used borrowed scenarios.	48
Number of children who had no ambivalence.	43
Number of children who showed no guilt.	43

Number of children who claimed independent thinking.	40
Number of children who reflexively aligned with alienating parent.	50
Number of children who extended animosity to alienated parents' family.	45
Number of children who instantaneously ceased PAS behaviors when their alienating parent ceased engaging in the PAS.	27 from 14 alienators
Number of children whose alienated parent was investigated by CPS.	37 w/35 unfounded

Number of children whose custody transferred or child now living with formerly alienated parent.	8
Number of children who had education issues.	19
Number of children who had behavioral issues.	51
Number of children with some degree of emotional issues.	51
Number of highly specious domestic violence allegations.	30

| Number of alienators who successfully co-opted a professional. | 23 of 32 |
| Number of the alienators who refused to participate in therapy and who had previously co-opted a professional. | 11 of 11 |

Number of children ages 2–4	5
Number of children ages 5–8	17
Number of children ages 9–11	11
Number of children ages 12–14	14
Number of children ages 15–16	5
Number of children ages 17–18	2
Number of children above 18 years	2

REFERENCES

Ackerman, N. W. (1958). *The psychodynamics of family life.* New York: Basic Books.

Ackerman, N. W. (1961). The emergence of family psychotherapy on the present scene. In M. I. Stein (Ed.), *Contemporary psychotherapies.* Glencoe, IL: Free Press.

Ackerman, N. W., & Franklin, P. (1965). Family dynamics and the reversibility of delusional formation: A case study in family therapy. In I. Boszormenyi-Nagy & J. Famo (Eds.), *Intensive family therapy* (Ch. 6.). New York: Harper and Row.

Ackerman, N. W. (1966). *Treating the troubled family.* New York: Basic Books.

American Psychiatric Association. (2002). *Diagnostic and statistical manual of mental disorders* (4th ed., text rev.). Washington, DC: Author.

Andolfi, M., Angelo, C., Menghi, P., & Nicolo-Corigliano, A. (1983). *Behind the family mask.* New York: Brunner/Mazel.

Andolfi, M., Angelo, C., & Nichilo, M. (1989). *The myth of atlas.* New York: Brunner/Mazel.

Andre, K., & Baker, A. (2009). *I don't want to choose: How middle school kids can avoid choosing one parent over the other.* New York: Kindred Spirits.

Baker, A. (2007). *Adult children of parental alienation syndrome.* New York: Norton.

Barden, R. C. (2006) Protecting the fundamental rights of children and families: Parental alienation syndrome and family law reform. In R. Gardner, R. Sauber, & L. Lorandos (Eds.), *International handbook of parental alienation syndrome* (pp. 419–432). Springfield, IL: Charles C Thomas.

Boscolo, L., Cecchin, G., Hoffman, L., & Penn, P. (1987). *Milan systemic family therapy.* New York: Basic Books.

Bowen, M. (1971). The use of family theory in clinical practice. In J. Haley (Ed.), *Changing families: A family therapy reader* (pp. 159–192). New York: Grune & Stratton.

Bowen, M. (1978). *Family therapy in clinical practice.* New York: Jason Aronson.

Burrill, J. (2002). *Parental alienation syndrome in court referred custody cases.* USA: Dissertation .Com.

Cartwright, G. (2006). Beyond parental alienation syndrome: Reconciling the alienated child and the lost parent. In R. Gardner, R. Sauber, & D. Lorandos (Eds.), *International handbook of parental alienation syndrome* (pp. 286–291). Springfield, IL: Charles C Thomas.

Clawar, S. S., & Rivlin, B. V. (1991). *Children held hostage: Dealing with programmed and brainwashed children.* Chicago, IL: American Bar Association.

Everett, C. (2006). Family therapy for parental alienation syndrome: Understanding the interlocking pathologies. In R. Gardner, R. Sauber, & D. Lorandos (Eds.), *International handbook of parental alienation syndrome* (pp. 228–241). Springfield, IL: Charles C Thomas.

Garbarino, J., & Scott, F. M. (1992). *What children can tell us: Eliciting, interpreting, and evaluating critical information from children.* San-Francisco, CA: Jossey-Bass.

Gardner, R. A. (1985). Recent trends in divorce and custody litigation. *Academy Forum* (a publication of the American Academy of Psychoanalysis), *29*(2), 3–7.

Gardner, R. A. (1998). *The parental alienation syndrome* (2nd ed.). Cresskill, NJ: Creative Therapeutics.

Gardner, R. A. (2001). *Therapeutic interventions for children with parental alienation syndrome.* Cresskill, NJ: Creative Therapeutics.

Gardner, R. A. (2002). Response to Kelly/Johnston Article. *Speak Out for Children* (a publication of the Children's Rights Council), *17*(2), 6–10.

Haley, J. (1963). *Strategies of psychotherapy* (1st ed.). New York: Grune & Stratton.

Haley, J., & Hoffman, L. (Eds.). (1968). *Techniques of family therapy.* New York: Basic Books.

Haley, J. (1971). *Changing families.* New York: Grune & Stratton.

Haley, J. (1973). *Uncommon therapy.* New York: Norton.

Haley, J. (1977). Toward a theory of pathological systems. In P. Watzlawick & J. Weakland (Eds.), *The interactional view* (pp. 37–44). New York: Basic Books.

Haley, J. (1990). *Strategies of psychotherapy.* Rockville, MD: The Triangle Press.

Hoffman, L. (1981). *Foundations of family therapy.* New York: Basic Books.

Jackson, D., & Weakland, J. (1971) Conjoint family therapy: Some considerations on theory, technique, and results. In J. Haley (Ed.), *Changing families* (pp. 13–35). New York: Grune & Stratton.

John A. v. Bridget M., V-01755-5/03. (Family Court, New York County, 2004).

John A. v. Bridget M., 16 A.D.3d 324; 791 N.Y.S.2d 421; Lexis 3374 (N.Y. App. Div. 2005).

Johnston, J. (7/9-9/10/2001). *Rethinking parental alienation and redesigning parent-child access service for children who resist or refuse visitation.* Paper delivered at the International Conference on Supervised Visitation, Munich, Germany.

Kempler, W. (1971). Experiential family therapy. In J. Haley (Ed.), *Changing families* (pp. 133–145). New York: Grune & Stratton.

Kopetski, L. (2006). Commentary: Parental alienation syndrome. In R. Gardner, R. Sauber, & D. Lorandos (Eds.), *International handbook of parental alienation syndrome* (pp. 378–390). Springfield, IL: Charles C Thomas.

Lorandos, D. (2006). Parental alienation syndrome: Detractors and the junk science vacuum. In R. Gardner, R. Sauber, & D. Lorandos (Eds.), *International handbook of parental alienation syndrome* (pp. 397–418). Springfield, IL: Charles C Thomas.

Lowenstein, L. (2006). The psychological effects and treatment of the parental alienation syndrome. In R. Gardner, R. Sauber, & D. Lorandos (Eds.), *International handbook of parental alienation syndrome* (pp. 292–301). Springfield, IL: Charles C Thomas.

Major, J. (2006). Helping clients deal with parental alienation syndrome. In R. Gardner, R. Sauber, & D. Lorandos (Eds.), *International handbook of parental alienation syndrome* (pp. 276–285). Springfield, IL: Charles C Thomas.

Maloney v. Maloney, 208 AD2d 603, 603–604. (New York).

Minuchin, S. (1974). *Families and family therapy.* Cambridge, MA: Harvard University Press.

Minuchin, S., Baker, L., & Rosman, B. (1978). *Psychosomatic families: Anorexia nervosa in context.* Cambridge, MA: Harvard University Press.

Minuchin, S., & Fishman, C. (1981). *Family therapy techniques.* Cambridge, MA: Harvard University Press.

Minuchin, S., & Nichols, M. (1993). *Family healing.* New York: The Free Press.

Minuchin, S., Lee, W., & Simon, G. (1996). *Mastering family therapy.* New York: John Wiley & Sons.

Minuchin, S., Nichols, M., & Lee, W. (2007). *Assessing families and couples: From symptom to system.* New York: Pearson.

Napier, A., & Whitaker, C. (1978). *The family crucible: The intense experience of family therapy.* New York: Harper Perennial.

Nichols, N. (1992). *The power of family therapy.* Lake Worth, FL: Gardner Press.

Nichols, M., & Schwartz, R. (2004). *Family therapy: Concepts and methods.* New York: Pearson.

Pruitt, K. (2000). *Fatherneed.* New York: Broadway Books.

Sauber, R. (2006). PAS as a family tragedy: Roles of family members, professionals, and the justice system. In R. Gardner, R. Sauber, & D. Lorandos (Eds.), *International handbook on parental alienation syndrome* (pp. 12–32). Springfield, IL: Charles C Thomas.

Steinberger, C. (2006). Father? What father? Parental alienation and its effect on children. *Law Guardian Reporter, 22*(3). New York, NY: Appellate Divisions of the Supreme Court of New York.

Young v. Young, No. 94/09240. (Supreme Court, Nassau County, NY. 1994).

Young v. Young, 212 A.D.2d 114; 628 N. Y. S.2d 957 (1995).

Wallerstein, J., & Kelly, J. (1980). *Surviving the breakup.* New York: Basic Books.

Warshak, R. (2001). Current controversies regarding parental alienation syndrome. *American Journal of Forensic Psychology, 19*(3), 29–59.

Warshak, R. (2006). Social science and parental alienation: Examining the disputes and the evidence. In R. Gardner, R. Sauber, & D. Lorandos (Eds.), *International handbook of parental alienation syndrome* (pp. 352–371). Springfield, IL: Charles C Thomas.

Warshak, R. (2010). *Divorce poison.* New York: Harper.

Whitaker, C. (1983). In M. Andolfi, C. Angelo, P. Menghi, & A. Nicolo-Corigliano, *Behind the family mask* (p. vi). New York: Brunner/Mazel.

Whitaker, C., & Bumberry, W. (1988). *Dancing with the family: A symbolic-experiential approach.* New York: Brunner/Mazel.

Williams, Frank. (1990). *Speak Out for Children,* Fall, 5(4).

INDEX

269

perverse, 4, 87, 158, 180, 207, 214, 222,
248–249, 254, 257, 258, 259
triangulation. *See* triangles

V

victimization of the alienated parent. *See* alienated parent
video recording sessions, 195
visitation/contact
highly effective for countering the alienation,
107–108, 109–110, 111, 133–134, 147,
148, 150, 234–238, 240, 241, 243, 246
obstruction, refusal, suspension of, ix, xv,
10–13, 15, 16, 19, 20, 24, 25, 26, 27, 28,
30, 31, 33, 34–35, 36–37, 38, 42–45,
46–50, 51–54, 58–59, 60–63, 61–65,
66, 67, 68, 69, 71, 73, 74, 75, 76, 84, 90,
91, 95, 96, 102, 105, 107, 110, 105, 114,
119–138, 183, 186, 187, 188, 192, 194,
196, 198, 200, 201, 205, 233, 234–237,
239, 242, 252, 258

sabotage during, 24–25, 28, 43–44, 45–53,
50–51, 54–55, 59–60, 108, 119–13

W

Wallerstein, J., 3
Warshak, R., 5–6, 7–8, 9, 150–151
Weakland, J., 156
Whitaker, C., 152–153, 154, 163
Williams, F., 210

Y

Young v. Young, 21, 221, 233, 235, 238, 246, 250

Z

Zarkadas, E., xx, 14–15, 25–26, 27, 54, 59, 213,
219, 221, 226–227, 233, 235, 240,
244–245

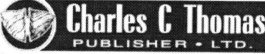

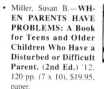
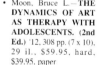
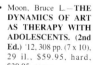

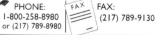
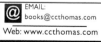
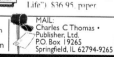